Mayo Clinic
MANUAL OF
PELVIC SURGERY

Second Edition

MAYO CLINIC MANUAL OF PELVIC SURGERY

Edited by

Maurice J. Webb, M.D.
Chairman, Division of Gynecologic Surgery
Consultant, Department of Surgery
Mayo Clinic and Mayo Foundation
Professor, Department of Obstetrics and Gynecology
Mayo Medical School
Rochester, Minnesota

With Contributions by
William A. Cliby • Bobbie S. Gostout
Darlene G. Kelly • Raymond A. Lee
Karl C. Podratz • Peter A. Southorn
C. Robert Stanhope • Tiffany J. Williams
Timothy O. Wilson

With 156 Figures

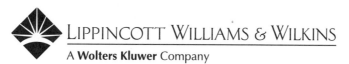
LIPPINCOTT WILLIAMS & WILKINS
A **Wolters Kluwer** Company
Philadelphia • Baltimore • New York • London
Buenos Aires • Hong Kong • Sydney • Tokyo

Acquisitions Editor: Lisa McAllister
Developmental Editor: Julia Seto
Production Editor: Melanie Bennitt
Manufacturing Manager: Kevin Watt
Cover Designer: Garry J. Post
Compositor: Maryland Composition
Printer: Maple Press

Lippincott Williams & Wilkins
530 Walnut Street
Philadelphia, PA 19106 USA
LWW.com

Cover: The background photograph is of the Mayo brothers operating at St. Mary's Hospital, probably in 1913. By permission of Mayo Historical Unit, Mayo Foundation, Rochester, Minnesota.

Printed in the USA

Library of Congress Cataloging-in-Publication Data

Mayo Clinic manual of pelvic surgery / edited by Maurice J. Webb; with contributions by William A. Cliby . . . [et al.].—2nd ed.
    p.; cm.
    Rev. ed. of: Manual of pelvic surgery. c1994.
    Includes bibliographical references and index.
    ISBN 0-7817-2592-5
    1. Pelvis—Surgery—Handbooks, manuals, etc. 2. Generative organs, Female—Surgery—Handbooks, manuals, etc. I. Title: Manual of pelvic surgery. II. Webb, Maurice J., 1941- III. Mayo Clinic
    [DNLM: 1. Pelvis—surgery—Handbooks. 2. Abdomen—surgery—Handbooks. 3. Genitalia, Female—surgery—Handbooks. 4. Surgical Procedures, Operative—methods—Handbooks. WP 39 M473 2000]
    RG104 .M35 2000
    617.5′5059—dc21
                                     99-054296

10 9 8 7 6 5 4 3 2 1

Contents

Contributing Authors

William A. Cliby, M.D. *Consultant, Department of Obstetrics and Gynecology and Surgery, Mayo Clinic and Mayo Foundation; Assistant Professor of Obstetrics and Gynecology, Mayo Medical School, Rochester, Minnesota*

Bobbie S. Gostout, M.D. *Consultant, Department of Obstetrics and Gynecology and Surgery, Mayo Clinic and Mayo Foundation; Assistant Professor of Obstetrics and Gynecology, Mayo Medical School, Rochester, Minnesota*

Darlene G. Kelly, M.D., Ph.D. *Consultant, Division of Gastroenterology and Hepatology and Internal Medicine, Mayo Clinic and Mayo Foundation; Assistant Professor of Medicine, Mayo Medical School, Rochester, Minnesota*

Raymond A. Lee, M.D. *Consultant, Departments of Obstetrics and Gynecology and Surgery, Mayo Clinic and Mayo Foundation; Professor of Obstetrics and Gynecology, Mayo Medical School, Rochester, Minnesota*

Karl C. Podratz, M.D., Ph.D. *Chairman, Department of Obstetrics and Gynecology, Consultant, Department of Surgery, Mayo Clinic and Mayo Foundation; Professor of Obstetrics and Gynecology, Mayo Medical School, Rochester, Minnesota*

Peter A. Southorn, M.D. *Consultant, Department of Anesthesiology, Mayo Clinic and Mayo Foundation; Associate Professor of Anesthesiology, Mayo Medical School, Rochester, Minnesota*

C. Robert Stanhope, M.D. *Consultant, Departments of Obstetrics and Gynecology and Surgery and Section of Medical Information Resources, Mayo Clinic and Mayo Foundation; Professor of Obstetrics and Gynecology, Mayo Medical School, Rochester, Minnesota*

Maurice J. Webb, M.D. *Chairman, Division of Gynecologic Surgery and Consultant, Department of Surgery, Mayo Clinic and Mayo Foundation; Professor of Obstetrics and Gynecology, Mayo Medical School, Rochester, Minnesota*

Tiffany J. Williams, M.D. *Emeritus Member, Departments of Obstetrics and Gynecology and Surgery, Mayo Clinic and Mayo Foundation; Emeritus Professor of Obstetrics and Gynecology, Mayo Medical School, Rochester, Minnesota*

Timothy O. Wilson, M.D. *Consultant, Departments of Obstetrics and Gynecology and Surgery, Mayo Clinic and Mayo Foundation; Assistant Professor of Obstetrics and Gynecology, Mayo Medical School, Rochester, Minnesota*

Preface

Writing the preface to a subsequent edition of a text is a distinct privilege. We are pleased that the audience accepted the first edition well enough to allow the second edition to be published. The preparation of this edition gave the authors the opportunity to reflect on the changes in medicine since the book was first published in 1994, and to note how these changes affect the way in which we care for our patients. This is a worthwhile experience.

During this time, we saw our surgical colleague, T.J. Williams, retire from active practice, and we recruited two new gynecologic oncologists, W.A. Cliby and B.S. Gostout, to our Division of Gynecologic Surgery at Mayo Clinic. The two new members of our team offer skills in the basic sciences, as well as superb surgical abilities, all of which will translate into a better understanding of the diseases we endeavor to treat, to the ultimate benefit of our patients. They both significantly contributed to this edition.

The surgical techniques described herein are the distillation of many years of experience by gynecologic surgeons at Mayo Clinic. That does not mean that variations in surgical technique or patient care have not occurred. The basic, standard techniques and principles of surgery that serve us well are preserved, while modifications in patient management are implemented. Examples include the now infrequent use of suction drainage after lymphadenectomy, fewer indications for the crossmatching of blood to cover surgical procedures, and an earlier start to suprapubic catheter clamping routines, dictated by the shorter length of hospital stay postoperatively. All the changes have been monitored closely through outcome analysis to be sure we are maintaining quality care for our patients.

Since the first edition, there also has been a cooperative effort within our group to standardize the postoperative care of our surgical patients. Clinical pathways have been developed for the more common operations, and all seven surgeons in the department adhere to these guidelines. A protocol has also been developed for postoperative analgesia. All patients are encouraged to attend a preoperative class where the daily care plans are discussed with them, and they are taught catheter and drain management and have their questions answered. These protocols, we believe, make it easier for the residents and nursing staff to provide excellent care for our patients and for the patients to become active partners in their postoperative management.

Also, since the first edition, endoscopic techniques and their indications are more standardized. All of our operating rooms are completely remodeled and outfitted with the latest endoscopic and audiovisual equipment. Thus, we added two new chapters on endoscopic techniques. The techniques described are those that we perform regularly and in considerable volume. We did not include endoscopic techniques that we regard as experimental or inappropriate. As we adopt newer techniques, we strive to follow the old Mayo principle that "the needs of the patient come first."

The reading list is updated to include new articles on surgical topics written by Mayo authors, and additional illustrations are included to provide further amplification from the illustrations of the first edition.

My thanks go to O. Eugene Millhouse, Ph.D., Roberta Schwartz, Marlené Boyd, and Dorothy Tienter in the Section of Scientific Publications, for their consummate professionalism and editing skills; to Robert Benassi, Emeritus Member of the Section of Visual Information Services, who produced numerous, outstanding new drawings; and to my colleagues at the Division of Gynecologic Surgery, for the way we work together as a team and enjoy each others' company as friends. My appreciation also goes to my secretary, Sherry Fields, who happily achieved the many deadlines, and to my wife, Val Webb, Ph.D., and my family, who are my never-ending source of optimism and encouragement.

Maurice J. Webb. M.D.

MAYO CLINIC
MANUAL OF
PELVIC SURGERY

CHAPTER 1

Preoperative Care

Maurice J. Webb, M.D.

I. Preoperative Assessment

Careful assessment of the patient preoperatively allows preventive measures to be taken to decrease surgical risk and morbidity.

A. Aims
1. To determine the risk/benefit ratio of the operation
2. To assess whether the operation is urgent or elective

B. History
1. Medical history
2. Surgical history
3. Family history
4. Current medications
5. Allergies
6. Tendency toward bleeding or thrombosis
7. Previous irradiation

C. Assessment of Organ Systems
1. Cardiovascular
2. Respiratory
3. Renal
4. Gastrointestinal
5. Nervous system

D. Assessment of Fluid and Blood Volume
1. Blood pressure and pulse rate
2. Weight
3. Tissue turgor
4. Edema
5. Ascites or pleural effusion
6. Jugular venous pressure
7. Hematocrit and hemoglobin

8. Serum electrolytes
9. Serum albumin
10. Urinary output and concentration

E. Assessment of Nutritional Status
1. Diet history
2. Weight loss
3. Muscle mass
4. Skinfold thickness
5. Anemia
6. Hypoproteinemia

F. Assessment of Risk Factors for Infection
1. Diabetes mellitus
2. Obesity
3. Malnutrition
4. Steroid drugs
5. Immunosuppressive drugs
6. Age
7. Malignancy
8. Previous irradiation therapy

II. Preoperative Routine Tests

A. General Principles
1. Preoperative testing depends on the patient's symptoms, history, examination results, disease process involved, and operation planned.
2. For uncomplicated pelvic surgical procedures in healthy patients, the following tests, dependent on the patient's age, are the minimum required.
   - < 40 years old: none required
   - 40 to 59 years old: electrocardiography, serum creatinine, and serum glucose levels
   - ≥ 60 years old: electrocardiography, chest radiography, complete blood count, serum creatinine, and serum glucose levels
   - A complete blood count in all patients who are typed and screened or crossmatched for a surgical procedure.

Maurice J. Webb: Chairman, Division of Gynecologic Surgery and Consultant, Department of Surgery, Mayo Clinic and Mayo Foundation; Professor of Obstetrics and Gynecology, Mayo Medical School, Rochester, Minnesota.

3. Serum potassium level should be measured in patients who are taking diuretics or undergoing bowel preparation.
4. Chest radiography is indicated for patients with a history of cardiac or pulmonary disease or recent respiratory symptoms or malignancy.
5. Other tests are performed at the discretion of the physician.

B. Preoperative Blood Crossmatch Orders
Suggested requirements for pelvic surgical procedures
1. Type and antibody screen only for
   - Laparoscopy
   - Bilateral salpingo-oophorectomy
   - Dilation and curettage
   - Total abdominal hysterectomy
   - Vaginal hysterectomy, with or without repair
   - Oophorectomy
   - Ovarian cystectomy
   - Tubal ligation
   - Cone biopsy
2. Blood crossmatch for
   - Radical hysterectomy, 1 U
   - Radical vulvectomy, 1 U
   - Hemicolectomy, 1 U
   - Small bowel resection, 1 U
   - Ovarian cancer debulking, 2 U
   - Splenectomy, 3 U
   - Exenteration, 4 U

C. Blood and Blood Components
Indications for
1. Whole blood
   - Acute hemorrhagic hypovolemic shock ($>$25% loss of blood volume)
   - Acute surgical blood loss
2. Erythrocytes
   - Symptomatic anemia
   - Acute hypovolemia (15% to 25% loss of blood volume)
3. Leukocyte-poor blood
   - Patients with granulocyte antibodies
   - Patients with repeated or severe febrile nonhemolytic transfusion reaction
4. Frozen erythrocytes
   - Storage of autologous blood
   - Storage of rare blood
   - Patients with anti-IgA antibodies who experience anaphylactic reactions to normal blood products
   - Patients with severe febrile nonhemolytic transfusion reactions not avoided by washed erythrocytes or leukocyte-poor blood
5. Autologous blood
   - Elective surgery in healthy patient: blood stored
   - Patients with multiple alloantibodies to high-frequency red blood cell antigens for whom it is difficult to find homologous donor blood

6. Granulocyte concentrate
   - Severe granulocytopenia ($<$500 neutrophils/mL) with severe infection not responding to antibiotics
7. Platelet concentrate
   - Chemotherapy-induced thrombocytopenia ($<$20,000/mL)
   - Before invasive procedure if platelet count is $<$50,000/mL
   - Actively bleeding patients with platelet count $<$50,000/mL
   - Patients with qualitatively abnormal platelets (rare)

   Note: In a 70-kg person, 1 U of platelet concentrate should increase platelet count by 5,000 to 10,000/mL.
   Note: Single donor (apheresis) platelets: patients refractory to platelet concentrates require HLA-matched platelets to achieve a clinical response.

8. Fresh frozen plasma
   - Replacement of isolated coagulation deficiencies, other than factor VIII and fibrinogen
   - Reversal of warfarin drug effect
   - Massive transfusion with dilutional coagulopathy
   - Antithrombin III deficiency
   - Primary and secondary aminodeficiency syndrome
   - Thrombotic thrombocytopenic purpura
9. Cryoprecipitated plasma (antihemophilic factor: contains factor VIII and fibrinogen)
   Factor VIII level $<$50% of normal
10. Factor VIII concentrate
    - Hemophiliac patients with circulating factor VIII inhibitors
    - Patients in whom cyroprecipitate is unsuitable
11. Cryoprecipitated fibrinogen (fibrin glue)
    - Selective embolization
    - Oozing surfaces, bleeding from suture holes
    - Presacral venous bleeding
    - Adhesive
12. Factor IX concentrate
    - Factor IX deficiency (Christmas disease)
    - Circulating factor VIII inhibitor in hemophiliacs
13. Normal serum albumin
    - Hypotension (shock)
    - Hypoproteinemia (temporary effect)

D. Criteria for Transfusion of Erythrocytes
1. Hemoglobin $<$8 g/dL in normal patients or $<$11 g/dL in patients with ischemic heart disease, cerebrovascular disease, and so forth
2. Anemia: causing symptoms such as
   - Tachycardia
   - Dyspnea
   - Angina
   - Mental status change
   - Electrocardiographic changes
3. Acute blood loss, causing the following:
   - $<$60 mm Hg diastolic pressure
   - $>$30 mm Hg decrease in systolic pressure

- Tachycardia >100/min
- Oliguria
- >15% loss of total blood volume
4. Pretreatment transfusion
- Before radiation therapy
- Aplastic anemia
- Preoperative severe anemia

III. General Preadmission Preparation

A. Instructions and Information for Patients

It is important to inform patients fully not only about the operative procedure but also about specific instructions necessary for adequate preoperative preparation.

1. Indications, risks, complications, and options related to the surgical procedure and success rates (if appropriate)
2. Preoperative fasting instructions
3. Preoperative bowel management (enemas, laxatives, etc.)
4. Instruction about taking or avoiding medications
5. Instruction about postoperative pain management (patient-controlled analgesia pump, epidural anesthesia, etc.)
6. Instruction about postoperative pulmonary toilet
7. Information about need for mobility and instruction in passive movements postoperatively, etc.
8. Information about anesthesia induction and recovery
9. Information about drains, catheters, and intravenous infusions
10. Information about thromboembolus-deterrent stockings and sequential calf compression devices

B. Steroid Preparation

1. Steroid suppression occurs if patient takes a quantity of adrenal steroids equal to or exceeding the normal adrenal gland output for ≥1 week.
2. Physiologic quantities per 24-hour period are as follows:
   - Cortisone, 25 mg
   - Hydrocortisone, 20 to 25 mg
   - Prednisone or prednisolone, 5 mg
   - Triamcinolone, 4 mg
   - Dexamethasone, 0.75 mg
   - Betamethasone, 0.6 mg
3. Suppression may persist for 2 months after stopping steroid therapy or for as long as 6 months if larger dosages are used or if prolonged treatment is given.
4. History must include
   - Duration of therapy
   - Dose
   - Mode of administration
   - Symptoms of hypercortisolism
   - Interval since steroid therapy was stopped
5. Treatment
   - Intramuscular route

— Dexamethasone, 4 mg i.m. on call to the operating room and every 12 hours on the day of the operation and then taper off
   or
— Prednisolone, 40 mg i.m. on call to the operating room and every 8 hours on the day of the operation, followed by 20 mg every 8 hours on the day after the operation and then taper off
   - Intravenous route (piggyback infusion)
— Dexamethasone, 5 mg i.v. every 6 hours
   or
— Prednisolone, 40 mg i.v. every 6 hours
   or
— Methylprednisolone, 40 mg i.v. every 6 hours and then taper off appropriately

C. Pulmonary Preparation

1. Is individualized for each patient but can involve the use of
   - Antibiotics
   - Mucolytic mists
   - Bronchodilators
   - Postural drainage
   - Intermittent positive pressure breathing
   - Incentive spirometry
   - Chest physiotherapy
2. Patients with severe pulmonary problems may benefit if admitted 48 hours preoperatively to undergo the above therapy.

D. Subacute Bacterial Endocarditis Prophylaxis

1. Standard regimen (see Dajani et al., 1997): Ampicillin, 2.0 g intravenously (i.v.) or intramuscularly (i.m.), plus gentamicin, 1.5 mg/kg i.v. or i.m. (not to exceed 120 mg), 30 minutes before the procedure, followed by amoxicillin, 1.0 g by mouth 6 hours after the initial dose or parenteral ampicillin 1 g 6 hours after the initial dose
2. Regimen for amoxicillin/ampicillin/penicillin-allergic patients: Vancomycin, 1.0 g i.v. administered over 1 to 2 hours plus gentamicin, 1.5 mg/kg i.v. or i.m. (not to exceed 120 mg), within 30 minutes of the procedure. May be repeated one time 8 hours after initial dose
3. Alternate regimen for low-risk patients: Amoxicillin, 2.0 g orally 1 hour before the procedure, or ampicillin, 2.0 g i.m. or i.v. within 30 minutes of starting the procedure

Note: Antibiotic regimens used to prevent recurrences of acute rheumatic fever are not adequate for the prevention of bacterial endocarditis. In patients with markedly compromised renal function, it may be necessary to modify the dose of gentamicin or vancomycin. Intramuscular injections of antibiotics may be contraindicated in patients receiving anticoagulants.

TABLE 1. *Two-day bowel preparation*

Two days preoperatively	One day preoperatively	Day of operation
Minimum residue diet	Clear liquid diet	Nothing by mouth after midnight
Two tap-water enemas (1,000 mL) after admission	Three tap-water enemas (1,000 mL) in a.m.	No enemas unless stool is not clear
	Three tap-water enemas (1,000 mL) in p.m.	
	Enemas until bowel return is clear, but maximum of eight. If not clear, notify physician.	
Phosphosoda, 15 mL by mouth on admission and 4 hours later	Phosphosoda, 15 mL by mouth 8 a.m.	
	Neomycin and metronidazole (Flagyl) base, 2 g each by mouth at 6 p.m. and 10 p.m.	

E. Bowel Preparation

1. For all patients in whom there is the possibility of intestinal surgery, preoperative bowel preparation should be administered (Tables 1 and 2). In patients with extensive pelvic malignancy (e.g., ovarian cancer) or postradiation problems or in whom severe adhesions are likely (e.g., ovarian remnant syndrome), the need for bowel surgery cannot be predicted by preoperative bowel radiography or by endoscopic examinations.

2. Bowel preparation is particularly important in patients with colostomy, ileostomy, Koch pouch, or bowel obstruction and/or severe inflammatory bowel disease.

3. Physical activity is important. The patient should be encouraged to take numerous walks during bowel preparation.

F. Parenteral Nutrition, Transfusions, and Fluids

1. Preoperative hydration with fluids given intravenously is required in some patients for the following reasons:
   - Intestinal obstruction
   - Acute fluid loss with gastrointestinal preparation
   - Septic states
   - Intestinal fistulas
   - Radiation- or chemotherapy-induced vomiting or diarrhea

2. Preoperative transfusions with erythrocytes may be indicated if a major procedure is contemplated and hemoglobin is <9 g/mL.

3. Patients in poor nutritional state may benefit from preoperative parenteral nutrition to aid healing of wounds and intestinal anastomoses (see Chapter 6).

G. Genital Preparation

1. Povidone-iodine douche is administered to all patients in whom entry into the vagina is planned.

2. Genital shave is performed as close to the time of the procedure as possible (preferably in the operating room or holding area and only in the area required) to reduce the risk of wound infection.

3. Types of genital and abdominal shaves
   - None: no shaving is necessary for dilation and curettage, cone biopsy, or other minor vaginal or cervical procedures.
   - Perineal shave: the posterior half of the vulva is shaved for minor surgical procedures around the posterior vulva, e.g., Bartholin abscess.
   - Vulvar shave: the whole of the vulva is prepared for vaginal hysterectomy, vaginal repairs, vulvectomy, etc.
   - Abdominal shave: the abdomen and mons pubis are shaved for all abdominal procedures.
   - Abdominal and vulvar shave: the abdomen and all the vulva are shaved for abdominoperineal procedures, e.g., pelvic exenteration, radical vulvectomy with inguinofemoral lymphadenectomy, retropubic bladder neck suspension, and others.

TABLE 2. *Polyethylene glycol 3350 (GoLYTELY) lavage, 1-Day preparation*

One day preoperatively	Day of operation
Clear liquid diet beginning at noon	Nothing by mouth after midnight
Polyethylene glycol electrolyte solution (GoLYTELY): drink 4–6 L commencing at 5 p.m.[a]	
Neomycin, 2 g at 6 p.m. and 10 p.m.	
Metronidazole (Flagyl), 2 g at 6 p.m. and 10 p.m. (after polyethylene glycol solution is finished)	
Bisacodyl, 10 mg at 10 p.m.	

[a] Feeding tube may be used.

H. Diabetic Preparation

When advising diabetic patients scheduled for outpatient or morning-admission procedures, the following guidelines should be followed:

1. Patients taking insulin should be scheduled for operation early in the day. It is not necessary that they be the first case. Sufficient preparation time for safe management of diabetic patients should be allowed.

2. Patients taking insulin who are scheduled for operation before 9 a.m. should be advised not to take their insulin before coming to the hospital the morning of the operation. They should be asked to bring their insulin with them to the hospital.

3. Patients taking insulin who are to take nothing by mouth after midnight and who are not admitted for operation until after 9 a.m. should be advised to test their blood glucose at 7 a.m. If the blood glucose level is >100 mg/dL, they should take one-half the usual dose of intermediate-acting insulin (no regular insulin) at that time. If the blood glucose level is <100 mg/dL, they should take 15 g of carbohydrate (i.e., ½ cup fruit juice or soda pop with sugar) and one-half the usual dose of intermediate-acting insulin (no regular insulin) at that time.

4. Patients taking insulin who are to take nothing by mouth after breakfast and who are scheduled for an operation later in the day should be advised to take one-half the usual dose of intermediate-acting insulin (no regular insulin) at breakfast instead of the full dose.

5. Patients taking hypoglycemic agents by mouth should be advised not to take the agents before coming to the hospital the morning of the operation.

I. Management of Cardiac Medications

A common concern is how to handle medications used for angina, heart failure, or arrhythmias. A major objective is to avoid, during anesthesia, severe hypotension or cardiac arrhythmias that might provoke an intraoperative infarction. Several recommendations that may be helpful in writing preoperative orders follow:

1. β-Blockers—atenolol (Tenormin), metoprolol (Lopressor), and propranolol (Inderal)
Patients taking β-blockers are subject to withdrawal hypersensitivity that begins as soon as doses of the drug are missed; this sensitivity may last for several days. Therefore, patients taking β-blockers should take this medication up to the morning of the operation; on the morning of the operation, the medication should be taken with a small sip of water. These medications should be resumed as quickly as possible postoperatively, providing that clinical circumstances (bradycardia or hypotension) do not militate against their use.

2. Calcium channel blockers—verapamil (Calan or Isoptin), diltiazem (Cardizem), and nifedipine (Procardia)
There is no evidence that calcium channel blockers aggravate hypotension intraoperatively, and because they help prevent ischemia, they should be continued up to the time of the operation and be resumed as quickly as possible postoperatively.

3. Long-acting nitrates: isosorbide dinitrate (Isordil)
As for calcium channel blockers, there is no evidence that long-acting nitrates aggravate hypotension intraoperatively. Thus, these drugs should also be continued up to the time of the operation and resumed as quickly as possible postoperatively. In the case of long-acting nitrates, transdermal administration of nitroglycerin can maintain protection when patients are unable to take medication orally. If a prolonged period of fasting is required, patients should be treated with transdermal nitroglycerin.

4. Antiarrhythmic drugs
Antiarrhythmic drugs may be prescribed for various disturbances of rhythm, ranging from benign and symptomatic atrial arrhythmias to the potentially life-threatening ventricular arrhythmias. Decisions about how to handle antiarrhythmia drugs should be made carefully after cardiologic consultation.

5. Digoxin
Digoxin should be given up to the day before the operation. Usually, it can be withheld safely until oral intake is possible; digoxin can be given intravenously during the time that oral intake is not possible.

6. Antihypertensive medications
It is important to continue antihypertensive medications up to the time of the operation, especially when these medications include β-blockers or clonidine given by mouth. The problem of clonidine withdrawal is significant but can be managed by conversion from oral to transdermal administration. It is best to make the conversion 2 to 3 weeks preoperatively.

Reading List

Pratt JH, Weisberg MG, Janes DR. Preoperative and postoperative care of the gynecologic patient. *J St Barnabas Med Center* 1970;7:98–106.

Dajani AS, Taubert KA, Wilson W, et al. Prevention of bacterial endocarditis. Recommendations by the American Heart Association. *JAMA* 1997;277:1794–1801.

CHAPTER 2

Intraoperative Management

Maurice J. Webb, M.D.

I. Intraoperative Preparation

A. Positioning Patient on Operating Room Table
1. Trendelenburg position
   - Trendelenburg position is useful in pelvic procedures (Fig. 1).
   - Ankle straps assist in maintaining the patient in this position.
   - Make sure that the break in the table corresponds to the flexion of the patient's knees.
   - Supports and restraints should be well padded.
   - Avoid a steep Trendelenburg position if there is a possibility of an intracranial lesion.
   - Avoid hyperextension of the patient's arms to protect against brachial palsy.
   - Avoid shoulder braces to protect against brachial palsy.
2. Lithotomy position
   - Lithotomy position is used for vaginal procedures.
   - If the patient has back or hip problems, elevate the legs while the patient is still awake.
   - Avoid pressure on the lateral aspect of the knee to prevent peroneal nerve palsy.
   - Hyperflexion of the hips may cause femoral nerve palsy.
3. Ski position (Fig. 2)
   - Ski position is used for combined abdominal and vaginal procedures, e.g., exenteration, radical vulvectomy with nodes, and laparoscopy.
   - The legs are supported in knee stirrups.
   - Adequate padding around the knees is necessary to prevent peroneal nerve palsy.

B. Deep Vein Thrombosis Prophylaxis
1. Use thromboembolus-deterrent stockings on all patients undergoing major surgical procedures.

Maurice J. Webb: Chairman, Division of Gynecologic Surgery and Consultant, Department of Surgery, Mayo Clinic and Mayo Foundation; Professor of Obstetrics and Gynecology, Mayo Medical School, Rochester, Minnesota.

2. Use sequential calf compression device intraoperatively and postoperatively for at least 72 hours in patients at high risk for deep vein thrombosis.
3. Consider subcutaneous heparin prophylaxis in high-risk patients (heparin, 5,000 U injected subcutaneously every 12 hours starting with on call to the operating room and continued until the patient is fully mobile). Alternatively, low-molecular-weight heparin (enoxaparin), 30 mg subcutaneously twice daily, can be used.

C. Preoperative Antibiotics
1. Principles
   - There should be a significant risk of infection before treating with antibiotics.
   - Drug should be present in the wound at incision.
   - Usage should be short-term.
   - Use broad-spectrum antibiotics.
   - Avoid drugs used for resistant organisms.
   - Low-cost drugs with low toxicity are preferred.
   - Treatment with antibiotics is not a substitute for good hemostasis and drainage.
2. Indications
   - Abdominal hysterectomy
   - Vaginal hysterectomy
   - Cesarean hysterectomy
   - Bowel operations
   - Oncologic operations
   - Postradiation procedures
   - All open abdominal procedures.
3. Dosage
   - Cefazolin, 2 g on call to the operating room

D. Skin Cleaning and Preparation
1. Shave the patient as close to the time of operation as possible and avoid abrasion of the skin.
2. Scrub the operative site with povidone-iodine solution.
3. Mop dry with a sterile towel.
4. Paint the operative site with povidone-iodine solution.
5. Drape the operative site.

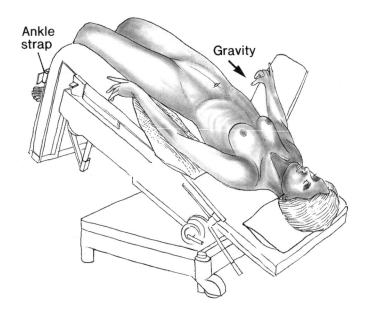

FIG. 1. Steep Trendelenburg position using ankle straps.

6. For abdominal procedures, swab the vagina with povidone-iodine solution and insert a Foley urethral catheter.

E. Urinary Catheter Drainage

1. Insert a Foley catheter in the bladder in the operating room before performing any abdominal procedures.
2. In all patients, the catheter is removed the next morning except under special circumstances, e.g., fistula repair and inadvertent cystotomy.
3. Advantages are
   * Bladder is kept empty during the operation, thus avoiding injury and improving exposure.
   * Urine output can be monitored closely during the operation.
   * Urine output can be monitored carefully during the postoperative period.
   * Urinary retention during the postoperative period is avoided.
4. If a suprapubic Foley catheter is used, insert it with the trocar before commencing a vaginal operation that involves anterior colporrhaphy or urethral surgery.

5. A suprapubic Foley catheter also is inserted through a cystotomy incision after a Marshall-Marchetti-Krantz operation, a radical hysterectomy, or a posterior pelvic exenteration.
6. A transurethral Foley catheter is used after simple vaginal hysterectomy without repairs or after vulvectomy.

II. Intraoperative Monitoring

A. Routine

Routine monitoring of vital signs such as pulse, blood pressure, skin color, urinary output, and blood loss

B. Other Techniques

Other monitoring techniques provide additional safety for the patient.

1. Swan-Ganz catheter
2. Pulse oximeter
3. Intraarterial pressure monitoring
4. Blood-gas monitoring

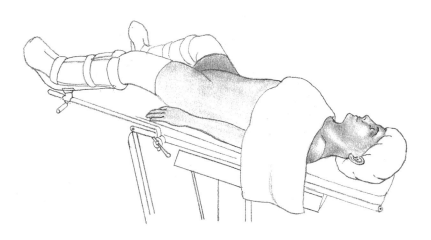

FIG. 2. Ski position.

III. Incisions

A. Principles
1. The type of incision is decided before draping.
2. Drape so the incision can be extended if necessary.
3. Exposure is of greater importance than cosmesis.
4. Intraoperative complications occur more frequently with small incisions because of poor exposure.
5. Note the presence of previous scars, and excise the scar if using the same incision location.
6. Midline or paramedian incisions give the best exposure and can easily be extended if necessary, especially if disease extends into the upper abdomen.

B. Types
1. Midline incision
   - Most commonly used incision
   - Fairly avascular
   - Easily extended
   - Most likely to develop hernia
2. Paramedian incision
   - Retracts rectus muscle, therefore stronger incision than midline
   - More bleeding from edges of incision
3. Pfannenstiel incision
   - Good cosmetic incision
   - Poor exposure
   - Cannot be extended into upper abdomen
   - Strong incision, unlikely to herniate
   - Suitable only for minor pelvic surgical procedures such as ovarian cystectomy, ectopic pregnancy, cesarean section
   - Hysterectomies that can be performed through Pfannenstiel incisions probably should be done vaginally.
4. Cherney and Maylard incisions (Figs. 3 and 4)
   - Muscle cutting or tendon cutting, transverse incisions
   - Good cosmesis and good exposure in lower abdomen and pelvis
   - Less exposure in upper abdomen and more difficult to extend
   - Muscle cutting weakens the incision.

IV. Suture Material

A. Principle
Synthetic absorbable sutures are preferred to catgut because they have greater tensile strength that is maintained for a longer time, cause less tissue reaction, and have a more predictable absorption pattern. Delayed absorbable synthetic sutures may be substituted if a longer lasting suture is desired.

B. Absorbable Sutures
1. 1-0 synthetic absorbable suture: used for
   - Abdominal and vaginal hysterectomy pedicles
   - Other large vascular pedicles
   - Reconstruction of the cervix after conization or trachelorrhaphy
   - Closure of vaginal vault in abdominal hysterectomy
   - Closure of abdominal wall fascia
   - McCall suture in vaginal hysterectomy enterocele prophylaxis
2. 2-0 synthetic absorbable suture: used for
   - Closure of peritoneum
   - Closure of vaginal mucosa in vaginal repairs
   - Approximation of fascial layers in vaginal repairs
   - Closure of vulvar skin incisions
3. 3-0 synthetic absorbable suture: used for
   - Ligation of small bleeding sites
   - Reconstruction of ovary after cystectomy
   - Subcuticular skin closure
   - Suturing of intestinal stomas to skin
   - Mucosal layer of intestinal anastomosis
   - Closure of cystotomy incisions in bladder
4. 4-0 synthetic absorbable suture: used for
   - Ureter/ureter, ureter/bladder, and ureter/bowel anastomoses (or substitute 5-0 delayed synthetic absorbable suture)

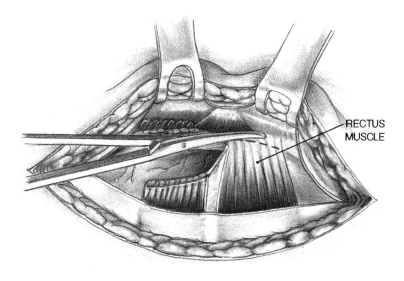

RECTUS MUSCLE

FIG. 3. Cherney incision.

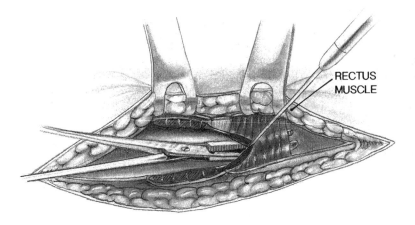

FIG. 4. Maylard incision.

RECTUS MUSCLE

- Bladder or rectal mucosal layer in repair of vesicovaginal or rectovaginal fistulas
- Mucosal layer in repair of urethra (diverticulum, fistula, etc.)

C. Nonabsorbable Sutures

Nonabsorbable sutures are used where prolonged tensile strength is required with minimal tissue reaction.

1. 0 polytef (Teflon)-coated polyethylene terephthalate (Dacron) (Ethibond, Ticryl): used for retropubic bladder neck suspension (Marshall-Marchetti-Krantz operation or paravaginal defect repair)
2. 3-0 silk or monofilament suture (Prolene): used for hernia fascial repair
3. 0 nylon or monofilament suture: used for abdominal incision with presence or risk of dehiscence and hernia repair
4. 3-0 nylon or monofilament or silk or staples: used for skin closure where subcuticular suture not used
5. 3-0 silk: used for seromuscular layer in intestinal anastomoses

V. Wound Closure

A. Principles

1. The wound dehiscence rate for gynecologic patients is probably <2/1,000 cases.
2. Predisposing factors are
   - Obesity
   - Malignancy
   - Advanced age
   - Diabetes mellitus
   - Malnutrition
   - Liver disease
   - Radiation therapy
   - Steroid therapy
   - Immunosuppression
   - Clean versus contaminated operation
   - Type of incision used
   - Wound infection
3. Preventive measures at the time of operation are

- Adequate preoperative cleansing and antisepsis
- Gentle tissue handling
- Meticulous hemostasis
- Obliteration of dead space
- Use of wound drains
- Prophylactic use of antibiotics
- Short operating time
- Correction of metabolic/nutritional problems preoperatively
- Selection of appropriate incision
- Irrigation of the incision before closure
- Selection of appropriate suture material
- Wound closure technique
- Use of gastrointestinal decompression if indicated
- Control of nausea and vomiting
- Adequate postoperative respiratory therapy to prevent infection

B. Standard Closure Technique

1. Peritoneum is closed with continuous 2-0 synthetic absorbable suture.
2. Fascia is closed with continuous 1 synthetic absorbable sutures supported by interrupted 1 synthetic absorbable sutures.
3. Skin is closed with subcuticular 3-0 synthetic absorbable suture (no fat sutures) or delayed absorbable suture (Monocryl).
4. A small 3-mm round suction drain is placed on top of the fascia for the full length of the incision before skin closure.

C. Smead-Jones Closure Technique

1. This technique is used to repair dehiscence or when wound dehiscence is likely, e.g., obese patient, malignancy, recent operation through the same incision, postradiation, etc.
2. Sutures are interrupted, 1 cm apart, and include at least 1.5 cm of the fascia on either side of the incision.
3. The wound is approximated but not tightly.
4. The suture includes fascia and peritoneum in one layer.
5. Nonabsorbable suture is best for the Smead-Jones type of closure (Fig. 5).

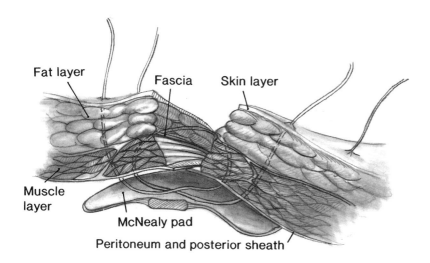

Fat layer

Fascia

Skin layer

Muscle layer

McNealy pad

Peritoneum and posterior sheath

FIG. 5. Smead-Jones far and near abdominal suturing.

TABLE 1. *Basic set of surgical instruments*

Mayo operating scissors 5½ in. curved and straight
Mayo long scissors 9 in. curved
Metzenbaum dissecting scissors 7 in. (vaginal repair)
Tissue forceps with teeth 6 in.
Adson tissue forceps 4¾ in. (skin closure)
CW Mayo Russian tissue forceps 9 and 6 in.
Halsted mosquito forceps 5 in. (fine clamping, ureteral anastomosis)
Kocher artery forceps 5½ in. straight (pedicle clamps with abdominal hysterectomy)
Allis intestinal tissue forceps 6 in. (bladder closure, intestinal surgery)
CW Mayo abdominal retractor (wound retraction)
Deaver retractors (vaginal and abdominal surgery)
Harrington-Pemberton springblade retractor (retract bladder during total abdominal hysterectomy)
Mayo-Collins retractor (wound fascial closure)
Balfour self-retaining retractor (abdominal procedure)
Right-angled gallbladder forceps 7¾ in. (ureteral dissection)
Doyen intestinal forceps 8¾ in. (small-bowel anastomoses)
Babcock intestinal forceps 6½ in.
Foss anterior resection clamp 11½ in. (rectosigmoid resection)
Pemberton sigmoid anastomosis clamp 9 in. (rectosigmoid resection)
Vein retractor (ureteral dissection, node dissection)
Stratte needle holder 9 in. (Marshall-Marchetti-Krantz operation)
Mayo-Hegar needle holders 8 and 12 in.
Auvard vaginal speculum (vaginal surgery)
Henrontin uterine vulsellum 8½ in. (cervical traction, vaginal vault traction in total abdominal hysterectomy)
Wylie uterine dilator (dilation and curettage)
Heaney hysterectomy forceps 8¼ in. (vaginal hysterectomy)
Suprapubic trocar and cannula (suprapubic catheter)

D. Delayed Wound Closure

1. This technique is used in a potentially contaminated wound.
2. The peritoneum and fascia are closed but skin sutures are not tied; the wound is packed open with gauze and changed daily.
3. If the wound is clean, skin sutures are tied on the third postoperative day.

E. Wound Dressings

1. A light occlusive sterile dressing is placed over the wound to avoid pressure on the wound.
2. The dressing should be removed the next morning so the wound can be inspected daily.

F. Wound Drains

1. Connected to suction device postoperatively
2. Can be irrigated with antiseptic solution if infection is likely
3. Are removed the morning after the operation if drainage is minimal, i.e., <20 mL/24 h

VI. Instrumentation

Instruments used depend on personal preferences. The ones listed in Table 1 are commonly used as part of the basic set of instruments at the Mayo Clinic.

Reading List

Souders JR, Pratt JH. Wound dehiscence and incisional hernia after gynecologic operations. *Clin Obstet Gynecol* 1962;5:522–539.

CHAPTER 3

Postoperative Care

Maurice J. Webb, M.D., Peter A. Southorn, M.D., Darlene G. Kelly, M.D., Ph.D.

I. Aim

The aim of postoperative care is to anticipate problems before they arise and to take preventive measures to avoid development of complications.

II. Postoperative Monitoring of Vital Signs

A. Pulse Rate, Blood Pressure, and Respiratory Rate
In the immediate postoperative period, the patient's pulse rate, blood pressure, and respiratory rate are monitored as follows:
1. Every 15 minutes for 1 hour *then*
2. Every 30 minutes for 2 hours *then*
3. Every 60 minutes for 8 hours *then*
4. Every 4 hours

B. Urine Output
Urine output is measured hourly until 6 a.m. the morning after the procedure and then every 4 hours, unless the output is low.

III. Respiratory Therapy

A. Aim
To avoid complications such as

Maurice J. Webb: Chairman, Division of Gynecologic Surgery and Consultant, Department of Surgery, Mayo Clinic and Mayo Foundation; Professor of Obstetrics and Gynecology, Mayo Medical School, Rochester, Minnesota.

Peter A. Southorn: Consultant, Department of Anesthesiology, Mayo Clinic and Mayo Foundation; Associate Professor of Anesthesiology, Mayo Medical School, Rochester, Minnesota.

Darlene G. Kelly: Consultant, Division of Gastroenterology and Hepatology and Internal Medicine, Mayo Clinic and Mayo Foundation; Assistant Professor of Medicine, Mayo Medical School, Rochester, Minnesota.

1. Atelectasis
2. Retained secretions
3. Pneumonia

B. High-Risk Patients
Particular care must be taken with patients at high risk, such as those with
1. Obesity
2. Advanced age
3. Asthma
4. Chronic obstructive pulmonary disease, emphysema, or other lung disease
5. Smoking history
6. Upper abdominal incision
7. Previous pulmonary embolus or deep vein thrombosis

C. Prophylaxis
Involves
1. Adequate hydration
2. Encouragement of deep breathing and coughing and incentive spirometry
3. Adequate pain relief
4. Early mobilization
5. Avoidance of abdominal distention

D. Adequacy of Oxygenation
If there is concern about adequacy of oxygenation, monitor with pulse oximeter or arterial blood gas analysis.

IV. Fluid and Electrolyte Balance

A. Principles
1. Careful monitoring and assessment of body fluid needs are essential postoperatively to prevent fluid and electrolyte imbalance.
2. Fluid and electrolyte orders should be written *after* the operation to take into account the losses intraoperatively.

B. Fluids and Electrolytes

1. Each of the following may influence fluid and electrolyte requirements:
   - Blood and fluid loss at operation and postoperatively
   - Body cavity drains
   - Intestinal suction
   - Intestinal fistula
   - Renal function
   - Drugs, e.g., diuretics
   - Fever
   - Respiratory losses
2. The fluids generally used postoperatively contain dextrose, sodium, and chloride. Potassium needs to be added to intravenous fluids; 40 to 60 mEq/L/day usually is sufficient.
3. Other electrolytes (calcium, magnesium, phosphorus, etc.) are also important but not in the first few days postoperatively; most patients usually are eating soon enough that they do not become deficient.

C. Measurement

1. In practice, hemoglobin and creatinine are measured on the first morning postoperatively.
2. Electrolytes are measured and then monitored at least daily in
   - Patients receiving prolonged administration of fluids intravenously
   - Patients with
     — Renal function abnormality
     — Ileus or bowel obstruction
     — Intestinal fistula
     — Intestinal resection or ileostomy
     — Intestinal suction drainage
     — Other excessive loss of body fluids
   - Patients taking
     — Cardiac medications
     — Diuretics
   - Patients who have had previous electrolyte disturbances such as syndrome of inappropriate antidiuretic hormone
3. It is essential to keep an accurate record of fluid intake and output and daily weight and to assess carefully hydration with tissue turgor, central venous pressure, lung auscultation, etc.

V. Mobilization, Deep Vein Thrombosis Prophylaxis, and Drain Management

A. Increased Risk of Deep Vein Thrombosis

1. Surgery
2. Malignancy
3. Immobilization
4. Estrogen use
5. Pregnancy
6. Hypercoagulable states
7. Previous deep vein thrombosis or embolus

B. Principles of Patient Mobilization

1. All patients are mobilized the morning after the procedure, except in specific circumstances (e.g., myocutaneous grafts).
2. On the first day postoperatively, the patient is walked around the bed and seated in a chair for a period; this is repeated four times daily. Leg exercises are encouraged.
3. Patients with vaginal reconstruction or vulval flaps are not allowed to sit for about 5 days but can stand or walk.
4. On the second day postoperatively, activity is extended to frequent (at least four) walks beyond the patient's room.

C. Principles of Deep Vein Thrombosis Prophylaxis

1. Knee-high thromboembolus-deterrent stockings are used on any patient undergoing a major surgical procedure until the patient is fully mobile.
2. Thromboembolus-deterrent stockings are removed twice daily for a 30-minute period and are washed every 3 to 4 days.
3. If sequential calf compression devices are used, they are placed preoperatively and kept on the patient for at least 72 hours postoperatively.
4. Sequential calf compression devices can be removed temporarily for ambulation and for bathing but not for >25 minutes each time.
5. Thromboembolus-deterrent stockings should also be used with the compression sleeves.
6. The compression sleeves should be removed if the patient experiences numbness, tingling, or pain.
7. Sequential calf compression devices are not recommended if the patient has any of the following:
   - Dermatitis
   - Gangrene
   - Recent skin graft on the leg
   - Recent stripping of varicose veins
   - Severe atherosclerosis
   - Massive edema of the leg
   - Suspected deep vein thrombosis
   - Leg deformity
8. Pillows under the calves and dangling of legs over the edge of the bed are not allowed.
9. Heparin (5,000 U subcutaneously two or three times daily) is given to patients at high risk for deep vein thrombosis or who have a history of pulmonary embolus.

D. Principles of Drain Management

1. Subcutaneous wound suction drains usually are removed on postoperative day 2.

2. Drains to a lymphadenectomy site (pelvis or groin) are removed when drainage is <50 mL/24 h on 2 consecutive days.

3. Drains inserted intraperitoneally because of oozing or a large raw area are removed on postoperative day 3. (Because these drains are intraperitoneal, they will continue to drain amounts of fluid if left in place.)

4. Drains inserted down to the level of a colonic anastomosis should be left until 24 hours after the bowels have opened to check that there has been no anastomotic leak.

5. The drain site is cleaned with soap and water three times daily, and povidone-iodine ointment is applied together with a gauze dressing.

VI. Pain Relief

A. Principles

1. Pain after a procedure is
   • Most severe immediately after the procedure
   • Aggravated by movement, coughing, etc.
   • Usually of minimal severity by the third postoperative day

2. Factors exacerbating pain include
   • Surgical incision extending into the upper abdomen
   • Patient anxiety
   • Lack of sleep
   • Presence of various noxious stimuli, including noise, tubes, drains, etc.
   • Complications such as wound hematomas

3. Benefits of pain relief include
   • Patient comfort
   • Improvement in patient mobility, thus decreasing the incidence of deep vein thrombosis
   • Allows patients to breathe deeply, to cough, etc., thereby improving pulmonary toilet and decreasing the incidence of atelectasis and pneumonia
   • Decrease in the metabolic response to pain, including hyperglycemia, hypercatecholemia, hypercortisolemia, etc.

4. Treatment of pain has two components
   • Supportive measures to decrease anxiety, to provide a pleasant environment, to control unpleasant symptoms, to ensure adequate sleep, etc.
   • Analgesia

B. Opiates

1. When the minimal effective blood analgesic concentration is exceeded, patients experience pain relief. Opiate dose required to provide pain relief varies among patients and is affected by factors such as
   • Age
   • Hepatic and renal function
   • Thyroid function
   • Psychological makeup
   • Nonsteroidal antiinflammatory drugs, which have an "opiate-sparing" effect
   • Concomitant use of sedatives and drugs

2. Side effects of opiates include
   • Respiratory depression (reversed by naloxone, 0.1 to 0.4 mg given intravenously, repeated as needed)
   • Pruritis
   • Nausea and vomiting
   • Ileus
   • Increased biliary sphincter tone

3. Many opiates exist, with no clear differences between them in terms of producing fewer side effects at equipotent analgesic doses. Physicians are advised to gain familiarity with one to two such drugs, e.g., morphine and meperidine (Demerol).
   • Morphine
     — Has a low lipid solubility
     — Is metabolized by the liver
     — Has effects that are considerably prolonged by renal failure
     — Has potential to cause bronchospasm
   • Meperidine
     — Has a sedative effect
     — Can cause hypotension
     — Has atropine- and quinidine-like effects
     — Can cause severe hypertension in patients taking monoamine oxidase inhibitors

4. Intramuscular administration
   • Least satisfactory method because it does not take into account patient variability and because of
     — The delay from the time pain is perceived to the time of relief
     — The fluctuating nature of pain relief
     — Irregular and occasionally poor absorption of opiate from the injection site
   • When opiates are given intramuscularly, it is appropriate to
     — Give the drug as needed and not according to a rigid schedule.
     — Shorten the time between doses rather than increasing dose of drug if pain relief is unsatisfactory.

5. Patient-controlled analgesia (PCA)
   This technology allows patients to give themselves intermittent doses of opiates intravenously with a preprogrammed pump. Preoperative education of patients about how to use the pump is important.
   • Controls available on the pump include
     — Dosage
     — Shortest interval between injections ("lock-out interval")
     — Maximal dose the patient can receive in a given time
     — Provision of a constant "background" opiate infusion, if desired

- Advantages include
  — Provides good pain relief
  — Can be adjusted to patient variability
  — Can be adjusted to change in the severity of pain with time and activities
- Compared with pain relief provided by opiates given intramuscularly, PCA
  — Increases spontaneous activity of patients
  — Produces less sedation
  — Increases sleep
  — Causes less respiratory depression
  — Usually allows total dose of opiate to be decreased
  — Allows earlier return of bowel function

6. Epidural administration of opiates
- This technique is very effective in relieving severe pain after major surgical procedures.
- The opiates usually are administered on a continuous basis through a catheter placed in the epidural space in the lumbar region.
- Disadvantages of epidural administration include
  — It requires trained personnel for insertion of catheter, monitoring, and maintenance.
  — It is time consuming.
  — It has potentially serious complications, including respiratory depression.
  — It requires continuous urinary catheterization when local anesthetics are given with opiates epidurally.
- Epidural administration has common minor side effects, including
  — Itching
  — Urinary retention
  — Nausea and vomiting
- Respiratory depression associated with epidural administration
  — Occurs particularly in elderly patients
  — Is more common in patients concomitantly receiving opiates systemically
  — Can have an onset delayed by several hours
  — Is more common with opiates of low lipid solubility, such as morphine, than for highly lipid-soluble drugs, such as fentanyl

Note: To detect and to treat respiratory depression, the respiratory rate should be monitored every half hour for the first 16 hours after starting administration of the drugs and then hourly from the 16th to the 24th hour.

Note: Naloxone, 0.1 to 0.4 mg (i.v.), should be available to reverse respiratory depression. Naloxone has a limited duration of effect, and repeat administration may be required.

C. Nonsteroidal Antiinflammatory Drugs (NSAIDs)

1. Ketorolac tromethamine (Toradol)
- A potent analgesic (30 mg is equivalent to 6 to 12 mg of morphine)
- Has "opiate-sparing" effect when given concomitantly with opioids immediately postoperatively. Good analgesia is obtained with a lower opiate dose and the

patient thereby experiences fewer opiate-related side effects.
- Potentially dangerous side effects have occurred, including gastrointestinal tract hemorrhage (particularly in the elderly), acute renal failure, asthma (particularly in patients sensitive to aspirin), and surgical bleeding when hemostasis is not secure.
- Contraindications to use include a previous history of peptic ulcer disease or gastrointestinal tract hemorrhage, poor renal reserve, and known hypersensitivity to NSAIDs. Other NSAIDs should not be given simultaneously with ketorolac.
- Administration should be limited to 5 days. Side effects increase after this time.
- Dose: 30 mg intramuscularly (i.m.) or i.v. every 6 hours. In patients older than 65 years or weighing <50 kg, the dose should be reduced to 15 mg. The drug should be used with caution—if at all—in patients who have renal impairment.

2. Other NSAIDs
Useful for managing the residual pain the patient may be experiencing on the second or third postoperative day. They include the following:
- Acetaminophen, 500 to 1,000 mg given orally
- Aspirin, 300 mg

VII. Catheter Management

A. Indications

1. Used to decompress the bladder after dissection in the region of the bladder or after operations on the bladder
2. Enables accurate measurement of hourly urine output (should be about 1 mL/kg/h) postoperatively

B. Urethral Catheter

1. Indications
Used for
- Vaginal or abdominal hysterectomy
- Paravaginal defect repair
- Vulvectomy
- Ureteral or bladder fistula repair
- Other intraperitoneal operations, e.g., oophorectomy, second-look laparotomy, myomectomy

2. Removal
- Removed the morning after the operation, except for patients undergoing retropubic suspension or vaginal repairs
- Removed on the second postoperative morning after paravaginal defect repair
- Removed on the third postoperative morning if used in association with anterior colporrhaphy
- Removed on the seventh postoperative morning after repair of a vesicovaginal fistula or cystotomy
- Removed 6 weeks postoperatively after repair of a vesicovaginal fistula or cystotomy in patients who have had pelvic irradiation

C. Suprapubic Catheter

1. Indications
   Used for
   - Anterior colporrhaphy
   - Bladder fistulas
   - Uretheral reconstruction and diverticulectomy
   - Marshall-Marchetti-Krantz operation
   - Radical hysterectomy
   - Posterior exenteration
2. Technique
   - Percutaneous technique
     — Fill the bladder with 500 mL of isotonic saline.
     — Palpate the bladder suprapubically.
     — Make a 0.5-cm incision in the skin suprapubically, approximately two fingerwidths above the symphysis.
     — Insert a Mueller-Hurwitz trocar until it enters the bladder.
     — Pass a 16-F Foley catheter into the bladder and inflate the balloon.
     — Remove the trocar, and suture the catheter to the skin.
   - Open technique: after an intraabdominal procedure has been completed
     — Free the bladder from the back of the symphysis by dissecting the retropubic space.
     — Grasp the dome of the bladder in an extraperitoneal position with two Allis clamps.
     — Make a small incision into the bladder with cautery or scissors.
     — Grasp the fascia of the anterior abdominal wall with a straight clamp, and make a small stab incision in the lower abdominal wall.
     — Insert large curved forceps from the retropubic space through the abdominal wall and the skin stab incision.
     — Grasp the tip of an 18-F Foley catheter in the teeth of the forceps, and draw the catheter through the skin and abdominal wall.
     — Insert the tip of the catheter into the cystotomy incision, and inflate the balloon.
     — Close the cystotomy around the catheter in two layers with continuous 3-0 synthetic absorbable suture.
3. Suprapubic catheter clamping schedule
   - Clamp catheter on the third postoperative morning after anterior colporrhaphy.
   - Clamp catheter on the seventh postoperative morning after Marshall-Marchetti-Krantz operation, cystotomy, nonirradiated fistula repair, urethral reconstruction, or diverticulectomy.
   - Clamp catheter on the 12th postoperative day after radical hysterectomy or posterior pelvic exenteration without previous irradiation.
   - Clamp approximately 6 weeks postoperatively in previously irradiated patients with partial cystectomy, fistula repair, radical hysterectomy, or posterior pelvic exenteration.
4. Clamping routine
   - On prescribed day, clamp catheter for 4 hours.
   - Have patient attempt to void every 1 to 2 hours.
   - Check residual urine after voiding at 4 hours.
   - When residual urine is <150 mL on two consecutive occasions, increase the clamping interval by 2 hours.
   - Intervals of clamping go from 4 to 6 to 8 to 10 to 12 hours and then to 24 hours.
   - The catheter is always unclamped any time the patient becomes distressed because of distention.
   - Once residual urine is <150 mL at 24 hours, the suprapubic catheter may be removed.
   - A pressure dressing is applied to the catheter site, and the patient is instructed to void frequently in the next 4 to 6 hours to allow the sinus to heal.

D. Maintenance of Indwelling Catheter

1. The catheter should be secured to the thigh with tape to avoid pulling or kinking.
2. The drainage tube should be looped and attached to the side of the bed with a clamp.
3. The drainage bag should be hung on the side of the bed at a level lower than the bladder to provide unobstructed flow of urine.
4. For urethral catheters, cleanse the perineum at least once daily with soap and water, washing away from the meatus.
5. Cleanse more frequently if vaginal discharge is present.
6. For suprapubic catheters, cleanse with soap and water three times daily; apply povidone-iodine ointment and split gauze dressing.

E. Self-Catheterization

1. For patients who are unable to void after removal of a urethral catheter or after clamping of a suprapubic catheter, intermittent self-catheterization may be preferred because of the lower risk of urinary tract infection.
2. Self-catheterization is contraindicated after urethral reconstruction, diverticulectomy, or fistula repair.
3. Technique
   - The patient is instructed at 7 a.m., 11 a.m., 4 p.m., and 9 p.m. initially or until the technique has been mastered.
   - The patient is instructed to try to void every 1 to 2 hours and just before self-catheterization.
   - The patient is instructed to wash hands thoroughly.
   - The catheter pack is opened, and the tip of the catheter is lubricated.
   - The labia are separated and pulled slightly upward to expose the meatus.
   - A washcloth held in the other hand is used to wipe the meatus with front to back strokes, rotating the cloth after each wipe.

- The catheter is inserted into the meatus slowly until urine drains.
- If no urine drains, the catheter is left in place, because it is probably in the vagina and is removed later. Another catheter is inserted in the correct position.
- The catheter is withdrawn slowly to drain the bladder completely.

4. Advancement routine

    The intervals between self-catheterization and the residual amounts required before advancement of the time intervals are the same as those for the suprapubic catheter clamping routine.

5. Cultures
   - A urine specimen is taken for culturing if the patient is symptomatic.
   - Antibiotics are not routinely administered for prophylaxis.

VIII. Gastrointestinal Tube Management

A. Nasogastric Tube
1. Indications
   - Ileus
   - Abdominal distention
   - Bowel obstruction
   - Intestinal surgery
   - Enteral feeding
   - Unable to take polyethylene glycol-electrolyte solution (GoLYTELY) bowel preparation orally
2. Insertion
   - Sit the patient upright.
   - Place a towel over the anterior chest.
   - Measure the length of tube to be inserted by stretching the tube from the tip of the nose and around the ear to the xyphoid process.
   - Lubricate the tube and insert it into the nostril until it reaches the back of the pharynx.
   - Encourage the patient to swallow ice chips or sips of water.
   - Advance the tube slowly to the required length.
   - Inject air into the tube, and auscultate the stomach to confirm placement.
   - Connect the tube to a suction device.
   - Secure the tube to the nose.

B. Long Intestinal Tube
1. Indication

    Small bowel obstruction
2. Insertion
   - The same as for nasogastric tube
   - Place the patient on her right side with the head elevated 12 in.
   - Advance the tube while the patient swallows a small amount of liquid.
   - Radiographically verify that the tube has advanced beyond the pylorus.

- Continue advancing and checking the progress radiographically.
- If there is difficulty getting the tube to pass through the pylorus, manipulation under fluoroscopy may be successful.
- Irrigate the tube as necessary with 30 mL of isotonic saline.

C. Management of Intestinal Tubes
1. Low intermittent suction is preferred.
2. Clamping and removal are individualized for each patient.
3. After flatus has been passed, clamp the tube for 3 to 4 hours and then place back on suction.
4. If nausea or vomiting does not occur and the return from reinstated suction is minimal, the tube can be removed.
5. Histamine receptor (H_2) blockers are used to prevent gastric ulceration.

IX. Bowel Management

A. Principles
1. Stool softeners may be given after oral intake has begun.
2. Laxatives should never be given after an intestinal anastomosis has been performed.
3. Enemas should not be given after colonic anastomosis or rectovaginal fistula repair.
4. Rectal suppositories are safe, but not after low rectal or anal anastomoses or rectovaginal fistula repair.

X. Parenteral and Enteral Nutrition

A. Nutrition Support
1. Indications: general
   - The patient is not expected to receive anything orally for >5 days.
   - Malnourished and/or stressed patient (see Chapter 6)
2. Indications: enteral (tube feeding)
   - Nasogastric or nasojejunal tubes and surgical gastrostomy or jejunostomy
     — No oral intake but gut works
     — Patient unwilling or unable to consume adequate diet
     — Ventilator-dependent patient
     — Dysphagia that precludes adequate intake
     — Surgical gastrostomy or jejunostomy indicated for longer term feeding
   - Surgically placed needle catheter jejunostomy
     — Allows very early postoperative feeding
3. Indications: parenteral (peripheral or central)
   - Use only when gut malfunctions:
     "If the gut works, use it."
     — Postoperative "ileus"
     — Short bowel

— Mechanical obstruction
— Enteric fistula
• Peripheral route
— Central venous access not possible or contraindicated
— Patient mildly to moderately stressed
— Short duration expected
• Central route
— Patient moderately to severely stressed
— Longer duration expected

B. Duration

1. Individualized
2. Tube feeding is safe for long period: duration depends on patient's ability and willingness to eat adequate diet.
3. Peripheral parenteral nutrition is usually inadequate calorically for long-term use and is indicated only for brief support, e.g., for ≤10 days.
4. Central parenteral nutrition is safe for long-term use, with close monitoring.

C. Nutrition Requirements

1. Calories based on Harris-Benedict (H-B) estimate of basal energy expenditure (see Chapter 6).
2. Protein needs are about 1.0 to 1.5 g/kg body weight (see Chapter 6).
3. Vitamins and minerals to meet recommended dietary allowances.
4. Fluids and electrolytes individualized on basis of laboratory data, weights, urine output, etc.
5. For modifications for obesity, sepsis, renal or hepatic failure, and extremes in hydrational status, see Chapter 6.

D. Diet Advancement

1. Individualized depending on
   • Duration of period without food
   • Bowel function
   • Patient cooperation
2. Progression of diets as tolerated
   • Clear liquid: broth, tea, gelatin, clear fruit juice
   • Full liquid: clear liquids plus milk-based liquids
   • Soft: solid foods excluding fresh fruits and vegetables
   • Mechanical soft (for edentulous patients or those with dysphagia): ground meats, fruits and vegetables, and liquids
   • General: no restrictions

XI. Diabetes Mellitus

A. General Considerations

1. Treatment must be individualized for each patient.
2. Successful postoperative management requires continuation of the preoperative and intraoperative attempts to sustain normal glucose levels and metabolism.
3. Poorly controlled diabetics have a higher perioperative mortality and morbidity.
4. End-organ disease associated with diabetes, including cardiovascular disease, myopathy, and nephropathy, deserve consideration. These patients are prone to small vessel coronary artery disease and have a two- to tenfold increase in incidence of myocardial infarction. Diabetic autonomic neuropathy can cause gastroparesis, painless myocardial ischemia, and perioperative cardiorespiratory arrest.
5. Diabetes is associated with poor formation of collagen and impaired tensile strength of deep surgical wounds.
6. When poorly controlled, diabetes impairs phagocyte function and increases the patient's susceptibility to infection.
7. Surgical procedures, trauma, and infection increase insulin requirements.
8. Both hyperglycemia and diabetic ketoacidosis can result in electrolyte disturbances.

B. Basic Objectives of Perioperative Management

1. Measure blood glucose level preoperatively.
2. Correct any acid-base, fluid, and electrolyte abnormalities preoperatively.
3. Provide adequate carbohydrates to inhibit catabolic proteolysis, lipolysis, and ketosis. (On average, 70 to 100 g of glucose are required for a 50-kg person daily during the operative period.)
4. Use insulin to prevent hyperglycemia and ketoacidosis, but take care to avoid hypoglycemia.
5. Avoid iatrogenic complications associated with diabetes.

C. Treatment

1. Noninsulin-dependent diabetes
   • Stop short-acting oral hypoglycemic agents on the day of the operation, and stop longer acting ones on the preceding day. Specifically, metformin has been associated with postoperative metabolic lactic acidosis and should be discontinued 24 to 36 hours before surgery.
   • For minor operations, insulin is rarely required.
   • For major operations, check blood glucose level hourly. Short-acting (soluble) human insulin may occasionally be required intraoperatively and postoperatively, depending on blood glucose levels (for dosage, see below).
2. Insulin-dependent diabetes
   • For minor operations, start 5% dextrose infusion, 100 to 150 mL/h, and give half the usual dose of insulin as intermediate-acting insulin subcutaneously.
   • Postoperatively, regular (soluble) human insulin may be required as a supplement, as indicated by blood glucose levels (for dosage, see below).
   • Postoperatively, check plasma glucose level every 6 hours for first 24 hours and then daily. When oral

fluids can be resumed, subcutaneous insulin injections can be resumed.

- For major operations, several different regimens exist. A continuous and adjustable intravenous infusion of insulin provides satisfactory control of blood glucose. To accomplish this
  — Start i.v. infusion of 5% dextrose, 50 mL/h.
  — Through a separate intravenous catheter with an infusion pump, give short-acting insulin, using a solution of 50 U of regular (soluble) insulin added to 250 mL of isotonic saline (i.e., 0.2 U/mL).

$$\text{hourly insulin units} = \frac{\text{blood glucose}}{100}$$

  (or divide by 150 if patient is thin or taking steroids)
  — Measure blood glucose hourly to allow insulin dosage adjustment.
  — All other fluids that are given intravenously to the patient should not contain dextrose or lactose.
  — If signs of hypoglycemia develop, i.e., tachycardia and sweating, immediately obtain a venous sample, stop insulin infusion, and give one ampule of 50% dextrose.

Note: β-Adrenergic blockers may mask these signs.

3. Emergency surgery and diabetic ketoacidosis (secondary to trauma or infection, etc.)
- If possible, delay the operation until the ketoacidosis has been brought under control and the patient has been resuscitated.
- Obtain arterial blood gas, acid-base analysis, serum levels of ketones and lactate, and urine and blood cultures. Measure electrolyte, creatinine, glucose, and serum phosphate levels. Acid-base balance and potassium and glucose levels should be rechecked frequently.
- Guided by monitoring of pulse rate, blood pressure, urine output, central venous pressure, and, if necessary, pulmonary capillary wedge pressure, correct volume depletion by infusion of isotonic saline: 1 L/h for 1 to 2 hours, then 1 L/2 h for 2 to 4 hours, and then 1 L/4 h. Patients typically have profound fluid deficits secondary to an osmotic diuresis. If not corrected, a lactic acidosis can be superimposed on the patient's existing ketoacidosis.
- Give 10 U of regular insulin i.v. and follow with an infusion of insulin at a dosage (units per hour) determined by the formula: blood glucose/150.
- Begin infusion of 5% dextrose when serum glucose reaches 250 mg/mL.

- Despite higher or normal initial serum levels of potassium, potassium depletion is often severe and should be closely monitored and corrected. Phosphate replacement is also required.
- Use of sodium bicarbonate to correct acidosis is not indicated unless acidosis is severe (i.e., pH <7.0). If given, stop use when pH is >7.2.

XII. Special Needs of Elderly Patients

A. Introduction
1. Elderly patients (>75 years old) have special needs in relation to gynecologic surgery because of the frequency of associated medical problems. Approximately 75% of patients older than 75 years have a concurrent medical problem.

B. Common Medical Problems
The medical problems likely to be encountered are, in descending order of frequency
1. Hypertension, 39%
2. Cardiac conditions, 20%
3. Hiatal hernia, 14%
4. Arthritis, 13%
5. Obesity, 11%
6. Cerebrovascular conditions, 4%
7. Phlebitis, 3%
8. Chronic obstructive pulmonary disease, 2.5%
9. Diabetes mellitus, 2.5%
10. Senility, 2%
11. Anemia, 2%
12. Other, 11%

C. Mortality Rate
Overall operative mortality in the Mayo Clinic series of elderly patients was 1.4%.

Reading List

Williams TJ. Preoperative and postoperative care in radical pelvic surgery. *Clin Obstet Gynecol* 1965;8:629–641.

O'Leary JA, Symmonds RE. Radical pelvic operations in the geriatric patient: a 15-year review of 133 cases. *Obstet Gynecol* 1966;28:745–753.

Stern BL, Williams TJ. Care of the bladder after gynecologic surgery. *Clin Obstet Gynecol* 1967;10:192–201.

Williams TJ. Care of the bladder in gynecologic surgery. In: Sturgis SH, Taymor ML, *Progress in gynecology*, vol 5. New York: Grune & Stratton, 1970:526–542.

Stanhope CR. Geriatric gynecologic oncology. In: Hofmeister FJ, ed. *Care of the postmenopausal patient*. Philadelphia: George F Stickley, 1985:67–73.

Williams TJ. Gynecologic surgery in the elderly female. In: Breen JL, Osofsky HJ, eds. *Current concepts in gynecologic surgery*. Baltimore: Williams & Wilkins, 1987:33–39.

Kinney WK, Egorshin EV, Podratz KC. Wertheim hysterectomy in the geriatric population. *Gynecol Oncol* 1988;31:227–232.

CHAPTER 4

Intraoperative Complications

Maurice J. Webb, M.D.

I. Introduction

Surgeons must be able to recognize and to deal appropriately with any complication that occurs during an operation. Even if definitive management of the complication is beyond the surgeon's expertise, the operator should still be familiar with the appropriate management of any situation that may arise so that the problem can be dealt with expeditiously.

II. Prevention of Intraoperative Complications

Several factors, apart from the experience of the surgeon, can have a direct effect on the prevention of intraoperative complications.

A. Preoperative Assessment
1. Treatment of any medical disorders
2. Imaging of urinary or gastrointestinal tract if necessary
3. Performing appropriate preoperative tests
4. Antibiotic prophylaxis if indicated
5. Bowel preparation if indicated
6. Availability of blood and blood products

B. Exposure
1. Incision
   - Must be adequate size
   - Should be made so it can be extended if necessary
2. Retractors
   - Self-retaining-type retractors are essential, e.g., Balfour.
   - Hand-held retractors should be available, e.g., Deaver, Harrington.

Maurice J. Webb: Chairman, Division of Gynecologic Surgery and Consultant, Department of Surgery, Mayo Clinic and Mayo Foundation; Professor of Obstetrics and Gynecology, Mayo Medical School, Rochester, Minnesota.

3. Packing
   The intestine should be packed out of the operative field.
4. Position
   A steep Trendelenburg position is useful for pelvic operations.

C. Assistants
1. Two knowledgeable surgical assistants are the optimal number.
2. Use of traction and countertraction provides the optimal state for dissection of tissue planes.

D. Lighting
1. Adequate lighting is essential.
2. It is best if lighting can be manipulated by the surgeon.

E. Anesthesia
1. Good anesthesia with adequate relaxation
2. Adequate vascular access
3. Careful monitoring of the patient's status, blood loss, urine output, etc.

III. Hemorrhage

Hemorrhage and sepsis are still the two major problems facing the surgeon, and patients still die of these complications. Anticipation of the problem is the initial step.

A. Preoperative Assessment
1. Determine whether the patient
   - Has a history of bleeding tendency
   - Has a liver disorder
   - Takes anticoagulation medication
2. Assess the coagulation profile
   - Hemoglobin concentration
   - Platelet count
   - Prothrombin time and international normalized ratio (INR)

- Partial thromboplastin time
- Bleeding time

B. Principles
1. Venous bleeding is always more troublesome than arterial bleeding.
2. Pressure controls bleeding.
3. Blind clamping is dangerous and may damage adjacent organs and further lacerate vessels.
4. Adequate lighting, exposure, assistance, and suction are essential.
5. Adequate venous access and availability of blood are important.
6. Sometimes, it may be best to insert a pack and to proceed with the dissection in another area to gain better exposure.
7. All veins in the pelvis can be ligated if necessary.
8. The major areas at risk for troublesome venous hemorrhage during pelvic surgery are on the pelvic sidewalls in the region of the internal iliac veins and in the presacral region.

C. Venous Bleeding
1. Options are to suture the defect, use hemostatic clips, or ligate the vein above and below the defect.
2. Compress the laceration with the fingers and suture beneath the fingers with 5-0 monofilament suture (Prolene) on a fine needle to pick up the vein wall (Fig. 1).
3. With traction on the suture and adequate suction, close the defect with a running suture.
4. Suture a piece of rectus muscle over the bleeding site if hemostasis is difficult.

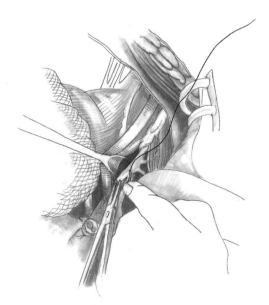

FIG. 1. Suturing bleeding veins in the obturator fossa by retracting internal iliac vessels medially and maintaining pressure on bleeding vein with a finger while suturing.

5. Use of topical thrombin or fibrin glue may help with hemostasis.
6. A sterile thumbtack pushed into the sacrum controls troublesome presacral venous bleeding.

D. Arterial Bleeding
1. Because arteries have thick walls, they do not tear as readily as veins, nor do they retract.
2. Cautery is useful for small arterial bleeders.
3. Visible arterial bleeders should be picked up with forceps, clamped, and then tied.
4. Ligation of a more major artery, e.g., the internal iliac artery, above the bleeding point may accomplish hemostasis.

E. Ligation of the Internal Iliac Artery
1. Used
   - To control bleeding:
     — From the vaginal cuff
     — In the broad ligament
     — From recurrent cancer
   - With a profusely bleeding uterus after confinement
   - Prophylactically
     — In the dissection of a complex pelvic mass
     — In the presence of an insecure uterine artery pedicle at abdominal hysterectomy
2. Principles
   - It is safer to ligate the anterior division of the internal iliac artery, because the internal iliac vein lies beneath the main trunk and is easily traumatized.
   - Ligation of the anterior division decreases bleeding from visceral branches.
   - The main trunk may be ligated bilaterally if there is extensive bleeding from pudendal branches, e.g., lacerated pelvic floor.
3. Technique
   - Open the pelvic peritoneum over the psoas muscle lateral to the ovarian vessels.
   - Trace the internal iliac artery down until the anterior division is reached, and then pass a ligature around the anterior division, using blunt dissection with right-angled forceps. Perform a bilateral ligation unless merely controlling bleeding from a unilateral uterine artery pedicle (Fig. 2).

F. Major Arterial Injury
1. Control bleeding with a vascular clamp or rubber slings.
2. Use a simple suture with 5-0 monofilament; otherwise polyethylene terephthalate (Dacron) or vein graft or patch reconstruction may be necessary.
3. Subsequent anticoagulation may be necessary.

G. Uncontrolled Bleeding
1. Persistence with attempts to control blood loss may jeopardize the patient. It may be best to insert a pack into the pelvis and to desist from further attempts.

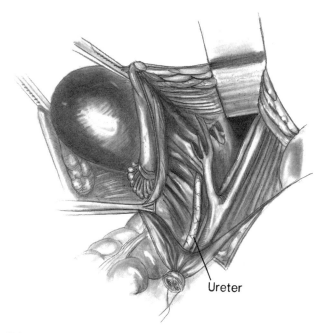

FIG. 2. Opened broad ligament showing anterior division of internal iliac artery before ligation.

2. If the blood loss is so great that the anesthesiologist is unable to keep up with replacement, apply pressure to the area and desist from further attempts at controlling the bleeding until the patient's condition has been stabilized and additional blood has been crossmatched.

3. A long pack can be inserted deep into the pelvis and brought out through the lower end of the incision.

4. The pack can be loosened or removed in 48 hours or later if the patient is stable clinically and coagulation variables are satisfactory.

5. For uncontrollable presacral bleeding, insert an umbrella pack, firmly filling the pelvis, and bring it out through the vagina.

6. A military antishock trousers (MAST) suit is useful in desperate situations to improve venous return, to increase peripheral resistance, and to maintain pressure on the pelvic pack.

IV. Urologic Trauma

A. Principle

Prevention of injury to the urinary tract (and loss of renal function or fistula formation) is an important part of all pelvic surgery.

B. Prevention

1. Adequate exposure
2. Identification of the ureter and bladder
3. Exposure and dissection of all contiguous structures
4. Visualizing the ureter through the peritoneum is not adequate. The ureter must be identified and palpated throughout its pelvic course.

C. Steps to Prevent Injury

1. Bladder
   - *Sharply* dissect the bladder off the cervix and vagina.
   - Expose 2 cm of vagina below the site of the transection of the vaginal cuff.
   - Retract the bladder during the operation with a Harrington retractor.
   - Use an indwelling catheter to keep the bladder empty during the operation.
   - Avoid excessive cautery to the back of the bladder.
2. Ureter
   - Divide the peritoneum lateral to the ovarian vessels and visualize the ureter crossing the bifurcation of the common iliac artery. It is attached to the broad ligament of the peritoneum (Fig. 3).
   - Palpate the ureter in the top of the cardinal ligament when applying parametrial clamps and ties. It can readily be palpated as a cord between the thumb and forefinger lateral to the cervix (Fig. 4).
   - Dissect the ureter throughout its pelvic course, using blunt dissection with a right-angled clamp if the ureter cannot be palpated or appears to be close to a clamp or ligature.
   - Open the bladder and pass a stent up the ureter if scarring or obesity makes identification of the ureter impossible.

D. Bladder Injury

1. Mark the defect with a suture, but do not repair until the operation has been completed.
2. Close the defect with two-layer closure, using 3-0 synthetic absorbable suture in a continuous fashion.
3. A flap of peritoneum, if available, may be sutured over the incision (Fig. 5).
4. Drain the bladder for 7 days with a catheter. (If the

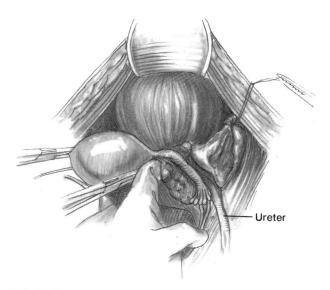

FIG. 3. Opened broad ligament showing ureter attached to medial leaf of broad ligament peritoneum.

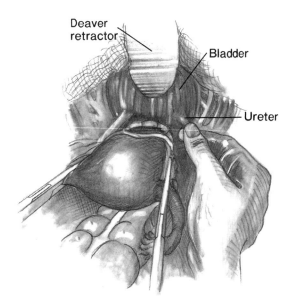

FIG. 4. Palpation of ureter at time of application of parametrial clamps at abdominal hysterectomy.

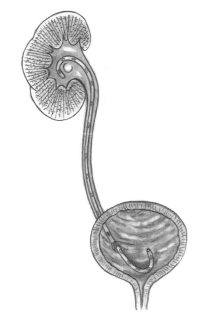

FIG. 6. Cystotomy with transvesical placement of double J ureteral stent.

pelvic area was irradiated previously, drain the bladder for 6 weeks.)

5. A similar technique is used if the injury is made during either an abdominal or a vaginal procedure.

E. Ureteral Injury

1. Damage to the adventitial layer: reapproximate with a few interrupted 3-0 synthetic absorbable sutures.
2. Crush injury with a clamp or ligature
   - Remove the clamp and inspect the ureter.
   - If the ureter segment is viable, approximate the adventitia, pass a double J stent transvesically, close the bladder incision, and leave a urethral catheter in place for 7 days. A suction drain is inserted down to the level of the ureteral injury site. Remove the stent and catheter in 7 days and the drain 24 hours later if no urine leakage occurs (Fig. 6).

   - If the ureter segment is not viable, resect and reanastomose.
3. Transection
   - If the injury is close to the bladder, perform ureteroneocystostomy.
   - Tunnel the ureter beneath the bladder mucosa and suture to the mucosa from within the bladder with a few interrupted synthetic absorbable 4-0 sutures. Drain the anastomosis with a suction drain through the abdominal wall and stent the ureter as before.
   - Mobilizing the bladder off the back of the symphysis and performing a "psoas hitch" (suturing the side of the bladder to the psoas muscle) gives more length and takes tension off the anastomosis (Fig. 7).
   - If the transected ureter is not long enough to reach the

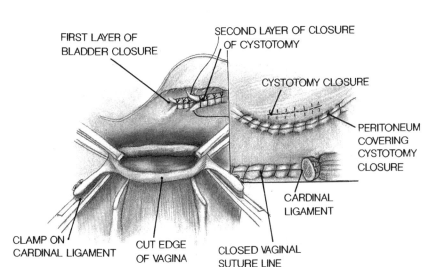

FIRST LAYER OF BLADDER CLOSURE

SECOND LAYER OF CLOSURE OF CYSTOTOMY

CYSTOTOMY CLOSURE

PERITONEUM COVERING CYSTOTOMY CLOSURE

CARDINAL LIGAMENT

CLAMP ON CARDINAL LIGAMENT

CUT EDGE OF VAGINA

CLOSED VAGINAL SUTURE LINE

FIG. 5. Two-layered closure of cystotomy, with flap of bladder peritoneum covering the suture line. (Redrawn from Lee RA. *Atlas of gynecologic surgery.* Philadelphia: WB Saunders, 1992:303, with permission.)

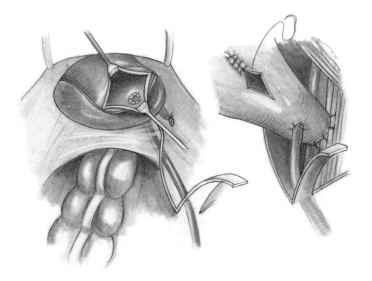

FIG. 7. Ureteroneocystostomy with psoas hitch to take tension off anastomosis. A peritoneal patch is shown that can be sutured over the site of anastomosis.

bladder, end-to-end anastomosis can be performed over a stent and drained as before. Ureteral ends are cut obliquely or fish-mouthed to give a wide anastomosis (Fig. 8).
- A bladder flap of the Demel or Boari type or interposition of a conduit of ileum may be useful if the ureter is too short to reach the bladder (Figs. 9 and 10).

- Transureteroureterostomy is another technique used when the ureter is too short to reach the bladder (Fig. 11).

Note: If the surgeon is not skilled in urologic procedures and a urologist is not available to assist in the management of a transected ureter, a single J stent should be passed up the

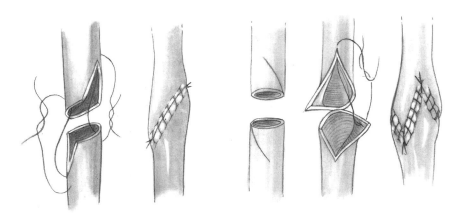

FIG. 8. Techniques for prevention of stenosis with ureteroureteral anastomosis.

Peritoneal flap

Bladder

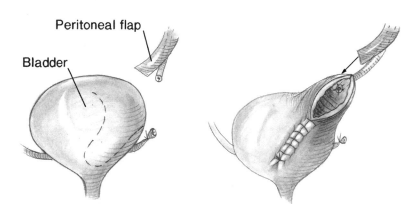

FIG. 9. Boari bladder flap in the presence of a short ureter.

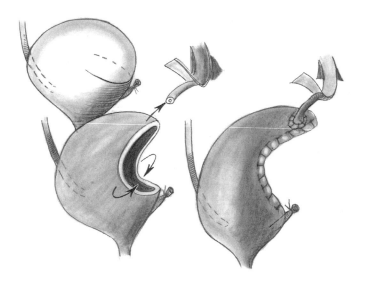

FIG. 10. Demel bladder flap.

ureter to the renal pelvis and brought out through the anterior abdominal wall. No attempt should be made to dissect the ureter to create a cutaneous ureterostomy, because this will make a subsequent reanastomosis difficult.

V. Gastrointestinal Trauma

A. Principle

If enterotomy or bowel resection is anticipated, full bowel preparation should be performed preoperatively. This is especially important in patients with suspected ovarian malignancy. It is impossible to predict which cases will require bowel resection; therefore, the bowel should be prepared preoperatively in all patients with suspected ovarian cancer.

B. Enterotomy

1. A serosal defect is repaired with a few 3-0 silk or synthetic absorbable sutures.
2. An enterotomy is repaired in a transverse fashion with continuous mucosal 3-0 synthetic absorbable suture and interrupted seromuscular 3-0 silk sutures (Fig. 12).
3. A transverse rather than a longitudinal closure does not constrict the bowel lumen.
4. A similar two-layered closure is performed for small-bowel or large-bowel injury (Fig. 13).
5. Antibiotics are used prophylactically.
6. Abdominal drains are necessary only if the left colon, sigmoid colon, or rectum is entered, because the intraluminal pressure is higher in these areas of the bowel.
7. Particular care should be taken to repair even minor defects in irradiated bowel, because fistula formation is more common in irradiated bowel.

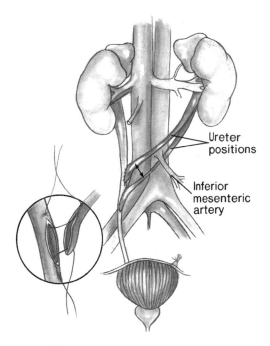

Ureter positions

Inferior mesenteric artery

FIG. 11. Transureteroureterostomy.

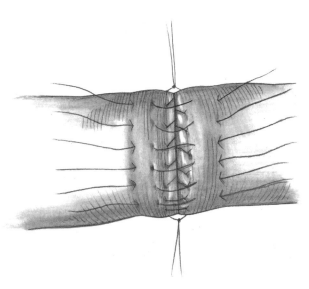

FIG. 12. Transverse two-layered repair of enterotomy.

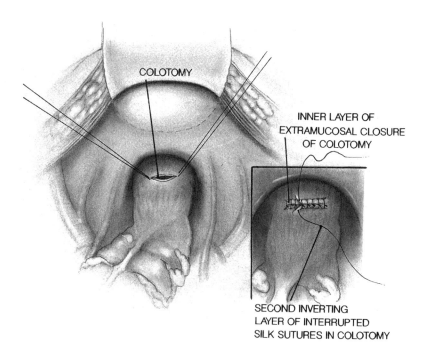

FIG. 13. Two-layered closure of injury to the rectum. (Redrawn from Lee RA. *Atlas of gynecologic surgery.* Philadelphia: WB Saunders, 1992:336, with permission.)

8. A nasogastric tube or other intestinal tube should be used in irradiated cases or after multiple repairs or extensive lysis of adhesions.
9. If a defect is produced in a patient who has numerous adhesions, delay repair until all the adhesions have been divided, because multiple defects often will be produced that may be managed better with segmental bowel resection.
10. Injuries to the large bowel do not require diverting colostomy, unless the bowel has been irradiated or there is significant bowel sepsis.
11. Copious peritoneal lavage should be performed at the conclusion of the operation.
12. The patient should be kept fasting until flatus has been passed.
13. If an intestinal tube has not been used, one should be inserted if any abdominal distention develops.

C. Intestinal Arterial Injury

1. Damage to the vascular supply of a segment of bowel may occur during a surgical procedure.
2. Any devascularized segment should be excised and reanastomosis performed.
3. If the superior mesenteric artery is injured, an arterial graft may be necessary.
4. The inferior mesenteric artery may be sacrificed with little likelihood of any sequelae developing.

VI. Vaginal Surgical Injuries

A. Principle

Principles similar to those mentioned above are applied to the prevention and management of complications of vaginal surgical procedures. However, a few special techniques need to be noted.

B. Cystotomy

Mark the defect with a suture, complete the hysterectomy, and then repair the defect with 3-0 synthetic absorbable suture in two layers. Drain the bladder with a catheter for 7 days.

C. Ureteral Transection

1. Reimplant by using a closed technique with pulley sutures to pull the ureter into the bladder and to anchor it in place.
2. Ureteral injury may be avoided by palpating the ureter routinely at vaginal hysterectomy. This is accomplished by inserting a finger into the peritoneal cavity anterior to the uterus and "snapping" the ureter against a Deaver retractor placed in the lateral vaginal fornix (Fig. 14).
3. Retraction of the bladder anteriorly and traction on the cervix help to keep the ureter away from the cardinal ligament clamps.

D. Urethral Trauma

1. Urethral trauma usually occurs during anterior colporrhaphy.
2. Repair the defect in two or three layers with interrupted 3-0 synthetic absorbable sutures.
3. Leave the catheter in the bladder for 7 days (suprapubic catheter placement is preferred to avoid urethral trauma).
4. A labial fat-pad flap can be interposed if further security is thought to be necessary (see Chapter 23).

VII. Nerve Injury

A. Principle

The most common nerve injuries are related to positional injury to the femoral nerves, peroneal nerves, or brachial plexus (see Chapter 5). Intraoperative injuries are less common.

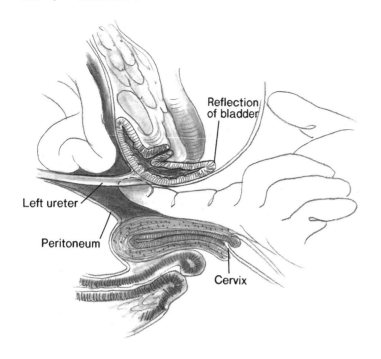

FIG. 14. Palpation of the ureter through the anterior cul-de-sac at time of vaginal hysterectomy.

B. Injuries Caused by Operational Dissection
1. Obturator nerve
   - May be avulsed at the time of pelvic node dissection
   - May be incorporated in suture during paravaginal defect repair
   - Injury causes some difficulty in abduction of the leg, but with time the patient is able to compensate by using other muscles.
   - Repair can be accomplished by careful reapproximation.
2. Sciatic plexus
   - May be traumatized during dissection of a pelvic sidewall tumor
   - May be incorporated in the suture during attempts at hemostasis on the pelvic sidewall
   - Resection may be necessary for removal of recurrent tumor.
   - The resultant defect depends on which nerve roots are injured.
3. Femoral nerve: may be injured during inguinal lymph node dissection
4. Genitofemoral and ilioinguinal nerves
   - Nerves may be incorporated in closure of transverse abdominal or groin incisions, resulting in chronic pain caused by nerve entrapment.
   - Minor sensory loss may occur in areas of the skin of the vulva or thigh.
5. Sympathetic plexus: may be severed during paraaortic lymph node dissection, with no significant sequelae

VIII. Splenic Trauma

A. Causes
The spleen may be traumatized during abdominal surgery by
1. Damage from abdominal retractors
2. Dissection during total omentectomy
3. Mobilization of splenic flexure during colectomy

B. Management
1. Splenectomy is usually necessary if there is any significant trauma (see Chapter 24).
2. The argon beam coagulator may successfully obtain hemostasis in small capsular tears.

IX. Diaphragmatic Trauma

A. Causes
The diaphragm is usually injured during attempts at debulking of diaphragmatic metastases of ovarian cancer or from diaphragmatic biopsy for staging purposes.

B. Treatment
1. Close the defect with sutures or, if the defect is large, with mesh.
2. Insert a thoracic drain to complete lung expansion.
3. Alternatively, the lung may be reinflated by inserting a suction catheter through the defect, applying suction and positive ventilatory pressure, and closing the defect with a purse-string suture of 3-0 monofilament suture as the catheter is removed.

Reading List

Pratt JH, Nelson GA, Wilcox CF III, et al. Blood loss during vaginal hysterectomy. *Obstet Gynecol* 1960;15:101–107.

Pratt JH: Ureteral injuries in pelvic surgery for benign lesions. *Minn Med* 1964;47:389–393.

Sinclair RH, Pratt JH. Femoral neuropathy after pelvic operation. *Am J Obstet Gynecol* 1972;112:404–407.

Williams TJ. Urologic injuries. In: Wynn RM, ed. *Obstetrics and gynecology annual.* Englewood Cliffs, NJ: Appleton Century Crofts, 1975:347–368.

Noller KL, Pratt JH, Symmonds RE. Bowel perforation with suprapubic cystostomy. *Obstet Gynecol* 1976;48[Suppl]:67S–69S.

Pratt JH. Common complications of vaginal hysterectomy: thoughts regarding their prevention and management. *Clin Obstet Gynecol* 1976;19:645–659.

Symmonds RE. Ureteral injuries associated with gynecologic surgery: prevention and management. *Clin Obstet Gynecol* 1976;19:623–644.

Symmonds RE. Urologic injuries: ureter. In: Scheefer G, Graber EA, eds. *Complications in obstetric and gynecologic surgery: prevention, diagnosis, and treatment.* Hagerstown, MD: Harper & Row, 1981:412–429.

Pratt JH. Acute posthysterectomy rectovaginal fistula. In: Nichols DH, ed. *Clinical problems, injuries, and complications of gynecologic surgery.* Baltimore: Williams & Wilkins, 1983:62–63.

Webb MJ, Weaver EW. Intestinal surgery in gynaecologic oncology. *Aust NZ J Obstet Gynaecol* 1987;27:299–303.

Lee RA, Symmonds RE, Williams TJ. Current status of genitourinary fistula. *Obstet Gynecol* 1988;72:313–319.

Webb MJ. Prevention and management of intraoperative complications in pelvic surgery. *Postgrad Obstet Surg* 1990;10:1–5.

CHAPTER 5

Postoperative Complications

Peter A. Southorn, M.D. and Maurice J. Webb, M.D.

I. Acute Emergencies: Circulatory Complications

A. Preoperative Considerations

1. Preexisting cardiovascular disease should be identified and treated before the operation.
2. All cardiovascular medications, including antihypertensive agents, should be continued throughout the perioperative period. For example:
   - Abrupt discontinuation of treatment with β-adrenergic blocking agents causes marked increase in perioperative myocardial oxygen demand.
   - Clonidine withdrawal is associated with rebound hypertension.

B. Postoperative Hypotension

1. Clinical evaluation
   - Verify the accuracy of the blood pressure measurement.
   - Evaluate for signs associated with hypotension, including:
     — Orthostatic hypotension
     — Pale, cold, clammy skin
     — Rapid thready pulse
     — Oliguria, <0.5 mL/kg/h of urine

   Note: These signs may be absent in the immediate postoperative period because of the residual effects of anesthesia.

2. Causes
   - Decreased ventricular preload is the most common cause and is produced by such factors as
     — Inadequate perioperative fluid volume replacement

Peter A. Southorn: Consultant, Department of Anesthesiology, Mayo Clinic and Mayo Foundation; Associate Professor of Anesthesiology, Mayo Medical School, Rochester, Minnesota.
Maurice J. Webb: Chairman, Division of Gynecologic Surgery and Consultant, Department of Surgery, Mayo Clinic and Mayo Foundation; Professor of Obstetrics and Gynecology, Mayo Medical School, Rochester, Minnesota.

     — Ongoing blood loss
     — Sequestration of fluids into the third space (after extensive intraabdominal or retroperitoneal operation or both)
     — Vigorous diuresis due to diabetes mellitus or to use of diuretics
     — Residual vasodilatory effects of anesthetic agents
   - Decreased myocardial contractility, which is associated with
     — Preexisting ventricular dysfunction
     — Myocardial ischemia or infarction
     — Drug-induced myocardial depression
     — Onset of cardiac arrhythmias
     — Profound acidosis
   - Massive decrease of systemic vascular resistance, which is associated with
     — Early sepsis
     — Anaphylaxis
     — Adrenal insufficiency (characterized by hypotension unresponsive to fluids or to pressors)
     — Vasodilator drug overdose, e.g., sodium nitroprusside
     — Sympathetic nervous system blockade produced by local anesthetics used for epidural or spinal anesthesia

3. Treatment
   - Place patient in the Trendelenburg position.
   - Administer 250 to 500 mL of crystalloid fluid challenge intravenously, monitoring the effect and repeating if blood pressure increases.
   - Reevaluate for accuracy of perioperative fluid replacement and possible blood loss intraoperatively and postoperatively.
   - If surgical bleeding is identified, initiate steps for reexploration.
   - Initiate crossmatch. (One unit of blood or packed cells increases hemoglobin level approximately 1 g/dL.)

   Note: Vasopressors, e.g., norepinephrine [0.1 to 0.5 μg/kg/min intravenously (i.v.)]

or

High doses of dopamine (>5 μg/kg/min i.v.) may be required initially in emergency management of severe hypotension.

Note: Invasive monitoring is particularly useful if hypotension persists despite adequate volume replacement. Pulmonary artery wedge pressure (Swan-Ganz) monitoring is usually preferred to central venous pressure, because the latter only reflects preload with *normal* left ventricular function.

4. Persistent hypovolemia is indicated by
   • Low pulmonary capillary wedge pressure
   • Low cardiac output
   • High systemic vascular resistance
5. Impaired myocardial contractility is associated with
   • High pulmonary capillary wedge pressure
   • Low cardiac output
   • High systemic vascular resistance
6. Conditions such as septic shock initially may be associated with
   • Low pulmonary capillary wedge pressure
   • High cardiac output
   • Low systemic vascular resistance

Note: Echocardiography is a useful noninvasive test for detecting abnormal left ventricular function and other cardiac abnormalities, e.g., tamponade.

C. Myocardial Infarction

1. Predisposing factors include
   • Coronary artery disease
   • Previous myocardial infarction
   • Hemodynamic instability in the perioperative period
2. Myocardial infarction in the past 6 months increases the likelihood of perioperative myocardial infarction.
3. Perioperative myocardial infarction often is silent, without angina pectoris. Diagnosis is suggested by
   • New onset of left ventricular failure with hypotension
   • Congestive heart failure
   • Pulmonary edema
   • Arrhythmias, e.g., premature ventricular contractions (PVCs) and conduction abnormalities
4. Confirmed diagnosis requires *both*
   • Serial, suggestive electrocardiographic findings (ST-segment elevation, T-wave inversion, and Q waves) on 3 successive days (by itself, a single electrocardiogram suggesting infarction does not confirm diagnosis)
   • Increase in the myocardial-specific isoenzyme fraction of creatine phosphokinase (CPK), serum glutamic-oxaloacetic transaminase (SGOT), or troponin
5. Management consists of
   • Bed rest for 2 or 3 days if uncomplicated
   • Continuous electrocardiographic monitoring for at least 48 hours, with antiarrhythmic therapy as indicated
   • Intravenous access
   • Analgesia with opiates (morphine) given intravenously

• Antiemetic agents given intravenously as needed
• High-flow oxygen
• Aspirin, 150 to 300 mg orally daily, improves survival.
• β-Adrenergic antagonist (e.g., metoprolol or atenolol) given intravenously and then orally. These relieve anginal pain, reduce the incidence of arrhythmias, and improve survival.
• Nitrates given sublingually or intravenously for persistent anginal pain and to treat left ventricular failure
• Left ventricular failure treatment may be assisted by pulmonary artery wedge pressure monitoring. Treatment may require nitroglycerin, diuretic therapy, and inotropes.
6. Coronary thrombolytic therapy is contraindicated after recent major surgical procedures, but transluminal coronary angioplasty or bypass grafting can be performed during this time.

D. Arrhythmias

1. Principles
   • Usually detected by electrocardiographic monitoring in postoperative recovery room.
   • Most arrhythmias are benign, but all warrant attention because some deteriorate into life-threatening abnormalities, e.g., ventricular tachycardia.
2. Sinus tachycardia
   The most common postoperative arrhythmia
   • Caused by
   — Pain
   — Hypoxia
   — Hypercapnia
   — Sepsis
   — Hypovolemia
   — Hypoglycemia
   — Vagolytic drugs, e.g., atropine
   • Treatment
   Correct the precipitating cause.
3. Premature ventricular contraction
   The second most common postoperative arrhythmia
   • Is frequently present preoperatively in the elderly and is usually benign
   • Associated with
   — Hypokalemia
   — Acid-base disturbances
   — Hypoxia
   — Myocardial ischemia
   — Myocardial infarction
   • Treatment
   — Manage the precipitating cause.
   — Lidocaine is indicated when there is evidence that the PVCs may degenerate into ventricular tachycardia or fibrillation:
   · >5 PVCs/min
   · Presence of bigeminy or trigeminy
   · Multifocal PVCs during the vulnerable period of ventricular repolarization (R-on-T phenomenon)

— Lidocaine is given intravenously as a bolus, 50 to 100 mg (1 to 1.5 mg/kg), followed by a maintenance dose of 2 to 4 mg/min. This maintenance dose is reduced 50% in elderly patients and in patients with heart failure or hepatic dysfunction.

— If lidocaine is ineffective, procainamide is given intravenously at a rate of 20 mg/min until one of the following occurs:

· The arrhythmia is suppressed.

· Hypotension develops.

· The QRS complex widens >50% of its original width.

· A total of 1 g has been given.

After the arrhythmia has been controlled, procainamide is given intravenously at a maintenance infusion rate of 1 to 4 mg/min.

4. Sinus bradycardia

• Most commonly associated with

— Pain

— Bladder distention

— Vasovagal stimulation

— Myocardial ischemia

— Myocardial infarction

— β-Adrenergic blockade

— High sympathetic nervous blockade due to epidural or spinal anesthesia

— Anticholinesterases (used to reverse effects of muscle relaxants)

— Hypothermia

• Treatment

— Used when patient is symptomatic, e.g., chest pain, decreased consciousness, decrease in blood pressure, heart failure, myocardial infarction

— Atropine, given intravenously, cautiously titrated for effect, 0.3 to 0.5 mg is usually adequate.

— Temporary pacemaker

E. Hypertension

1. Common in the immediate postoperative period

2. Patients at particular risk include those with preexisting hypertension, particularly when

• The hypertension was poorly controlled or untreated.

• The antihypertensive treatment was stopped before the operation.

• Other factors are

— Pain

— Urinary retention

— Hypoxia

— Carbon dioxide retention

— Fluid overload

— Hypothermia

— Interaction between monoamine oxidase inhibitors and other medications, especially meperidine

3. Hypertension induces myocardial ischemia, particularly when associated with tachycardia. It also can cause heart failure and cerebrovascular accidents and increased surgical bleeding.

4. Treatment should be aggressive and immediate:

• Correct underlying cause, e.g., inadequate analgesia, hypothermia, hypoxia, hypercapnia.

• Review previous hypertension control.

• Exclude drug-induced hypertension reaction.

• Antihypertensive agents are given to correct blood pressure >200/100 mm Hg, especially if associated with tachycardia. Treatment should be consistent with previous drug therapy and according to whether tachycardia is present.

• Labetalol produces a combination α_1- and β-adrenergic blockade: 0.5 to 2 mg/min i.v. infusion with dose reduction as blood pressure decreases.

• Hydralazine, a direct-acting arteriolar vasodilator, 5- to 10-mg i.v. bolus; it may require coadministration of a β-adrenergic blocker, e.g., propranolol (0.5 to 2 mg i.v.) to control reflex tachycardia.

• Sodium nitroprusside, a direct-acting smooth muscle relaxant, initial dose 0.5 μg/kg/min; it decreases preload and, to a lesser extent, afterload.

II. Acute Emergencies: Respiratory Disorders

A. General Considerations

1. Abdominal surgery is associated with

• Decreased lung volumes

• Impaired ability to cough

• Pain when taking deep breaths

2. These effects, which persist for several days, are normally of little consequence, but in certain patients, they can lead to retention of airway secretions, atelectasis, and bacterial invasion and proliferation, causing pneumonia.

3. Patients particularly at risk for developing respiratory complications include those

• Undergoing operations requiring upper abdominal incision

• With preexisting lung disease, particularly obstructive lung disease

• Who smoke

• Who are obese

• Who are elderly

• Who have neuromuscular disorders such as myasthenia gravis and Guillain-Barré syndrome

4. Pulmonary complications in patients at risk can be markedly decreased by

• Preoperative pulmonary function studies and pulmonary preparation for 48 hours in patients with severe preexisting lung disease

• Encouraging and supervising patients to cough and to breath deeply postoperatively

• Encouraging mobilization

• Use of incentive spirometry

• Good analgesia to accomplish the above goals

B. Carbon Dioxide Retention
1. Ventilatory failure results from
   • Respiratory center depression due to
     — Persistent effect of anesthetic agents in the immediate postoperative period until these drugs are excreted, metabolized, or pharmacologically reversed.
     — Opiates used for postoperative pain relief.
   • Respiratory muscle weakness resulting from residual effect of muscle relaxants used in anesthesia or disease, e.g., Guillian-Barré syndrome.
   • Chronic lung disease
2. Diagnosis
   • Often associated with few clinical signs or symptoms
   • Arterial blood gas analysis revealing a carbon dioxide tension >50 to 60 mm Hg
3. Treatment
   • Intubate airway and artificially ventilate.
   • Reverse drug-induced depression of respiratory center, e.g., use naloxone to treat opiate overdose.
     — Give naloxone cautiously (i.e., 0.1 to 0.2 mg i.v.) to avoid intense stimulation of the sympathetic nervous system. Repeat as needed.
     — The effect of naloxone may last for a shorter time than the effect of the opiates, resulting in redevelopment of respiratory failure.
   • Take care with giving uncontrolled high concentrations of oxygen in patients with chronic lung disease who may depend on a hypoxic respiratory drive.

C. Hypoxemia
1. Can occur any time in the first 2 weeks postoperatively
2. There are multiple causes, including
   • Atelectasis (most common cause)
   • Pneumonia
   • Pneumothorax (diagnosed by chest examination and radiography)
   • Bronchospasm (often associated with a history of wheezing)
   • Massive pulmonary embolus (suggested when respiratory distress is of sudden onset)
   • Pulmonary edema (due to either increased pulmonary capillary hydrostatic pressure produced by myocardial infarction, fluid overload, mitral stenosis, etc., or increased capillary permeability produced by aspiration pneumonitis, adult respiratory distress syndrome, etc.)
3. Diagnosis
   • Dyspnea
   • Tachypnea
   • Tachycardia
   • Cyanosis
   • Hypoxemia is confirmed by arterial blood gas analysis.
4. Treatment
   • Treat cause
   • Oxygen therapy

It is difficult to increase patients' inspired oxygen percentage > 60% by using a mask.
   • Mechanical ventilation and positive end-expiratory pressure (PEEP)
   Use these methods if supplemental oxygen by mask fails to restore arterial oxygen to safe levels, e.g., oxygen tension >60 mm Hg.

D. Atelectasis and Retained Secretions
   The most common postoperative respiratory complication
1. Prevention
   Postoperatively, patients, particularly those at risk (see above), should
   • Be provided with good pain relief to permit their cooperation
   • Be encouraged to cough and to take deep breaths
   • Use incentive spirometry (to be effective, this should be performed at least five to ten times each hour while patient is awake)
   • Be mobilized and ambulant as soon as possible
2. Treatment
   Consists of the above plus
   • Gravity postural drainage in combination with chest percussions
   • Fiberoptic bronchoscopy to aspirate secretions
   • PEEP
   • Airway intubation and mechanical ventilation to allow safe and repeated tracheal suctioning
   • Oxygen therapy as adjunct to prevent hypoxemia

E. Nosocomial Pneumonia
1. Diagnosis
   May be difficult to distinguish from atelectasis and retained secretions. The following suggest the diagnosis:
   • Fever
   • Dyspnea
   • Productive cough producing purulent sputum
   • Leukocytosis
   • Increasing or new lung infiltrates on chest radiography
   • Sputum Gram stain and culture (to be diagnostic, sputum sample from the lower respiratory tract should be obtained with deep coughing)
   • Bronchoalveolar lavage—indicated in immunocompromised patients susceptible to unusual opportunistic infections such as *Pneumocystis, Candida,* or *Aspergillus*
   • If bronchoalveolar lavage fails to provide a diagnosis, lung biopsy is indicated.
   • Blood cultures, at least two 30 minutes apart, are only occasionally positive but do provide specific information about causative organisms.
2. Treatment
   • Antibiotics are initiated once adequate sputum samples and blood cultures have been obtained.
   • The regimen can be changed when culture results and antibiotic sensitivities become available.

3. Causes
   Organisms most commonly responsible for nosocomial pneumonia are
   - *Pseudomonas aeruginosa*
   - *Staphylococcus aureus*
   - *Klebsiella*
   - *Enterobacter*
   - *Escherichia coli*
   - *Serratia*
   - *Proteus*
4. Supportive therapy
   - Oxygen therapy
   - Chest physiotherapy

F. Aspiration Pneumonia
1. Associated with
   - Altered conscious state, e.g., anesthesia
   - Impaired laryngeal reflexes, e.g., elderly patients
   - Passive regurgitation, e.g., obstetric patients, bowel obstruction, hiatal hernia, increased intraabdominal pressure, nasogastric tube
2. Can result in acid aspiration (Mendelson syndrome)
   - Occurs with aspirate pH <2.5
   - Diffuse severe damage of the pulmonary capillary membranes causes low-pressure pulmonary edema.
   - This condition may produce
     — Severe dyspnea
     — Cyanosis
     — Bronchospasm
     — Shock
3. Treatment
   - Admit patient to intensive care unit.
   - Clear airway with suctioning.
   - Administer 100% oxygen to ensure safe Pao_2.
   - Use mechanical ventilation to relieve respiratory failure: PEEP may improve oxygenation.
   - Bronchodilators may relieve bronchospasm.
   - Bronchoscopy is indicated for
     — Particulate aspiration
     — Focal pulmonary collapse
   - Give cardiovascular support as needed.
   - Antibiotics are indicated if infection develops.

III. Acute Emergencies: Renal Failure

A. Acute Renal Failure
1. Features
   - Defined as acute inability of the kidneys to maintain the volume and/or composition of the internal environment
   - May be superimposed on chronic kidney disease
   - Often occurs as part of a disease process involving multiple organs, e.g., sepsis
2. There are three types of acute renal failure, all of which can occur postoperatively.
   - Prerenal oliguria

   — Most common type of renal failure
   — Due to inadequate renal perfusion caused by low cardiac output or extracellular fluid deficit, e.g., shock, dehydration
   - Postrenal failure
     Obstruction of urine flow due to surgical procedure, retroperitoneal process, uterine/ovarian mass, urolithiasis, etc.
   - Intrinsic renal failure
     Caused by acute tubular necrosis; this is more likely to occur in patients with preexisting renal disease and in the elderly
   - Acute tubular necrosis has numerous causes, including
     — Unrelieved severe prerenal oliguria (the most common cause)
     — Septicemia
     — Congestive heart failure
     — Acute hemorrhage
     — Cirrhosis of the liver, bile duct obstruction
     — Nephrotoxic agents, e.g., gentamicin and cyclosporine
     — Nonsteroidal antiinflammatory drugs, e.g., ketorolac
     — Radiographic contrast media
     — Intravascular hemolysis or myoglobinuria
3. Diagnosis of acute renal failure
   - Be alert to situations in which it is likely to occur.
   - Diagnosis is suggested by oliguria: urine output < 30 mL/h.
   - Perform physical examination to
     — Assess state of hydration (neck veins, postural hypotension)
     — Rule out urinary tract obstruction
       · Obstruction is suggested by sudden, rather than gradual, cessation of urine.
       · History and physical examination findings may suggest cause.
       · If obstruction still cannot be ruled out clinically, pelvic ultrasonography and retrograde pyelography are indicated.
     — Differentiate prerenal oliguria and acute tubular necrosis by urine analysis (results are often invalid after diuretics have been administered), as indicated in Table 1.
4. Treatment of acute renal failure varies with cause, which should be ascertained as soon as possible.
   - Prerenal
     — Correct hypovolemia. Type of fluid depends on the source of the hypovolemia, i.e., isotonic saline or blood may both be appropriate.
     — Prolonged prerenal failure can produce acute tubular necrosis. Therefore, fluids should be discontinued if diuresis is not achieved.
     — Diuretics, furosemide (0.5 to 10 mg/kg i.v. or 50 to 100 mL 20% mannitol i.v.) may establish diuresis in fluid-repleted patients.
     — Low dose of dopamine (e.g., 2 to 4 μg/kg/h) may

TABLE 1. *Differentiation of prerenal oliguria from acute tubular necrosis by urine analysis*

Factor	Prerenal oliguria	Acute tubular necrosis
Urine osmolarity	High, >500 osm/L	Isomolar with plasma
Urine sodium	Low, <20 mmol/L	High, >40 mmol/L
Specific gravity	High, 1.020	Typically fixed, 1.010–1.012

also help initiate and sustain diuresis after volume replacement.

- Postrenal
  Early removal of source of obstruction or bypassing of obstruction is required to avoid intrinsic renal damage.

B. Acute Tubular Necrosis

1. The clinical course of acute tubular necrosis typically consists of three phases.
- Oliguric/anuric phase
  — Usually lasts 10 to 14 days
  — Associated with
    · Progressive increase in serum levels of creatinine and urea
    · Risk of hyperkalemia
    · Metabolic acidosis
    · Risk of fluid overload and pulmonary edema
    · Susceptibility to infection
    · Uremic enterocolitis, stress ulcers, and gastrointestinal bleeding
    · Disseminated intravascular coagulation
    · Bleeding tendency
    · Pericarditis
- Diuretic phase
  — Urine output seldom exceeds 4 L/day.
  — Renal function remains poor.
  — Associated with
    · Fluid/electrolyte losses
    · Continuation of symptoms of uremia
    · Continued susceptibility to infection.
- Recovery phase
  Gradual recovery of renal function, including ability to concentrate urine
2. Treatment of acute tubular necrosis
- Fluid balance
  Fluid intake is restricted in oliguric phase. (Drugs are administered in concentrated solutions, etc.)
- Electrolyte control
  — Hyperkalemia (>6 mEq/L)
    · Potentially life-threatening: ventricular fibrillation and cardiac arrest can occur.
    · Potassium intake should be restricted.
    · Effects of high potassium levels on heart are exaggerated by hypocalcemia.
    · Acute medical treatment consists of 1 g calcium gluconate or 0.5 g chloride (given i.v. over 1 to 3 minutes with electrocardiographic monitoring), correction of acidosis with 50 mL 8.4% sodium

bicarbonate given intravenously, glucose [25 g (500 mL D_5W) to 50 g (500 mL $D_{10}W$ or 1 L D_5W)] plus 5 to 10 U regular human insulin given intravenously.
    · Longer term management consists of 30 to 60 g of sodium polystyrene sulfonate enemas and/or dialysis.
  — Hyponatremia
    · Common, particularly when 5% dextrose in water is used for management of acute renal failure (5% dextrose in 0.5 isotonic saline preferred)
    · Treated with sodium bicarbonate given intravenously and dialysis if persistent
  — Hypermagnesemia
    Dangerous. It can be avoided by not using magnesium-based antacids/cathartics.
- Metabolic acidosis
  Rarely a problem, but if severe, it can be managed by dialysis.
- Adequate nutrition
  Important: A high-calorie nitrogen-sparing diet (30 g protein/day) is used to decrease catabolism.
- Drugs
  When drugs are excreted by the kidney, e.g., digoxin and aminoglycosides, the dosage should be decreased appropriately.
- Infection control
  Patients with acute tubular necrosis are prone to infection.
- Stress ulcer prophylaxis
  Use antacids and H_2 antihistamine blockers (avoid magnesium-containing antacids).
- Dialysis
  Indications are
  — Uncontrolled hyperkalemia, >6 mEq/L
  — Uncontrolled acidosis, pH <7.2
  — Pulmonary edema
  — Development of symptoms of uremia (drowsiness, coma, seizures, pericarditis, pruritis, nausea/vomiting, gastrointestinal bleeding, etc.) or blood urea >100 mg/dL

IV. Acute Emergencies: Septic Shock

A. Features

1. Clinical course is determined by the host and is not unique to any specific microorganisms.
2. Septic shock has high mortality, >50%.

B. Clinical Presentation

Variable

1. In classic early "warm shock," the patient is
   - Vasodilated
   - Hypotensive
   - Tachypneic
   - Tachycardic
2. "Cold shock" may follow or be the initial presentation
   - Severe hypotension
   - Vasoconstriction
   - Peripheral cyanosis
   - Renal failure
   - Liver failure
   - Respiratory failure caused by the adult respiratory distress syndrome
   - Coagulopathy (disseminated intravascular coagulation)
   - Glucose intolerance
   - Metabolic acidosis

C. Treatment

The aim is to identify and to eradicate the source of infection.

1. Blood cultures
   Blood should be drawn for three sets of cultures before antibiotics are started. Each set consists of 6 bottles (3 aerobic and 3 anaerobic), with 5 mL of blood in each bottle.
2. Gram stain and culture
   Urine, peritoneal fluid obtained by culdocentesis, pus from the vaginal apex, etc., are sent for aerobic and anaerobic culturing, Gram staining, and microscopy.

Note: Infections that occur after vaginal and abdominal hysterectomy or ones associated with a ruptured tubo-ovarian abscess are usually polymicrobial, consisting of normal microflora of the vagina and cervix.

Note: Septic shock associated with abortal infection usually results from endotoxin-producing aerobic gram-negative bacilli: *E. coli* is the organism most commonly involved.

3. Antibiotics
   - Treatment should be prompt and empiric until culture results are available. Antibiotic choices are based on the likely organisms and the site of entry. Coverage against gram-negative bacteria and gram-positive cocci is warranted, and coverage against anaerobes deserves consideration. With immunosuppressed patients, infection may be endogenous or exogenous in origin and is often difficult to diagnose. An infectious disease specialty consultation is advisable. The publication *Medical Letter* regularly reviews suitable antibiotic therapy.
   - Trovafloxacin, 200 to 300 mg i.v. once daily, is active against both aerobic and anaerobic cocci and bacilli and, currently, is one of the drugs of choice to begin therapy.
4. Surgery

To remove or to drain infected tissue. Laparotomy is sometimes useful if the source of infection cannot be identified.

5. Supportive measures
   - Admit the patient to the intensive care unit for close monitoring.
   - Monitor
     — Heart rate and blood pressure (invasive monitoring is indicated)
     — Urine output
     — Central venous pressure, pulmonary capillary wedge pressure, cardiac output
     — Daily chest radiograph
     — Laboratory tests, including arterial blood gases and acid-base status, electrolytes, liver function tests, creatinine, blood glucose, hemoglobin, platelet and leukocyte counts, and coagulation status
6. Hemodynamic support
   - Preload
     Isotonic saline or colloid is given to produce a low normal pulmonary capillary wedge pressure. Excess fluids must be avoided.
   - Cardiac output
     If this is low after normalizing preload, administration of inotropes, e.g., dobutamine (1 to 20 μg/kg/min), may be indicated. (The ability of the patient to sustain a high cardiac output may be associated with improved survival.)
7. Respiratory support
   - Oxygen therapy
     Hypoxia is common and is usually relieved initially with an oxygen mask.
   - Mechanical ventilation and PEEP
     Required if adult respiratory distress syndrome develops; it is suggested by tachypnea, worsening hypoxemia, and later, diffuse lung infiltrate seen on chest radiographs.
8. Nutritional support
   - Parenteral nutrition is required to counter the hypercatabolic state and negative nitrogen balance associated with sepsis.
   - Insulin: given according to a sliding scale, may be required to manage the hyperglycemia that occurs occasionally with sepsis.
9. Preservation of renal function
   - Acute renal failure is common and increases the morbidity of septic shock.
   - Aminoglycosides used to treat sepsis are potentially nephrotoxic.
   - Preventing oliguric renal failure requires maintaining urine output and optimizing cardiorespiratory function. Continuous infusion of dopamine (2 to 4 μg/kg/min) and intermittent furosemide (10 to 40 mg i.v.) may be of value.
10. Gastrointestinal bleeding
    Antacids plus H^2 receptor blockers are effective in

reducing the incidence of gastrointestinal bleeding, a common complication of sepsis.

11. Disseminated intravascular coagulation
Also seen in sepsis; treatment consists of
- Removal of septic source
- Correcting shock
- Platelets and fresh frozen plasma as needed to correct coagulopathy

12. Metabolic acidosis
Most commonly due to lactic acidosis caused by anaerobic metabolism; treatment consists of
- Correcting hypoxemia
- Improving cardiac output
- 50 mL of 8.4% sodium bicarbonate if metabolic acidosis is severe (pH < 7.2)

V. Acute Emergencies: Psychiatric and Central Nervous System Disorders

A. Psychiatric Disorders
1. Postoperative agitation/delirium is associated with
- Alcohol or drug addiction and/or acute withdrawal
- Neurologic disease
- Chronic systemic disease
- Old age
- Visual and/or auditory impairment
2. Contributing factors include
- Unfamiliar hospital environment
- Pain and other noxious stimuli
- Sleep deprivation
- Anxiety
- Inability to communicate
3. Treatment
- Psychiatric medications should be continued throughout the perioperative period.
- Alcoholics should receive thiamine [50 to 100 mg daily i.v. or intramuscularly (i.m.)] until dietary intake can be resumed.
- Haloperidol: currently, the drug of choice for treating agitation. In emergency situations, the dose is 2 to 5 mg i.m. or orally, repeated hourly for desirable effect. For milder agitation, 0.5 to 5 mg given orally two or three times daily may suffice.

B. Altered Conscious State and Coma
Coma postoperatively is rare.
1. Causes include
- Intracranial events, e.g., hemorrhage, infection, ischemic insult (global anoxic episode associated with cardiac arrest or anesthetic mishap)
- Extracranial factors, e.g., hypoglycemia or hyperglycemia, liver and renal failure, drug effects, etc.
2. Treatment
Altered mental states, including coma, require emergency evaluation and treatment as follows:

- Check airway patency and intubate if compromised.
- Confirm adequacy of respiration. If inadequate, initiate artificial ventilation.
- Stabilize cardiac output and circulation. (This is important with myocardial infarction and shock states.)
- Metabolic status. Glucose, electrolytes, creatinine and urea, blood count, and prothrombin and partial thromboplastin times should be urgently measured. Because of the risk of producing hyperglycemic metabolic acidosis, the historical practice of giving 50 mL of 50% dextrose i.v. immediately, before laboratory results are available, is no longer recommended unless the likelihood of hypoglycemia (with type 1 diabetes mellitus) is high.
- Control seizures if present. Diazepam (2 mg/min i.v. until seizures stop or until a maximal dose of 30 mg is reached) is given together with an infusion of phenytoin (18 mg/kg i.v. at a rate *not* faster than 50 mg/min).

Note: Diazepam may cause apnea, and phenytoin can produce bradycardia and hypotension.

3. Further management
The ultimate extent of neurologic injury depends not only on the primary injury but also on the secondary neurologic injury that occurs in the subsequent minutes, hours, and days. The patient should be admitted to an intensive care unit as soon as possible.
4. Ongoing management consists of
- Detailed and ongoing neurologic assessment. The Glasgow Coma Scale is used to assess the depth of coma; it has prognostic value.
- Computed tomography (CT) of the head is used to rule out a mass effect, including intracranial bleeding.
- Lumbar puncture is appropriate if bacterial meningitis is suspected. Clinical examination and CT of the head must first have excluded the possibility of increased intracranial pressure before lumbar puncture is performed.
- Electroencephalography is rarely needed except to identify coma associated with status epilepticus.
- Treatment of the precipitating cause, if feasible, and prevention of secondary injury associated with increased intracranial pressure, cerebral vasospasm, etc.
- Supportive nursing and medical care, including prevention of
  — Eye injury
  — Pressure sores
  — Performing bronchial toilet
  — Bladder care
- Nutritional support

VI. Acute Emergencies: Anaphylaxis

A. Principles
1. Once initiated, serious anaphylaxis (IgE antibody mediated) and anaphylactoid reactions (non-IgE

antibody mediated) can produce the following conditions within minutes:

- Cardiovascular collapse
- Severe bronchospasm
- Laryngospasm
- Various associated cutaneous and gastrointestinal effects

2. Anaphylaxis and anaphylactoid reactions follow exposure to the provoking agent, are caused by a sudden release of a large number of mast cell and basophil mediators, particularly histamine, and can be fatal if not treated immediately.

3. Agents that commonly cause anaphylaxis on repeat exposure include
- Intravenous contrast media
- β-Lactam antibiotics
- Sulfonamides
- Ester local anesthetics
- Blood products

4. Anaphylactoid reactions can occur on first-time exposure to some compounds, e.g., iodinated contrast media.

B. Symptoms and Signs
1. Often within minutes, the patient experiences *symptoms* including
- Choking sensation
- Metallic taste
- Paresthesias
- Coughing
- Apprehension

2. Clinical signs may include
- Tachycardia, hypotension, and shock
- Rhinitis, dyspnea, bronchospasm, and laryngeal obstruction
- Erythema, generalized urticaria, angioneurotic edema, and conjunctivitis
- Nausea, vomiting, abdominal cramps, and diarrhea

C. Management
1. Principles
- Treatment must be initiated immediately to prevent life-threatening circulatory collapse and airway obstruction.
- It is appropriate to summon help by calling the hospital cardiopulmonary resuscitation team.

2. Epinephrine: the mainstay and most important component of treatment
- Give 0.3 to 0.5 mL of 1/1,000 solution subcutaneously (s.c.) or i.m., repeated two to three times at 15-minute intervals.
- If the patient is already in shock, give 1 mL/min of 1/10,000 solution (2 μg/min) i.v., with electrocardiographic monitoring.

3. Circulatory collapse
- Place patient in the Trendelenburg position.

- Administer fluid challenges with crystalloid (large volumes may be required).
- Central venous pressure monitoring is helpful.
- If blood pressure is not sustained by these means, give vasopressor, e.g., norepinephrine (0.1 to 0.5 μg/kg/min).

4. Airway obstruction
- Administer 100% oxygen through a face mask.
- If the patient is severely dyspneic (respiratory rate >40 breaths/min), intubate with an endotracheal tube (a smaller tube than normal, e.g., a 5-mm tube may be appropriate).
- If endotracheal intubation is technically impossible because of laryngeal spasm or edema, perform needle (12 to 14 gauge) cricothyroidotomy, surgical cricothyroidotomy, or tracheostomy.
- Mechanical ventilation is required to treat respiratory failure, severe bronchospasm, and apnea.
- Aminophylline (5 to 6 mg/kg i.v. at a rate not exceeding 25 mg/min, followed by an i.v. infusion of 0.5 to 1.0 mg/kg/h) may help relieve bronchospasm.

5. Ancillary medications
- Corticosteroids are not of immediate clinical benefit but help reduce bronchospasm and laryngeal edema; they also reduce the late recurrences of anaphylaxis. Hydrocortisone succinate 200 mg is given i.v. every 6 hours for 24 to 48 hours.
- Antihistamines are not part of the primary management of anaphylaxis. H_1 blockers, e.g., diphenhydramine 25 to 50 mg i.v., may help histamine-induced cardiopulmonary effects and cutaneous manifestations such as urticaria; H_2 blockers such as cimetidine may help reverse refractory anaphylaxis.

Note: After anaphylaxis, it is important to identify the drug or agent responsible.

VII. Specific Complications: Deep Vein Thrombosis

A. Prevention
1. Recognition of patients at high risk is essential.
2. Risk factors are
- Specific factors following surgery
  — Old age
  — Obesity
  — Previous deep vein thrombosis
  — Malignancy
  — Prolonged surgery
  — General anesthetic compared with regional
- Venous stasis
  — Immobility (surgery, bed rest, limb paralysis)
  — Heart failure
  — Varicose veins
- Increased coagulability

— Dehydration
— Polycythemia
— Oral contraceptives/estrogen use
— Pregnancy/puerperium
— Inflammatory bowel disease
— Nephrotic syndrome
• Deficiency of anticoagulants
— Antithrombin III
— Protein C
— Protein S
• Antiphospholipid antibody
— Lupus anticoagulant
3. Measures to prevent occurrence of deep vein thrombosis involve
• Correction of risk factors if possible
• Avoiding constriction of legs by straps or other restraining devices
• Trendelenburg position
• Graduated compression stockings applied preoperatively
• Sequential compression devices
• Short operating time
• Low dose of heparin, 5,000 U given every 12 hours s.c., or low-molecular-weight heparin (dose varies with the preparation)
• Early postoperative mobilization

B. Diagnosis
1. Clinical examination (unreliable in 50% of cases)
• Leg swelling
• Calf or thigh tenderness
• Calf or thigh pain
• Venous congestion
• Homans sign
2. Impedance plethysmography: measures variations of the volume of blood in the calf that normally occur with respiration or the Valsalva maneuver
• False-negative rate, approximately 10%
• False-positive rate, approximately 20%
• Not useful if chronic venous insufficiency is present
3. Doppler ultrasonography: the normal change in the frequency of the reflected ultrasound beam is not present or is lowered if veins are clotted and blood is either not flowing or flowing sluggishly.
• More useful for large proximal veins
• Less useful in detecting clots in calf veins
• Most useful before collaterals develop
• Accuracy as high as 90% or more
4. Venography: contrast material is injected into foot veins, and radiographs are examined for evidence of obstruction in the venous system.
• Invasive procedure with risks and side effects
• Most reliable method for detecting deep vein thrombosis
5. ^{131}I Fibrinogen: fibrinogen labeled with ^{131}I is injected intravenously, and the limbs are scanned to detect areas of increased activity, which signify a thrombus.
• Can be repeated at daily intervals to detect propagation of a clot
• Active clot formation is necessary; old clots are not detected.
• More useful for calf vein thrombosis than for femoral thrombosis

C. Treatment
1. Hospitalize patient.
2. Bed rest with legs elevated
3. Heparin: 5,000 U i.v. as a bolus, then continuous infusion of 1,000 U/h
4. Monitor partial thromboplastin time, maintaining it at about 1.5 to 2 times the normal value by adjusting the heparin dosage.

Note: Complications of heparin include bleeding, intracranial hemorrhage, and thrombocytopenia.

5. Start treatment with sodium warfarin (orally) after symptoms improve.
6. Cease intravenous heparin once prothrombin time is twice normal value or INR is 2.0.
7. Continue warfarin treatment for a minimum of 3 months.
8. Check prothrombin time daily until it is twice normal value, then check it weekly for 4 weeks, and then every 2 weeks.
9. Wearing of compression stockings for 3 months

VIII. Specific Complications: Pulmonary Embolus

A. Usually Results from Thrombi Dislodged from Ileofemoral Venous System

B. Prevention
Same as for deep vein thrombosis

C. Diagnosis
1. Clinical diagnosis (not always accurate)
• Pleuritic chest pain
• Syncope
• Cyanosis
• Dyspnea
• Cough/hemoptysis
• Apprehension
• Tachycardia
• Fever
• Cardiopulmonary arrest
• Pleural rub
• Rales and wheezes
• Loud pulmonary second sound
2. Diagnostic tests
• Chest radiography

- Electrocardiography: QRS and ST-segment changes
- Complete blood count: increased leukocyte count
- Arterial blood gases: P_{O_2} low, P_{CO_2} increased, pH <7.4
- Lung perfusion scan: segmental perfusion defects
- Ventilation/perfusion scan (eliminates other causes of poor perfusion of lungs)
- Imatron fast CT lung scan is highly sensitive and specific for pulmonary embolism.
- Pulmonary arteriography: definitive test if other test findings are equivocal; useful in pregnant women in whom isotopes are contraindicated; can have significant complications.

D. Treatment
1. Support cardiopulmonary function with inotropes, oxygen, and mechanical ventilation as needed.
2. Same as for deep vein thrombosis: use heparin given intravenously.
3. Maintain heparin treatment for at least 7 days.
4. Use vena caval umbrella or filter if there are repeated emboli.
5. Thrombolytic agents (urokinase, streptokinase) may be useful and should be considered with any hemodynamic compromise, but may cause surgical bleeding.
6. Continue warfarin treatment for 6 months.

IX. Specific Complications: Postoperative Bleeding

A. Principles
1. Hemorrhage during the postoperative period can occur despite meticulous attention to hemostasis intraoperatively.
2. Bleeding may be arterial or venous in origin or may be due to a coagulation disorder.
3. Bleeding may occur within the first 24 hours or occasionally later as a secondary hemorrhage.

B. Diagnosis
1. Hypotension
2. Tachycardia
3. Oliguria
4. Tachypnea
5. Decreasing hemoglobin and hematocrit
6. Vaginal bleeding
7. Abdominal distention
8. Increased drain output

C. Management
1. Principles
- Resuscitate patient (see Hypovolemic Shock).
- Crossmatch blood.
- Provide adequate venous access.
- Monitor vital signs.
2. Vaginal bleeding
- Inspect vagina: need adequate assistance and good lighting.
- If there is cuff bleeding after abdominal hysterectomy or vaginal wall bleeding after vaginal surgery, oversew bleeding point with figure-of-eight 2-0 synthetic absorbable sutures.
- If there is bleeding after cone biopsy, cauterize or suture-ligate bleeding point and insert a vaginal pack and catheter for 12 hours and hospitalize patient.
3. Abdominal bleeding
  If significant intraperitoneal bleeding occurs after vaginal or abdominal hysterectomy, laparotomy is necessary because attempts to ligate the bleeding point through the vaginal cuff are rarely successful and put the urinary tract at risk.
- Remove all blood from the peritoneal cavity.
- Irrigate with copious amounts of isotonic saline.
- Inspect all pedicles for active bleeding.
- Most intraperitoneal bleeding after abdominal or vaginal hysterectomy is from the uterine artery and occasionally from the ovarian vessels.
- If the uterine artery pedicle is the site of bleeding, oversew bleeding point after identifying ureter and then ligate the anterior division of the internal iliac artery on that side, lateral to the ureter, or dissect and ligate the uterine artery itself.
- If there is generalized bleeding from the hysterectomy site, attempt to oversew or to cauterize all bleeding areas and then ligate the anterior division of the internal iliac arteries bilaterally.
- If ovarian pedicles are bleeding, dissect the vessels proximally by dividing the peritoneum parallel to the vessels until above the bleeding point, and then clamp and religate the pedicle, keeping the ureter under direct vision.
- Always check all areas of the abdomen and pelvis, even though the site of bleeding appears to be obvious.
- If there is a large raw area with generalized oozing, use topical clotting agents and leave a large intraperitoneal suction drain in place.
- Occasionally an intraperitoneal pack may be needed as a life-saving measure.
4. Wound bleeding
- Bleeding from the skin edge can be controlled by
  — Pressure dressing
  — Suture
  — Application of skin staples
  — Cautery
- Bleeding from deeper in the wound, forming a wound hematoma, requires evacuation of the hematoma by opening the incision and ligating or cauterizing the bleeding site. A wound drain should then be placed before resuturing.

X. Specific Complications: Disseminated Intravascular Coagulation

A. Principle

Disseminated intravascular coagulation can be initiated by massive blood loss, gram-negative sepsis, or pregnancy complications.

B. Diagnosis

Is made by assessment of
1. Thrombocytopenia
2. Prolonged prothrombin time
3. Prolonged partial thromboplastin time
4. Low fibrinogen levels
5. Presence of fibrin split products
6. Presence of fibrin monomer

C. Treatment

1. Treat cause of disseminated intravascular coagulation.
2. If there is bleeding, give blood products to correct the identified coagulation abnormality, e.g., platelets, cryoprecipitate.

Note: Other supportive measures such as oxygen, vasopressors, packs, and military antishock trousers (MAST suit) may be indicated.

XI. Specific Complications: Hypovolemic Shock

A. Definition

Shock refers to hypoperfusion of vital organs and secondary dysfunction.

B. Causes

1. Trauma
2. Postoperative complications
   - Bleeding pedicle
   - After extensive dissection, e.g., ovarian cancer, pelvic exenteration

C. Clinical Presentation

1. Hypovolemic shock usually develops soon after a surgical procedure (primary hemorrhage) but may be delayed (secondary hemorrhage).
2. Indications of severe bleeding include
   - Hypotension
   - Tachycardia
   - Pallor
   - Sweating
   - Cyanosis
   - Hyperventilation
   - Confusion
   - Oliguria
3. The source of bleeding is usually obvious, but the true extent of the bleeding may often be underestimated.

D. Treatment

Resuscitation and surgical management should proceed simultaneously.
1. Place large-bore peripheral intravenous catheters.
2. Institute resuscitation with isotonic crystalloid solutions, giving 500-mL boluses until patient is hemodynamically stable and/or until blood is available.
3. Transfuse erythrocytes when available to restore the hemoglobin to 10 g/mL and to achieve a hematocrit of 30%.
4. Surgical treatment may be required to stop the bleeding: urgent preparation for it should be initiated.
5. MAST suit—a controversial ancillary aid that may tamponade intraabdominal bleeding in special circumstances.
6. Ongoing monitoring of heart rate, blood pressure, respiratory rate, mental status, urine output, and central venous pressure (or, better, pulmonary artery wedge pressure) should be initiated to guide fluid replacement.
7. Urine output should improve if blood volume is rapidly replenished.
8. Low dose of dopamine (2 to 4 μg/kg/min i.v.) and small doses of furosemide (10 to 40 mg i.v.) after restoration of blood volume may help initiate diuresis.
9. Metabolic acidosis, hyponatremia, and hypokalemia are common and respond to resuscitation.
10. Sodium bicarbonate is given only with severe metabolic acidosis (pH <7.2) because it exacerbates intracellular acidosis, causes hypokalemia, and creates a sodium load.
11. Dopamine (5 to 20 μg/kg/min) and/or norepinephrine (0.1 to 0.5 μg/kg/min) or other intravenously given vasopressors may be required temporarily while intravascular volume is being restored.

Note: Hypotension not responding to fluid replacement suggests continued bleeding or other complications, such as tension pneumothorax, pericardial tamponade, congestive heart failure, pulmonary embolus, and sepsis.

E. Arterial Embolization

1. Rarely used method but useful for controlling postoperative arterial bleeding
2. Arteriography performed with the Seldinger technique through the femoral artery
3. Bleeding vessel identified under fluoroscopy
4. Bleeding vessel embolized with various agents, including
   - Gelatin sponge (Gelfoam)
   - Cellulose (Oxcel)
   - Wire coils
   - Autologous blood clot
   - Balloon catheters
5. Vasopressor infusion has been used to control bleeding from intestinal anastomosis sites.

12

6. Indications for embolization rather than operation include
   - Hemodynamically stable patient
   - Recurrent cancer with bleeding
   - Radionecrosis
   - Debilitated patient
   - Distorted pelvic anatomy

Note: A patient in shock from acute blood loss is not an ideal candidate for embolization because a surgical approach with ligation is usually much quicker.

XII. Specific Complications: Ileus and Bowel Obstruction

A. Principles
1. Ileus is common after pelvic surgery; obstruction is less frequent.
2. Differentiation of ileus from obstruction is often difficult.

B. Diagnosis
1. Nausea and vomiting
2. Distended abdomen
3. No or minimal flatus
4. Silent abdomen (ileus or late obstruction)
5. Hyperactive bowel sounds (obstruction)
6. Intestinal succussion splash (ileus and obstruction)
7. Radiography of abdomen
   - Ileus: diffuse large- and small-bowel distention
   - Obstruction: localized and progressive distention

C. Management
1. Insert a nasogastric tube (nothing by mouth without a tube may be adequate for ileus with no distention or vomiting).
2. Administer fluids intravenously and monitor fluid balance closely.
3. Perform complete blood count and serum electrolytes and correct abnormalities as indicated.
4. Closely monitor abdominal signs and distention (measure girth).
5. Prescribe rectal suppositories.
6. Encourage active mobilization.

Note: Progressive distention, fever, and leukocytosis associated with constant pain may indicate bowel necrosis from strangulation or perforation. Immediate surgical treatment is required.

7. After flatus has been passed, clamp the nasogastric tube for 4-hour intervals, give a limited amount of clear fluids, and then reaspirate tube.
8. If nasogastric tube return is minimal (<100 mL) and nausea or distention does not recur, remove the tube and slowly advance the diet.
9. A long intestinal tube may be more effective than a nasogastric tube in the management of obstruction, but there is disagreement about this.
10. Acute obstruction occurring in the immediate postoperative period should be managed surgically.
11. Volvulus of the sigmoid, cecum, or transverse colon is rare and requires immediate operation.
12. Pseudo-obstruction of the colon is also rare and causes acute colonic dilation down to the rectosigmoid. It is treated by decompression using colonoscopy or, if unsuccessful, cecostomy.
13. A cecal diameter of 12 to 13 cm on radiographs signifies imminent rupture.

XIII. Specific Complications: Wound Infection

A. Principles
1. Wound infection rates should be monitored closely.
2. Abdominal hysterectomy, because of entry into the vagina, is classed as a clean-contaminated case with regard to the wound.

B. Causes
1. Debilitated patient, e.g., diabetes, cancer
2. Wound hematoma or collection
3. Contaminated operation (bowel, personnel)
4. Prolonged surgical procedure
5. Obesity
6. Prolonged preoperative hospitalization
7. Drainage through wound
8. Early preoperative shaving

C. Preventive Measures
1. Prophylactic treatment with antibiotics
2. Preoperative correction of any medical problem, e.g., diabetes
3. Shaving patient in operating room immediately before operation
4. Preoperative skin scrub
5. Short operating time
6. Meticulous hemostasis and surgical technique
7. Wound suction drainage
8. Delayed closure of contaminated wounds

D. Management
1. If cellulitis only, culture and treat with antibiotics.
2. If obvious collection is present
   - Open wound widely.
   - Drain pus.
   - Culture.
   - Irrigate with half-strength hydrogen peroxide.
   - Pack with saline-moistened gauze three times daily.
   - Antibiotics are not usually necessary unless there is adjacent cellulitis.
3. Removal of dried dressings debrides wounds and promotes healing.

4. Secondary reapproximation of skin edges may be performed for large defects after they are clean and granulating.

XIV. Specific Complications: Wound Dehiscence

A. Occurrence
1. Usually occurs in patients with
   - Malignancy
   - Poor nutritional status
   - Obesity
   - Chronic cough
   - Postradiation
   - Abdominal distention (obstruction or ileus)
2. Is less common now because of use of synthetic absorbable sutures rather than catgut
3. Occurs most commonly about the seventh to tenth postoperative days
4. Often preceded by profuse serosanguineous wound drainage

B. Diagnosis
Made by opening skin wound and inspecting fascia to see if intact

C. Treatment
1. Apply saline dressings and binder and take patient to the operating room.
2. Reopen the wound.
3. Replace the intestine in the peritoneal cavity.
4. Close the wound with Smead-Jones-type closure with interrupted synthetic nonabsorbable sutures.
5. Prophylactic treatment with antibiotics.
6. Drain the wound.

XV. Specific Complications: Necrotizing Fasciitis

A. Features
1. Caused by a combination of aerobic and anaerobic bacteria
2. Occurs in the vulva, perineum, groin, or abdominal wall
3. Soft tissue crepitation is present.
4. Very rapid spread of necrosis, with blistering cellulitis and dusky skin
5. Turbid offensive fluid drainage from wound
6. Often associated with diabetes
7. Patient's condition rapidly becomes very toxic.
8. Gas may be seen in the involved tissues on radiography.

B. Diagnosis
1. Gram stain
2. Blood cultures, aerobic and anaerobic
3. Wound cultures, aerobic and anaerobic

C. Treatment
1. Early surgical debridement is critical.
2. Adequate fluid resuscitation
3. Antibiotics, if Gram stain and cultures show only *Streptococcus* pyrogens and clostridia; high-dose penicillin G is the agent of choice.
4. Hyperbaric oxygen has been used for treating clostridial infection.
5. Mortality rate is high unless the condition is treated early, urgently, and aggressively.

XVI. Specific Complications: Intraabdominal or Pelvic Hematoma

A. Prevention
1. Adequate hemostasis
2. Postoperative suction drainage

B. Diagnosis
1. Decrease in hemoglobin concentration or hematocrit
2. Localized pain
3. Fever
4. Abdominal or pelvic mass
5. Ultrasonographic or CT scan demonstrates collection

C. Location
Usually retroperitoneal, in the broad ligament, above the bladder and vault or in lymphatic spaces after lymphadenectomy

D. Treatment
1. Transfusion, if hemoglobin concentration is low or the patient is hemodynamically unstable
2. Antibiotics, to prevent abscess formation
3. Observation, unless hematoma becomes infected, is enlarging, or is significantly symptomatic
4. If progressively enlarging or if patient becomes hemodynamically unstable, laparotomy is required for hemostasis.
5. If infected, consider CT or ultrasonographically guided percutaneous catheter drainage.

XVII. Specific Complications: Pelvic or Abdominal Abscess

A. Diagnosis
1. May be difficult to localize and to diagnose
2. Unexplained fever and chills (exclude other causes)
3. Leukocytosis
4. Localized pain
5. Usually occurs ≥1 week postoperatively
6. CT especially but also ultrasonography or gallium scan may localize the abscess.

B. Treatment
1. CT-guided or ultrasonographically guided percutaneous drainage is the preferred surgical treatment.

2. It must be a unilocular abscess with close contact to the abdominal wall to be suitable for percutaneous drainage.

3. Culture the abscess contents and start triple antibiotic therapy with gentamicin, clindamycin (or metronidazole), and penicillin (or ampicillin).

4. Perform sinography through the drain to confirm complete resolution of abscess cavity before removing the drain.

5. Transvaginal, transrectal, or laparotomy drainage is alternative to percutaneous drainage.

XVIII. Specific Complications: Peritonitis

A. Causes
1. Rupture of viscus
2. Leak from gastrointestinal anastomosis
3. Urinary leakage
4. Ischemic viscus from volvulus, obstruction, or thrombosis
5. Rupture of pelvic abscess
6. Pelvic inflammatory disease
7. Postoperative appendicitis, cholecystitis, or diverticulitis

B. Diagnosis
1. Abdominal pain, nausea, and vomiting
2. Guarding and rebound tenderness
3. Fever and chills
4. Abdominal distention
5. Ileus
6. Septicemia

C. Tests
1. Leukocytosis
2. Air under diaphragm on erect radiographs
3. CT and/or ultrasonographic scan is useful if abscess is present.
4. Laparoscopy is useful for diagnosis of pelvic inflammatory disease.

D. Treatment
1. Intravenous fluids, nasogastric suction
2. Correction of metabolic disturbances
3. Systemic antibiotics (triple antibiotics)
4. Correction of cause of peritonitis, e.g., repair of perforated viscus
5. Drainage of abscess, if present

XIX. Specific Complications: Pseudomembranous Colitis

A. Causes
1. Caused by toxin produced by *Clostridium difficile*
2. Develops after antibiotic treatment (cephalosporins, clindamycin, gentamicin, and ampicillin)

B. Diagnosis
1. Toxin assay of stool specimens
2. Sigmoidoscopic examination

C. Treatment
1. Metronidazole, 250 mg every 6 hours orally for 7 days *or*
2. Vancomycin, 125 mg every 6 hours orally for 7 days
3. Relapses may occur and require retreatment.

XX. Specific Complications: Lymphocyst

A. Features
1. Cystic swelling that develops after lymphadenectomy
2. Usually asymptomatic

B. Diagnosis
1. By palpation
2. Confirmed with ultrasonographic scan

C. Prevention
1. Adequate postoperative suction drainage
2. Heparin given subcutaneously increases the incidence.
3. If drains are not used, do not close the peritoneum over the lymphadenectomy site.

D. Treatment
1. The majority disappear without treatment after a few months
2. Indications for treatment include
   • Obstructed ureter
   • Infected lymphocyst
   • Pain
   • Increased bladder pressure
3. Treatment includes
   • Percutaneous suction drainage with use of sclerosing agents, e.g., povidone-iodine
   • Laparotomy or laparoscopy with marsupialization into the peritoneal cavity for pelvic or abdominal lymphocysts

XXI. Specific Complications: Anastomotic Leak from Intestinal Tract

A. From Small Bowel
1. Administer intravenous fluids and nasogastric suction.
2. Perform laparotomy to resect and reanastomose the bowel.
3. If a fistula develops through the wound or vagina and no peritonitis is present, try conservative management with total parenteral nutrition and intestinal suction and, possibly, fistula suction.
4. A postradiation fistula is less likely to heal spontaneously.

B. From Large Bowel

1. If leakage is through the suction drain only, maintain suction and add total parenteral nutrition, nasogastric suction, and antibiotics.
2. If a fistula develops, perform a proximal diverting colostomy to allow spontaneous healing.
3. Check healing of anastomosis site with colon radiography in 3 months, and if there is no leakage, close the colostomy.

XXII. Specific Complications: Urinary Fistula

A. Features

1. Fistulas usually occur within a few days after the operation.
2. Late fistulas usually result from radionecrosis or recurrent malignancy.

B. Vesicovaginal Fistula

1. Insert a tampon in the vagina, and fill the bladder with methylene blue through a urethral catheter.
2. A stained tampon verifies the presence of a vesicovaginal fistula.
3. Cystoscopy may confirm and locate the fistula.
4. Intravenous pyelography is essential to exclude associated ureteral obstruction.
5. If confirmed, insert a large (20-F) urethral catheter to allow continuous drainage and add antibiotics.
6. With good drainage, most small fistulas generally heal.
7. If healing is not present in 4 weeks, surgical repair is necessary.
8. Repair the fistula after 3 months, when postoperative healing is complete (see Chapter 15).

C. Ureterovaginal Fistula

1. If there is no leakage after filling the bladder, inject 1 ampule of indigo carmine intravenously.
2. A stained tampon verifies the presence of a ureteral fistula.
3. Perform intravenous pyelography to exclude ureteral obstruction.
4. If obstruction is present, perform percutaneous nephrostomy and attempt to pass a stent in an anterograde fashion.
5. If there is no obstruction, perform cystoscopy and attempt to pass a stent in a retrograde fashion.
6. If stenting is successful, leave for 6 weeks, repeat intravenous pyelography, and remove stent if there is no leakage.
7. If stenting is unsuccessful, repair ureteral fistula in 3 months if tissues are well healed (see Chapter 15).

XXIII. Specific Complications: Ureteral Obstruction

A. Prevention

1. Visualize the ureter by opening the broad ligament during intraabdominal operations.
2. Palpate the ureter lateral to the cardinal ligament clamps before ligating the pedicles.
3. Palpate the ureter between the index finger and the vaginal retractor during parametrial clamping at vaginal hysterectomy.

B. Causes

1. Ligature around ureter
2. Kinking of ureter from nearby suture
3. Obstruction from postoperative hematoma, lymphocyst, etc.

C. Diagnosis

1. Transient increase of serum creatinine level 24 to 72 hours postoperatively should be investigated.
2. Costovertebral angle pain may or may not be present.
3. Patient may become febrile.
4. Renal mass may be palpable.
5. Frequently, patients are asymptomatic.
6. Intravenous pyelography shows hydronephrosis and a dilated ureter, with delayed or no subsequent drainage.
7. Ultrasonography may reveal a dilated ureter and renal pelvis.

Note: It is important to investigate the possibility of ureteral obstruction if symptoms or signs are suggestive or if creatinine levels increase from the preoperative level.

D. Treatment

1. Percutaneous nephrostomy
2. Anterograde placement of ureteral stent (double J stent)
3. Retrograde stenting via cystoscopy (less successful unless performed with ureteroscope)
4. If stenting is successful, remove nephrostomy and leave stent in place for 6 weeks (prophylactic treatment with antibiotics).
5. Repeat intravenous pyelography within 1 week after removal of stent to check ureteral drainage.
6. If stenting is unsuccessful, alternatives are immediate removal of obstructing suture or delayed repair.
7. Opening of the vaginal vault and removing the uterosacral plicating sutures after vaginal hysterectomy may be successful, because these sutures are commonly the cause of ureteral obstruction.
8. Reopening the abdomen to release sutures should not be contemplated after 3 days postoperatively or if there is any urine leakage or infection, because the tissues are too edematous for reanastomosis.
9. Under the above circumstances, the kidney is protected by percutaneous nephrostomy, and the operation to alleviate the obstruction can be delayed for 8 to 12 weeks.
10. If obstruction is due to a mass, e.g., lymphocyst or hematoma, percutaneous aspiration of the collection is performed under ultrasonographic guidance. If this is not successful, incision and drainage may be necessary.

XXIV. Specific Complications: Urinary Infection

A. Principle

Ascending infection through the urethra is the most common mode of introduction of urinary infection.

B. Postoperative Factors Predisposing to Infection

1. Diabetes
2. Poor urinary volume
3. Incomplete bladder emptying
4. Bladder trauma from surgical procedure
5. Indwelling catheter

C. Prophylaxis

In the presence of an indwelling catheter, prophylaxis includes

1. Insertion of catheter under aseptic conditions and use of lubricant
2. Maintenance of good urine output
3. Closed-system gravity drainage
4. Introital hygiene (see Chapter 3)
5. Removal of catheter as soon as possible
6. No data support the use of suppressive antibiotic therapy in the presence of an indwelling catheter.
7. Significant bacteriuria should be treated after the catheter has been removed.

XXV. Specific Complications: Neurologic Injuries

A. Principle

Neurologic injury can occur from positioning of the patient on the operating table or from direct operative trauma. Positional injuries have become more common with prolonged laparoscopic procedures.

B. Causes of Specific Neurologic Injuries

1. Brachial palsy
   - Use of shoulder rests in the Trendelenburg position should be avoided.
   - Forced abduction of the arm
   - Both obese and diabetic patients are especially at risk.
2. Femoral palsy
   - Exaggerated lithotomy position
   - Pressure from abdominal wall retractor
3. Peroneal palsy
   Prolonged pressure from lithotomy stirrups
4. Sciatic nerve trauma
   Lithotomy position with prolapsed disk (elevate legs before anesthesia is induced in patients with back problems)
5. Lumbosacral plexus trauma
   Intraoperative damage, e.g., with node dissection or control of bleeding
6. Obturator nerve trauma
   May be avulsed, resected, or traumatized during pelvic lymphadenectomy; no significant sequelae apart from difficulty with leg abduction

C. Decreasing Risk

In the lithotomy position, the risk of nerve injury is decreased by
1. Elevating and flexing both legs simultaneously
2. Flexing the thighs no more than 90 degrees before rotating the stirrups laterally
3. Using proper padding between legs and stirrups

XXVI. Specific Complications: Cautery or Chemical Burns

1. Carefully apply cautery pad.
2. Avoid contact between the patient and the metal parts of the operating table.
3. Avoid use of flammable antiseptic solutions.
4. Avoid cautery contact with metal retractors and instruments.
5. Check the temperature of hot packs and irrigating solutions.
6. Determine whether the patient is allergic to antiseptic solutions.
7. Avoid pooling of antiseptic solutions between the patient and the operating table.

CHAPTER 6

Principles of Surgical Nutrition

Darlene G. Kelly, M.D., Ph.D.

I. Nutritional Assessment

A. Definition
Malnutrition is defined as the depletion of body stores. Various methods have been used to determine the degree of malnutrition.

B. Traditional Methods for Determining Nutritional Status
The following are useful in selected cases but misleading in others:
1. Diet history
2. Weight for height
3. Creatinine-height index
4. Triceps skin-fold thickness
5. Arm muscle circumference
6. Delayed hypersensitivity reactivity
7. Lymphocyte count
8. Albumin (or other short half-life protein) level
9. Grip strength
10. Recent (past 3 months) unintentional weight loss: most useful indicator in euvolemic patients
   • >20% loss from usual body weight: severe protein calorie malnutrition
   • 10% to 20% loss of body weight: moderate protein calorie malnutrition
   • <10% loss of body weight: mild protein calorie malnutrition

C. Stress and the Metabolic Response to Injury, Inflammation, or Infection
1. Alter nutritional requirements
2. Are mediated by cytokine stimulation or counterregulatory hormones (epinephrine, cortisol, glucagon, growth hormone) that cause
   • Anorexia
   • Skeletal muscle breakdown
   • Negative nitrogen balance
   • Increased lipolysis
   • Impaired water excretion and sodium retention
3. Resulting biochemical changes
   • Hypoalbuminemia due to
     — Increased albumin clearance
     — Shift of albumin from intravascular to extravascular compartment
     — Shift of hepatic synthesis
       · Decreased albumin synthesis (independent of nutritional status)
       · Increased acute phase protein synthesis
   • Trace element changes (usually independent of nutritional status)
     — Decreased serum iron
     — Decreased serum zinc
     — Increased serum copper (due to increase in ceruloplasmin)
   • Increased urea nitrogen excretion
   • Neutrophilia
   • Gluconeogenesis
4. Disease states responsible for severe stress (*most surgical procedures* produce *minimal* stress)
   • Sepsis
   • Head injury
   • Severe burns
   • Polytrauma
   • Anorexia nervosa
   • Some cancers

II. Preoperative Nutrition Support

A. Why?
Increased mortality and morbidity are associated with severe malnutrition.

Darlene G. Kelly: Consultant, Division of Gastroenterology and Hepatology and Internal Medicine, Mayo Clinic and Mayo Foundation; Assistant Professor of Medicine, Mayo Medical School, Rochester, Minnesota.

B. Who?

1. Elective or semielective cases only
2. No consensus
3. No specific cutoff point for malnourished patients who will benefit
4. Patients who are not malnourished will not benefit, and expense/risks cannot be justified.

C. How?

1. Enteral (either oral or through feeding tube) if gut functions
2. Parenteral if gut malfunctions

D. How Much?

1. Follow the same guidelines as for other patients.
2. Excessive calories and protein offer no added benefit.

E. How Long?

1. Depends on degree of malnutrition and urgency of operation
2. Usually 1 to 2 weeks
3. <7 days is not beneficial

F. Expectations?

1. Response varies and depends on the duration of nutrition support.
2. Albumin changes generally do not occur, especially in severely stressed patients.
3. Positive nitrogen balance generally does not occur in critically ill immobilized patients.
4. There is weight gain (major component is water).
5. Possible important effects are
   - Increased glycogen stores
   - Normalization of membrane function
   - Induction of enzymes
   - Improved synthesis of interleukins by monocytes or macrophages, thus improved immune response

III. Nutrition Requirements

A. Calories (kcal)

1. Calories based on Harris-Benedict (H-B) estimate of basal energy expenditure (BEE)
   - Female: H-B (kcal) = 655 + (1.7 × height in cm) + (9.6 × weight in kg) − (4.7 × age in years)
   - For intensive care unit patients, provide kcal at level equal to H-B.
   - For ward patients, provide kcal at level ranging from H-B to H-B + 20% to provide for increased activity.

B. Protein

1. For intensive care unit patients, 1.5 g/kg of body weight (for obese patients, base requirement on estimated lean weight)
2. For ward patients, 1.0 to 1.5 g/kg: based on estimated lean weight (estimated lean weight = 100 pounds + 5 pounds/in. above 5 ft for females)

C. Vitamins and Minerals

To meet Recommended Dietary Allowances

D. Fluids and Electrolytes

Individualized on basis of laboratory data, weight, etc.

E. Modifications

1. For severely stressed or septic patients, use measured indirect calorimetry (oxygen uptake, carbon dioxide expired) to determine resting energy expenditure.
2. For extremely overweight or cachectic patients, use indirect calorimetry.
3. For renal or hepatic failure, restrict protein intake in some patients.
4. For severe overhydration or dehydration, use estimated euvolemic weight to calculate calories and protein.
5. For a few selected patients, 24-hour urinary nitrogen may be measured to estimate protein needs.
6. For complicated cases, consult Nutrition Support team if available.

IV. Routes of Administration

A. Enteral Route

1. Requires functioning gut
2. Preferred for maintenance of gut integrity and possibly for decreased bacterial translocation from gut lumen to mesenteric lymph nodes and organs
3. Fewer serious complications

B. Oral Route

1. Requires patient cooperation
2. Requires adequate dentition
3. Limited by postoperative nausea and emesis
4. Usually progress from liquids to solids, as tolerated by the patient

C. Tube Feedings

1. Gastric tube
   - Normal gastric emptying mechanism controls entry into the duodenum
   - Usual nasogastric tube: polyurethane; 8, 10, or 12 F; > 90 cm in length
   - Usual surgical gastrostomy tube: rubber, 16 to 18 F
   - Check placement of nasogastric tubes radiographically before using
   - Check intragastric residual volumes
     — In continuous feeding, check every 6 hours
     — In gravity feeding, check immediately before infusion
     — If volume is greater than twice the hourly feeding rate or >100 mL, stop infusion and recheck in 1 hour
2. Postpyloric tubes
   - Principles
     — Assumed to decrease risk of aspiration

— Preferred in critically ill patients and in others with unprotected airways
- Infusion port at the ligament of Treitz
- Usual nasoenteric tube: polyurethane; 8, 10, or 12 F; > 110 cm in length
- Usual surgical jejunostomy tube: rubber, 16 F
- Caliber: depends on viscosity of formula and medications to be infused
- Check placement of nasoenteric tubes radiographically before using
- No need to check residual volumes

3. Specialized postpyloric tubes: needle catheter jejunostomy
- Principles
  — "Ileus" represents postanesthetic absence of gastric and colonic (but not small bowel) motility
  — Feeding begins as early as in the recovery room
    · Very slow infusion
    · Optimal formula yet to be determined: elemental versus polymeric?
    · Minimal fiber initially
- A 16-gauge polyurethane catheter placed at operation through the bowel wall and abdominal wall
- Catheter removed when eating is resumed

4. Formula and administration (gastric and jejunal feedings)
- Most patients use polymeric (intact protein) isotonic formula, which supplies 1 to 1.2 kcal/mL.
- Commence with full-strength isotonic formula at slow infusion rate (10 to 20 mL/h), advancing by 10 to 20 mL every 12 to 24 hours, as tolerated until goal rate is reached.
- Flush tube with water, 30 to 60 mL, four times daily.
- Specialized formulas: use as guided by Nutrition Support Service. Special formulas available include fiber-containing, elemental, branched-chain amino acid-enriched, glutamine-containing, nucleic acid- and arginine-enriched, and renal-failure formulas.

D. Parenteral Nutrition

1. Principle
Use parenteral nutrition only if gut cannot be used.
2. Central parenteral nutrition
- Subclavian or internal jugular vein is the usual site for venous access.
- Single-lumen catheters are preferred, but generally this is not possible because of limited venous access.
- Confirm catheter placement in superior vena cava radiographically before use.
- Formulas are individualized
  — General approach includes amino acids to provide 1 to 1.5 g/kg estimated lean weight
  — Lipids given over 24 hours to provide ≤30% of kcal
    · 250 mL of 20% lipid = 500 kcal
    · 500 mL of 10% lipid = 550 kcal

- Dextrose (as 10% to 25% solution) to provide balance of calories
- Volume is dictated by renal, cardiac, and fluid status.
- Standard intravenous vitamin packet:
  — Vitamin K not included, to avoid interference with warfarin therapy
  — Patients not taking anticoagulant medication should receive vitamin K (5 mg intramuscularly each week).
- Electrolytes are given as indicated by serum levels and acid-base data.
- Trace elements
  — Standard: zinc, 4 mg; copper, 0.8 mg; manganese, 0.4 mg; chromium, 8 μg; and selenium, 48 μg
  — Altered doses are based on serum levels (interpreted with consideration of albumin level)
- Monitoring
  — Initially, monitor twice daily with peripheral glucose meter to keep blood glucose 100 to 200 mg/dL in critically ill patients and 100 to 150 mg/dL in others
  — Chemistry panel, weekly
  — Hematology group (complete blood count), initially
  — Electrolyte panel, weekly; sodium and potassium, first 4 days.
  — Essential element screen (zinc, magnesium), weekly
  — Prothrombin time, weekly
  — Selenium, every 4 weeks
  — Triglycerides, initially
  — Calcium and phosphorus as indicated
  — Adjustments to formula as indicated by results of laboratory tests and guided by Nutrition Support Service

3. Peripheral parenteral nutrition
- Principle
At best, peripheral parenteral nutrition is a temporizing approach and generally should not be used for >10 days.
- Achieving adequate caloric level without excessive fat is difficult.
- Caloric density is limited by osmolality and venous tolerance: most formulas, > 800 mOsm/L (<1,000 mOsm/L is desirable).
- Usual formula (dextrose, 5%, and amino acids, 4.25%) provides 340 kcal/L.
- To achieve adequate caloric level without providing excessive amino acids, it is usually necessary to give more than 50% of calories as fat.
- Monitoring is the same as for central parenteral nutrition.

E. Home Parenteral Nutrition

1. Indications: gut failure
- Short bowel
- Motility/obstructive disorders (radiation changes)
- Fistulas (goal is *temporary* bowel rest)

2. Relative contraindications
   - Recurrent cancer (risks outweigh benefits)
   - Patient or designee unable to perform the technique safely
3. Cost
   In United States, $75,000 to $200,000 per year, plus costs of laboratory tests, examinations, and hospitalization for complications
4. Management team
   - Physician/nutritionist
   - Nurse coordinator
   - Pharmacist
   - Dietitian
   - Social worker
   - Nurse instructors
   - Home care company
5. Education
   - Inpatient program with one-on-one teaching by knowledgeable nurse and pharmacist
   - Protocolized teaching program
   - Patient must demonstrate sufficient knowledge and performance
6. Monitoring
   - Body temperature
   - Weight
   - Urine output
   - Laboratory studies
7. Duration
   - For many patients, home parenteral nutrition is permanent.
   - For patients with fistulas, failure to heal within 6 to 8 weeks suggests that surgical repair is necessary.

V. Risks and Complications

A. Enteral Route
1. Diarrhea
   - Minimized by isotonic formulas and slow progression of infusion
   - Avoid sorbitol-containing medications
   - Gut atrophy from lack of enteral feeding: reverses with time
2. Tube discomfort: decreased by small-caliber polyurethane tube
3. Binding of some medications, e.g., phenytoin, by formula
4. Clogged tube: minimized by using tube of proper caliber and water flushes following medications
5. Esophageal damage: decreased with current feeding tube design (and avoidance of regular nasogastric tubes)

B. Parenteral Route
1. Mechanical
   - Pneumothorax during insertion of line

   - Air embolus
   - Hemorrhage
   - Venous thrombosis
2. Infectious: catheter sepsis
   - Prevention
     — Decreased by meticulous care of site and daily inspection of site
     — Transparent dressing or gauze and tape.
     — Dressing change and site care: use aseptic technique with alcohol and povidone-iodine every 48 hours or more often if indicated.
     — Minimize interruption of line.
     — Restrict use of lumen to nutrition only.
     — Routine timing for changing of lines is not established, although there is increase in infection rate with triple lumen catheters in place for more than 10 to 14 days.
   - Treatment
     — In febrile patient, change catheter over wire.
     — Culture catheter tip.
     — If tip culture is positive, abandon site.
     — Use of antibiotics is guided by culture and sensitivity results.
3. Metabolic
   - Overfeeding contributes to
     — Hyperglycemia
     — Fluid retention
     — Electrolyte disturbances
     — Fatty infiltration of the liver
   - Hyperglycemia: in absence of overfeeding, may require insulin
   - Liver function abnormalities: wide range of abnormalities
     — Asymptomatic increase in liver enzymes, often self-limited
       · Transaminases within first 2 weeks
       · Alkaline phosphatase and bilirubin within 2 to 3 weeks
     — Fatty infiltration of liver
     — Intrahepatic cholestasis
     — Gallbladder sludge and stones
     — Cirrhosis reported with long-term use
     — Treatment
       · Resume enteral nutrition as soon as possible.
       · Rule out other causes of liver abnormalities.
       · Reassess formula that is being used.
   - Nutrient deficiency or excess
   - Fluid and electrolyte imbalance
   - Acid-base derangements

VI. Selected Diets

A. Low Residue
1. Avoids fiber
2. Indications

- Partial mechanical bowel obstruction
- Pseudo-obstruction
- Diverticulitis (acute)

B. Diabetic
1. Controls caloric and free sugar intake
2. Indication: diabetes mellitus

C. High Fiber
1. Includes undigestible carbohydrate from unrefined grain products, fruits, and vegetables
2. Indications
   - Constipation
   - Some implications for anticarcinogenic effect, especially in breast and colorectal cancer

D. For Renal and Liver Failure
Individualized for patient by dietitian and Nutrition Support Service

VII. Specific Nutritional Problems

A. Short-Bowel Syndrome
1. Amount resected
   - Resection of >50% of the small bowel causes malabsorption.
   - If there is <50 cm of remaining bowel (i.e., >90% resection), central parenteral nutrition is essential.
   - If <50% of the bowel is resected, nutritional deficiency with normal diet is rare.
   - If 50% to 90% of the bowel is resected, fluid, divalent cations, and electrolyte balance are most problematic; nutritional route is individualized.
2. Remarkable ability of intestine to adapt by villous hypertrophy and hyperplasia, with associated improved absorptive capacity
   - Luminal nutrients important for adaptation
   - Begins within 48 hours after resection
   - Peaks at about 12 days
   - Continues for up to 2 years
3. Initial parenteral nutrition often required, with gradual ability to maintain nutrition orally
4. Resection of distal ileum is a special situation because vitamin B_{12} and conjugated bile salts are absorbed exclusively at this site.
   - Replace with vitamin B_{12}, 100 μg given intramuscularly (or intravenously, if patient is on parenteral nutrition) every month.
   - Cholestyramine (bile-salt binding agent), given 4 g three times daily to patients *with intact colon* who have cholestatic diarrhea. Drug is useless after colectomy.
   - Give antidiarrheal agents as needed.

B. Enteric Fistulas
1. Spontaneous closure rate depends on cause.
   - Radiation-induced fistulas
     - Poor response to treatment
     - Low rate of spontaneous closure
     - High mortality rate
   - Cancer-related fistulas: slightly better response to treatment
   - Surgical fistulas
2. Nutrition support is primarily intended to improve nutritional status in preparation for surgical procedure.
3. Best route for nutrition support is uncertain: parenteral feeding versus very low residue tube feeding.
   - Spontaneous closure rate is probably higher with parenteral nutrition, but effect on mortality is uncertain.
   - Fistulas not closing within 4 to 6 weeks of conservative treatment are unlikely to close spontaneously.

C. Radiation-Induced Gut Injury
1. The critical dose for injury to the small bowel is 4,500 cGy.
2. The epithelium is most sensitive because of rapid turnover and suppression of cell proliferation by radiation.
3. Mesenchymal tissue changes are responsible for long-term sequelae.
4. Early changes, in first or second week, include nausea and vomiting or diarrhea or constipation.
   - Bile salt malabsorption if ileal mucosa is involved
     - Cholestatic diarrhea
     - Mild malabsorption of fat
   - Nutritionally significant malabsorption is unusual; manage conservatively.
5. Later changes, i.e., 3 months to decades
   - Malabsorption, especially with severe ileal involvement
   - Fat malabsorption with steatorrhea
     - Cholestyramine: 4 to 12 g/day as needed for diarrhea
     - Trial of medium-chain triglycerides in polymeric versus elemental supplements
     - Some patients may require home parenteral nutrition
   - Bowel obstruction from extensive adhesions or strictures: often complicated by bacterial overgrowth and resulting disaccharide and lipid malabsorption and vitamin B_{12} deficiency
     - Some patients require temporary or long-term parenteral nutrition.
     - In some, enteral formulas are tolerated.

Reading List

Fleming CR, Nelson J. Nutritional options. *In:* Kinney JM, Jeejeebhoy KN, Hill GL, Owen OE, eds. *Nutrition and metabolism in patient care.* Philadelphia, WB Saunders, 1988:752–772.

Pemberton CM, Moxness KE, German MJ, Nelson JK, Gastineau CF. *Mayo Clinic diet manual,* 6th ed. Toronto: BC Decker, 1988.

Sarr MG, Mayo S. Needle catheter jejunostomy: an unappreciated and misunderstood advance in the care of patients after major abdominal operations. *Mayo Clin Proc* 1988;63:565–572.

National Research Council, Food and Nutrition Board Subcommittee on the Tenth Edition of the RDAs. Recommended dietary allowances, 10th ed. Washington, DC: National Academy Press, 1989.

McMahon MM, Bistrian BR. The physiology of nutritional assessment and therapy in protein-calorie malnutrition. *Dis Mon* 1990;36:375–417.

Kelly DG, Burns JU. Home nutrition support. *Gastroenterologist* 1996;4[Suppl]:S29–S39.

Kelly DG, Stanhope CR. Postoperative enteral feeding: myth or fact? (editorial) *Gynecol Oncol* 1997;67:233–234.

CHAPTER 7

Surgery of the Uterus

Maurice J. Webb, M.D.

I. Dilation and Curettage

A. Indications
1. Abnormal uterine bleeding
2. Postmenopausal bleeding
3. Persistent vaginal discharge
4. Retained products of conception
5. Pyometra, hydrometra, or hematometra
6. Investigation of infertility, pelvic pain, dysmenorrhea, etc.
7. Prior to vaginal hysterectomy
8. When office sampling of endometrium is not possible in patients taking estrogens

B. Preoperative Investigations
1. Nothing apart from Pap smear if patient is younger than 40 years, is in good general health, and has no significant bleeding
2. Complete blood count if significant bleeding
3. Electrocardiography and serum chemistry for patients 40 to 59 years old
4. Serum chemistry, complete blood count, electrocardiography, and chest radiography if patient is older than 60 years or if indicated by medical history

C. Preoperative Preparation
1. Perineal shaving not necessary
2. Povidone-iodine douche

D. Surgical Technique
1. Place the patient in the lithotomy position.
2. Use general anesthesia or paracervical block.
3. Scrub the vagina and vulva with povidone-iodine and then paint with povidone-iodine and drape.

4. Examine vagina bimanually to assess the pelvis and the position and size of the uterus.
5. Grasp the anterior lip of the cervix with a tenaculum.
6. Sound the depth of the endometrial cavity.
7. Dilate the cervix with curved forceps and then with the dilator.
8. Perform hysteroscopy depending on indications.
9. Curette the endocervical canal and note the consistency, cavitation, etc.
10. Curette the endometrial cavity in a stepwise fashion in a clockwise direction.
11. Search for polyps with Desjardins gallstone forceps or curved forceps.

E. Intraoperative Complications
1. Perforation of the uterus
   - If it is recognized before any curettage is performed, bowel damage is unlikely and the patient can be observed. No antibiotics are given.
   - If it is recognized late and bowel damage is likely or if bowel muscle is found on curetted material, exploration is indicated.
2. Laceration of the cervix
   - This occurs with forceful dilation.
   - Repair with interrupted 2-0 synthetic absorbable suture.
   - If tear extends to involve the uterine body and bleeding is excessive, either hysterectomy or ligation of the uterine artery via laparotomy may be required.
   - The surgeon may attempt to mobilize the vaginal wall and expose the laceration and repair it through the vagina.
3. Inability to probe the canal
   First start with a fine silver probe, and after the track is found, dilate with fine sharp-pointed curved forceps and proceed as before.

F. Postoperative Management
No restriction of activities

Maurice J. Webb: Chairman, Division of Gynecologic Surgery and Consultant, Department of Surgery, Mayo Clinic and Mayo Foundation; Professor of Obstetrics and Gynecology, Mayo Medical School, Rochester, Minnesota.

G. Specific Postoperative Complications

1. Infection
   - Culture cervix and start treatment with broad-spectrum antibiotics.
   - If there is uterine collection, probe the cervix to drain adequately.
2. Peritonitis
   Suspect intestinal injury and perform laparotomy.
3. Bleeding
   - Because many dilation and curettage procedures are performed for dysfunctional uterine bleeding, bleeding may persist postoperatively and require hormonal manipulation for control.
   - Excessive bleeding as a result of dilation and curettage alone is uncommon, except in the presence of malignancy or gestational trophoblastic disease.

II. Suction Curettage

A. Indications

1. Termination of pregnancy
2. Evacuation of retained products of conception
3. Evacuation of hydatidiform mole

B. Preoperative Investigations and Preparation

1. The same as for dilation and curettage
2. Prophylactic treatment with antibiotics

C. Surgical Technique

1. Position, anesthesia, and preparation are the same as for dilation and curettage.
2. Start intravenous infusion with 20 U of oxytocin (Pitocin) added.
3. Gently dilate the cervix with Hegar dilators.
4. An 8- to 10-mm suction curette is adequate for most cases.
5. Insert the suction curette gently until it reaches the fundus.
6. Start suction and rotate the curette gently around the endometrial cavity in a clockwise direction.
7. Occasionally withdraw the tip of the curette from the cervix to allow products of conception to be aspirated along suction tubing.
8. Gently recurette the cavity with a sharp curette.
9. Give 0.02 mg of methylergonovine (Methergine) intramuscularly.
10. Reaspirate the cavity with the suction curette.
11. Massage the uterus to get it to contract to diminish bleeding.

D. Intraoperative Complications

1. Perforation of the uterus
   If performed with a suction curette, laparotomy or laparoscopy is necessary because the bowel may have been aspirated into the tip of the curette and damaged.

2. Laceration of the cervix
   - This is much easier to do in pregnant women, and the laceration bleeds more freely.
   - Suture the laceration with interrupted sutures.

E. Postoperative Management

1. Methylergonovine tablets: 0.02 mg orally three times daily for 2 days
2. With gestational trophoblastic disease, measure the serum levels of β-human chorionic gonadotropin (β-HCG) weekly until they are normal, and then measure them monthly.

F. Postoperative Complications

1. Infection
   - Culture the cervix and start treatment with broad-spectrum antibiotics.
   - Consider whether retained products of conception are still present; if so, repeat dilation and curettage.
2. Hemorrhage
   - Massage the uterus and give oxytocic agents.
   - If bleeding persists, consider that there are still retained products and repeat dilation and curettage.
3. Amenorrhea
   Consider Asherman syndrome

III. Total Abdominal Hysterectomy

A. Indications

1. Endometrial malignancy
2. Tubal malignancy
3. Ovarian malignancy
4. Uterine sarcoma
5. Symptomatic fibroid uterus
6. Asymptomatic fibroids larger than 12 weeks of gestation size.
7. Benign adnexal mass in postmenopausal woman
8. Dysfunctional uterine bleeding when vaginal hysterectomy is contraindicated or not feasible
9. Endometriosis, chronic pelvic inflammatory disease, pelvic pain syndromes

B. Preoperative Investigations

1. Complete blood count
2. Serum chemistry
3. Urinalysis
4. Pap smear
5. Electrocardiography for patients older than 40 years
6. Chest radiography for patients older than 60 years or if indicated by medical history

C. Preoperative Preparation

1. Povidone-iodine douche
2. Abdominal shave
3. Microenema

4. Thromboembolus-deterrent stockings
5. Prophylactic treatment with antibodies

D. Surgical Technique
1. Swab the vagina.
2. Insert an indwelling urethral catheter.
3. Make a lower midline incision.
4. Explore the abdomen.
5. Collect peritoneal washings from the cul-de-sac and the right paracolic gutter if there is an adnexal mass, endometrial cancer, or tubal cancer.
6. Insert a self-retaining Balfour retractor.
7. Place the operating table in a steep Trendelenburg position.
8. Pack away the intestine with a long pack.
9. Grasp the uterus with straight Kocher clamps on either side to include the round ligament, utero-ovarian ligament, and broad ligament.
10. Clamp the round ligament on the right side with a straight Kocher clamp and divide it, opening up the retroperitoneal space (Fig. 1).
11. Extend the peritoneal incision caudally along the vesicouterine fold, and extend it cranially parallel to the ovarian vessels.
12. Display the ureter as it crosses the bifurcation of the common iliac artery and runs down into the pelvis, attached to the medial leaf of the broad ligament.
13. Place the index finger beneath the ovarian vessels, and perforate the peritoneum of the broad ligament (Fig. 2).
14. Clamp across the utero-ovarian ligament and tube, if conserving the ovary, or across the infundibulopelvic ligament, if salpingo-oophorectomy is to be performed.
15. Ligate the ovarian vessels and the round ligament with a free tie.

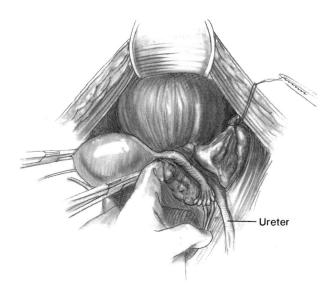

FIG. 2. The right ureter is exposed and palpated before perforating the peritoneum and clamping the ovarian vessels.

16. Repeat a similar dissection on the left side.
17. With traction maintained on the uterus by an assistant, elevate the vesicouterine fold of the peritoneum with long forceps and divide with scissors.
18. By using sharp dissection with scissors, dissect in the avascular space between the bladder and cervix until a point 2 cm below the external os of the cervix is reached (Fig. 3).
19. Insert a Harrington retractor to retract the bladder away from the cervix.
20. Clamp the right parametrium with straight Kocher forceps, with the tip at the level of the external cervical os.
21. Palpate the ureter between the thumb and forefinger lateral to the clamp and adjust the clamp as necessary if it is close to the ureter (Fig. 4).
22. Divide the parametrium between the clamp and the uterus/cervix (Fig. 5).
23. Repeat the parametrial clamping and transection on the left side.
24. Develop a layer of endopelvic fascia on the front of the vagina with scissors (Fig. 6).
25. Divide the uterosacral ligaments on each side with scissors just below the cervix (Fig. 7).
26. Divide the cul-de-sac peritoneum between the uterosacral ligaments, and push the rectum off the back of the cervix and upper vagina approximately 2 cm (Fig. 8).
27. Open into the vagina at the right lateral angle of the vault; cut around the anterior fornix, left angle, and then posterior fornix, placing Henrontin tenacula on the cuff at the 3, 12, 9, and 6 o'clock positions (Fig. 9).

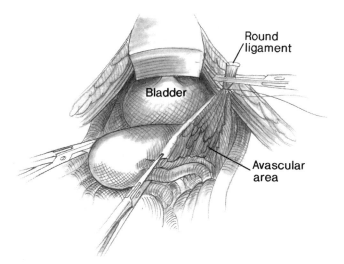

FIG. 1. Opening the retroperitoneum by dividing the round ligament.

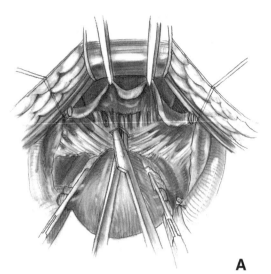

FIG. 3. A: The bladder is sharply dissected away from the front of the cervix. *(continues)*

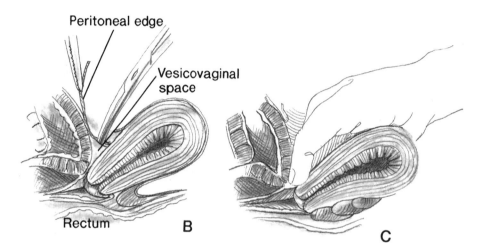

Peritoneal edge

Vesicovaginal space

Rectum **B**

C

FIG. 3. *(continued)* **B** and **C:** The bladder is sharply dissected approximately 2 cm below the cervix.

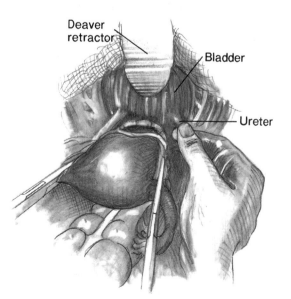

Deaver retractor

Bladder

Ureter

FIG. 4. The ureter is palpated between the thumb and fore-finger lateral to the clamp.

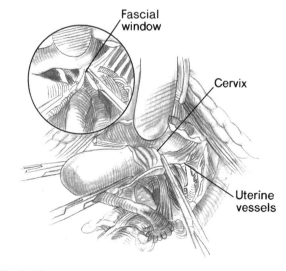

Fascial window

Cervix

Uterine vessels

FIG. 5. The parametrium is clamped with a single straight clamp and transected, opening up a fascial window at the tip of the clamp.

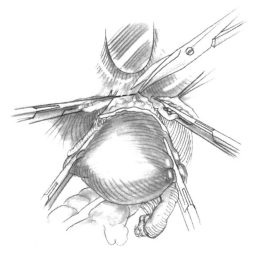

FIG. 6. The endopelvic (pubocervical) fascia is divided anterior to the cervix.

28. Remove the uterus and swab the vagina with povidone-iodine swabs.
29. Insert a large sponge into the pelvis to cover the two cardinal ligament clamps.
30. Suture the vaginal vault edges together with running no. 1 synthetic absorbable suture in a submucosal fashion, starting at the right angle of the vault, coming across to the left angle, and then running the suture back again to incorporate the endopelvic fascia layer anteriorly and the uterosacral ligaments posteriorly (Fig. 10).
31. Check hemostasis of the vault, using light cautery if necessary.

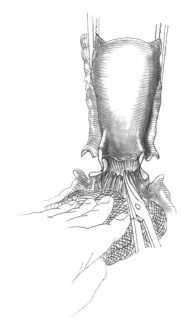

FIG. 8. The rectum is dissected off the upper part of the vagina.

32. Suture-ligate the left parametrial pedicle with no. 1 synthetic absorbable suture. Doubly ligate with a second free tie, checking by palpation that the ureter is free of all ties before tying the sutures.
33. Repeat a similar ligation of the right parametrial pedicle. The ureter is again palpated before tying these ligatures.
34. Inspect the back of the bladder and the rest of the pelvis for hemostasis.

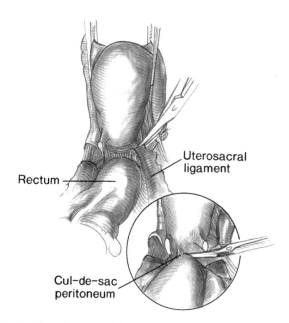

Rectum

Uterosacral ligament

Cul-de-sac peritoneum

FIG. 7. The uterosacral ligaments are transected, and the cul-de-sac peritoneum is divided.

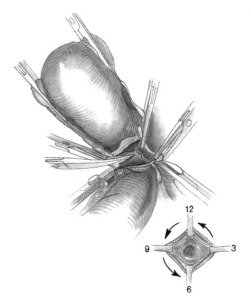

FIG. 9. The vagina is opened at the 3 o'clock position, and the dissection is continued around the cuff in an anticlockwise direction. The vaginal cuff is clamped with tenacula.

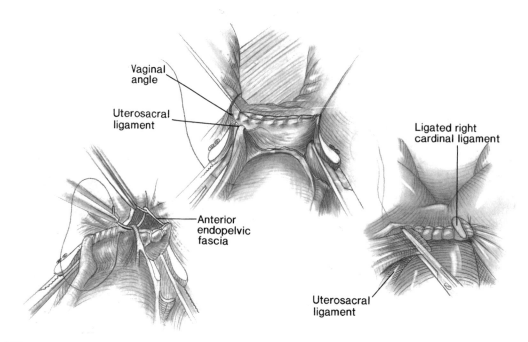

FIG. 10. The vaginal cuff is closed in two layers in a submucosal fashion, incorporating the endopelvic fascia and the uterosacral ligaments in the second layer.

35. Closure of the pelvic peritoneum is not usually performed. If it is, the ovarian vessels are incorporated in the suture, giving these vessels double ligatures.

36. If there is any concern about the proximity of the ureter to the parametrial ligatures, the parametrial pedicle should be grasped with a long curved clamp and traction applied medially. By using a right-angled forceps, the ureteral tunnel is opened to display the ureter as it courses in the top of the cardinal ligament (Fig. 11).

37. In the presence of a potential or actual enterocele, a wedge of redundant posterior vaginal fornix can be excised and reapproximated before closing the vault (Fig. 12), thereby approximating the uterosacral ligaments.

E. Intraoperative Complications

1. Enterotomy: usually occurs in the small intestine during the opening of the incision in patients operated on multiple times or may occur into the rectosigmoid with division of severe pelvic adhesions, e.g., endometriosis. Repair as in Chapter 24.

2. Cystotomy: mark the defect with a suture, complete the hysterectomy, and then close the bladder defect in two layers with 2-0 synthetic absorable suture. Drain the bladder with a urethral catheter for 7 days.

3. Crush injury or transection of ureter: see Chapter 4.

4. Bleeding from vascular pedicle: open the broad ligament, identify the ureter, and ligate the anterior division of the internal iliac artery or uterine artery on the appropriate side.

F. Postoperative Management

1. Measure urine output hourly with the indwelling catheter, with notification of the medical staff if there is < 30 mL of output per hour for 2 hours.

2. Allow intravenous fluids only, apart from ice to suck, on the day of the operation.

3. Mobilize the patient the day after the operation, and start oral fluids.

4. Remove the urethral catheter on the first morning postoperatively.

5. Check the hemoglobin and serum creatinine levels on the first morning postoperatively.

6. Advance diet as tolerated.

G. Specific Postoperative Complications

1. Urinary retention
   Reinsert the urethral catheter and remove again in 48 hours.

2. Vaginal bleeding
   • Inspect the vault, and suture the bleeding point if possible.
   • If no bleeding site is visible, pack the vagina firmly and insert an indwelling catheter.

3. Intraabdominal bleeding
   • Reopen the abdomen, remove the blood and clot, and ligate the specific bleeding point.
   • If no actual bleeding vessel is found, ligate the anterior division of the internal iliac artery bilaterally.

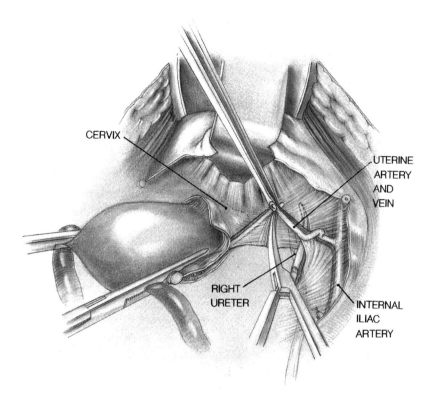

FIG. 11. Right-angled forceps tunneling beneath the uterine artery during dissection of the ureter from the cardinal ligament.

4. Pelvic abscess
 • Drain with percutaneous computed tomographically guided suction drainage.
 • Treat with appropriate antibiotics.
5. Ureteral obstruction: see Chapter 5.
6. Urinary fistula: see Chapter 5.
 Note: For other complications, see Chapter 5.

IV. Modified Radical Hysterectomy

This operation is similar to total abdominal hysterectomy except that the medial one-third of the cardinal ligament, the upper part of the uterosacral ligaments, and a 1.5- to 2-cm cuff of vagina are taken with the specimen. To accomplish this, the uterine artery is ligated lateral to the ureters, and the

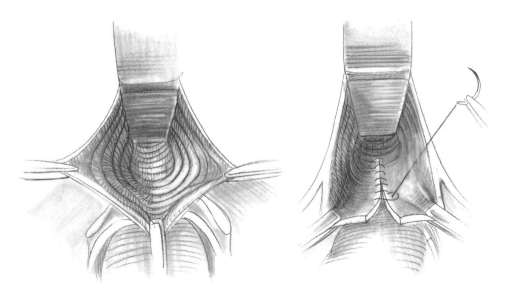

FIG. 12. If an enterocele (actual or potential) is present, a wedge of posterior vaginal fornix mucosa is excised to narrow the vault.

ureters are dissected out of their tunnels and pushed laterally. The procedure is not as extensive as a full radical hysterectomy, which divides the cardinal ligaments flush with the pelvic sidewalls.

A. Indications

1. Early invasive cervical cancer (stage IA[2])
2. Endometrial cancer with minimal cervical involvement
3. Endometrial cancer with extensive lower segment involvement
4. Small recurrence of cervical cancer after radiation therapy

B. Preoperative Investigations

1. Complete blood count
2. Serum chemistry
3. Urinalysis
4. Electrocardiography for patients older than 40 years
5. Chest radiography
6. Intravenous pyelography

C. Preoperative Preparation

1. Povidone-iodine douche
2. Abdominal shave
3. Microenema
4. Thromboembolus-deterrent stockings
5. Prophylactic treatment with antibiotics

D. Surgical Technique

1. Use the same technique as for total abdominal hysterectomy up to where a Harrington retractor is used to retract the bladder away from the cervix and vagina.
2. Dissect the ureter free of its attachment to the broad ligament peritoneum.
3. With traction on the uterus, tunnel above the right ureter with a sharp-pointed right-angled clamp.
4. Clamp, divide, and ligate the uterine artery just lateral to where it crosses the ureter.
5. Continue unroofing the ureter by using right-angled forceps and tunneling, then clamping, dividing, and ligating the tissue in the roof of the ureteral tunnel down to where the ureter enters the bladder (Fig. 13).
6. By using a vein retractor to elevate the ureter, free it inferiorly from the cardinal ligament in the avascular tissue plane beneath the ureter.
7. Do not dissect the web of tissue lateral to the lower 2 cm of the ureter.
8. Push the ureter downward and laterally to expose the medial one-third of the cardinal ligament (Fig. 14).
9. Clamp the cardinal ligament with curved forceps and divide it approximately 2.5 to 3 cm lateral to the edge of the cervix, extending down lateral to the vaginal fornix approximately 2 cm.
10. Repeat the ureteral dissection and division of the cardinal ligament on the left side.
11. Divide the cul-de-sac peritoneum behind the cervix, and push the rectum off the posterior aspect of the vagina and off the uterosacral ligaments laterally.
12. Divide the uterosacral ligaments approximately 2 cm below the cervix.
13. Open the vagina at the right lateral angle of the vault, and remove the uterus with a cuff of vagina, as with total abdominal hysterectomy.
14. Close the vaginal vault, as for total abdominal hysterectomy, in a submucosal fashion.
15. Suture-ligate the parametrial pedicles and stick-tie into the angles of the vault; there is no need to doubly ligate because the uterine artery has been ligated independently.
16. Suture-ligate the uterosacral ligaments and stick-tie into the angles of the vault.
17. Inspect for hemostasis.
18. Closure of the pelvic peritoneum is optional.

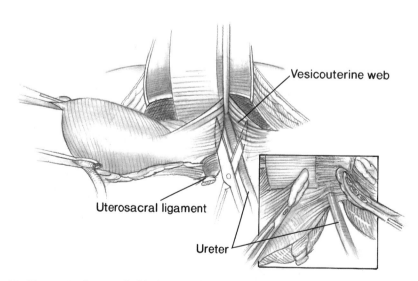

FIG. 13. The ureter is unroofed in its tunnel in the superior aspect of the cardinal ligament.

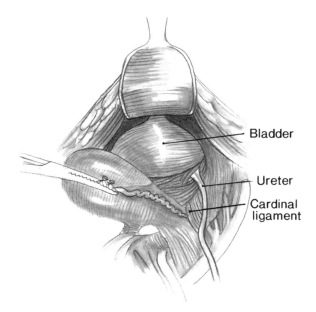

Bladder

Ureter

Cardinal ligament

FIG. 14. After the ureter is freed up throughout its pelvic course, the cardinal ligament can be clamped and divided.

E. Postoperative Management

The same as for total abdominal hysterectomy, except leave the Foley catheter in place for 4 days, because of more extensive bladder and ureteral dissection.

F. Specific Postoperative Complications

1. Urinary fistula formation is slightly more likely than with total abdominal hysterectomy but is very rare if the dissection is performed carefully.
2. In previously irradiated patients with residual or small recurrence of cervical cancer, a modified radical hysterectomy rather than a full radical hysterectomy must be performed to avoid ureteral fistulas.

V. Radical Hysterectomy

Radical hysterectomy involves resection of the cardinal ligaments flush with the pelvic sidewall, the uterosacral ligaments well posteriorly lateral to the rectum, and a 2- to 3-cm cuff of vagina. A larger vaginal cuff is excised for stage IIA cervical cancer or vaginal cancer in the upper vagina. Pelvic lymphadenectomy is normally performed in association with radical hysterectomy (see Chapter 22).

A. Indications

1. Cervical cancer, stage IB or IIA
2. Endometrial cancer, stage II
3. Vaginal cancer, stage I or II in the upper one-half of the vagina

Note: For recurrent cervical cancer located in the cervix after full pelvic irradiation, a modified radical hysterectomy is performed for small lesions and a pelvic exenteration for large lesions. A full radical hysterectomy after full irradia-

tion produces an unacceptably high rate of urinary fistula formation.

B. Preoperative Investigations

1. Complete blood count
2. Serum chemistry
3. Urinalysis
4. Electrocardiography for patients older than 40 years
5. Chest radiography
6. Computed tomographic or magnetic resonance imaging scan of the abdomen and pelvis: useful for ruling out distant metastases and ureteral obstruction (if not available, intravenous pyelography at least should be performed)
7. Cystoscopy and proctoscopy, as indicated by the extent of the lesion on the cervix

C. Preoperative Preparation

1. Povidone-iodine douche
2. Abdominal shave
3. Microenema
4. Thromboembolus-deterrent stockings
5. Heparin given subcutaneously (optional)
6. Prophylactic treatment with antibiotics

D. Surgical Technique

1. Use the same technique as for total abdominal hysterectomy up to where the broad ligament is opened, displaying the ureter attached to the medial leaf of the broad ligament peritoneum.
2. By using blunt dissection with the index finger and long forceps, open up the avascular pararectal space between the peritoneum and ureter medially and the internal iliac artery laterally.
3. Extend the dissection downward along the curve of the sacrum.
4. With blunt dissection, open the paravesical space by dissecting similarly between the external iliac vessels laterally and the obliterated hypogastric artery medially (Fig. 15).
5. Extend this dissection down to the floor of the pelvis, exposing the levator and obturator muscles.
6. With the index finger, perforate the broad ligament beneath the ovarian vessels.
7. Clamp across the utero-ovarian ligament and tube, if conserving the ovary, or across the infundibulopelvic ligament, if salpingo-oophorectomy is being performed, and ligate the pedicle.
8. Elevate the peritoneum beneath the inguinal ligament, and insert a Deaver retractor to expose the full length of the external iliac vessels.
9. Insert a second Deaver retractor into the paravesical space, and retract the bladder medially.
10. Proceed to perform pelvic lymphadenectomy, removing all the lymph node tissue up to the aortic bifurcation (see Chapter 22).

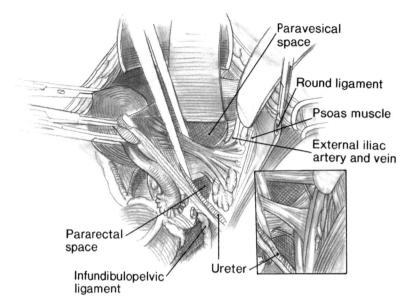

FIG. 15. The cardinal ligament is exposed between the paravesical and pararectal spaces just before crossclamping.

11. Clamp the anterior division of the internal iliac artery at its origin with right-angled forceps, and divide and ligate.
12. Clamp, divide, and ligate the obliterated hypogastric artery up near the anterior abdominal wall.
13. With traction on the uterus to the opposite side, insert a thumb into the pararectal space and an index finger into the paravesical space, and, with fingers beneath the cardinal ligament, gently tunnel in the avascular space.
14. Double clamp across the cardinal ligament flush with the pelvic sidewall using long curved clamps, extending down to the space already created beneath the ligament (Fig. 16), and divide the ligament.

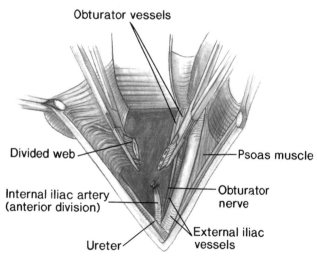

FIG. 16. The anterior division of the internal iliac artery and the cardinal ligament (web) have been clamped and divided.

15. Pull the cardinal ligament web medially and ligate the lateral pedicle by oversewing it with a continuous no. 1 synthetic absorbable suture.
16. Ligate the medial pedicle of the cardinal ligament and leave the ends of the suture long for identification purposes.
17. Repeat the node dissection and cardinal ligament transection on the opposite side.
18. Dissect the lower ureter from its attachment to the broad ligament peritoneum on both sides.
19. Divide the cul-de-sac peritoneum between the uterosacral ligaments, and dissect the rectum from the back of the upper vagina anteriorly and the medial aspect of the uterosacral ligaments laterally.
20. Clamp each uterosacral ligament with a right-angled clamp well back, lateral to the rectum, and divide the ligaments; this allows the uterus to be lifted high up into the abdominal wound (Fig. 17).
21. With upward traction on the uterus, divide the vesicouterine fold of peritoneum by elevating it with long forceps and incising with scissors.
22. By using sharp dissection with scissors, dissect in the avascular space between the bladder and the cervix to 3 to 4 cm below the external os of the cervix.
23. Insert a Harrington retractor to retract the bladder away from the cervix and vagina.
24. With traction on the uterus to the opposite side, grasp the uterine artery pedicle with long curved forceps, pull it medially with the uterus, and grasp the cardinal ligament pedicle with long curved forceps and pull it laterally.
25. The ureter can now be visualized in its tunnel, traversing the top of the cardinal ligament.
26. With sharp-pointed right-angled forceps, unroof the

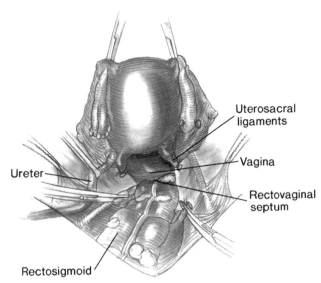

FIG. 17. The uterosacral ligaments are clamped and transected well back lateral to the rectum, and the rectum is dissected away from the posterior aspect of the vagina.

ureter in its tunnel down to its insertion into the bladder (Fig. 13).

27. The ends of the sutures used to ligate the tissue over the top of the ureter should be left long and should be held on the abdominal wall with forceps.

28. Lift up the ureter with a vein retractor, and free it from the top of the cardinal ligament by sharp dissection in the avascular plane.

29. Remove the curved clamp from the cardinal ligament pedicle, pull the ligament beneath and medial to the ureter, and reapply the clamp.

30. Clamp, divide, and ligate the posterior portion of the vesicouterine web medial to the ureter by clamping it with curved forceps just inferior and medial to the ureter. Leave the suture long, and use this suture to retract the ureter laterally (Fig. 18).

31. Repeat the same dissection on the other side, freeing up the left ureter.

32. Lift the uterus and right cardinal ligament upward to the opposite side, and, retracting the bladder inferiorly and the ureter laterally with a Harrington retractor, clamp with a large curved clamp across the paracolpium beneath the cardinal ligament at the level of the intended transection of the vagina.

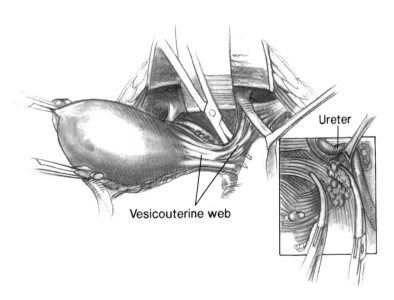

FIG. 18. The web of tissue on the floor of the ureteral tunnel is clamped and divided; the ureter is retracted laterally, and the cardinal ligament is brought medially beneath the ureter.

33. Divide the paracolpium up to the edge of the vagina.
34. Repeat this step on the left side.
35. Open into the vagina on the right side at the level of these paravaginal clamps and cut around the vagina, removing the uterus and applying tenacula to the vaginal cuff, as in performing a simple hysterectomy.
36. Swab the vagina with povidone-iodine swabs.
37. Insert a corner of a large sponge into the cul-de-sac, and cover the two uterosacral ligament clamps and the two paravaginal clamps with the sponge.
38. Close the vault in a submucosal fashion with a no. 1 synthetic absorbable suture, checking hemostasis when completed.
39. Suture-ligate the paravaginal pedicles into the corners of the vault with a no. 1 synthetic absorbable suture.
40. Suture-ligate the uterosacral pedicles into the corners of the vault.
41. Inspect the pelvis for hemostasis.
42. The pelvic peritoneum is not closed, and no suction drains are used.
43. Open the bladder in an extraperitoneal fashion, and insert an 18-F Foley catheter brought through a stab incision in the anterior abdominal wall.
44. Close the cystotomy in two layers with a continuous 3-0 synthetic absorbable suture.

E. Intraoperative Complications
1. Hemorrhage
   - The most likely site of bleeding is on the pelvic sidewall, after division and ligation of the insertion of the cardinal ligament.
   - Another likely site of bleeding is from laceration and retraction of the lumbar or gluteal veins during node dissection.
   - Bleeding from both of these sites may be excessive and should be managed according to the principles outlined in Chapter 4.
2. Cystotomy
   - Mark the defect with a small suture, and complete the operation.
   - Repair the defect with two layers of 3-0 synthetic absorbable sutures.
3. Ureteral damage
   Manage according to the principles set out in Chapter 4.

F. Postoperative Management
1. It is the same as for simple abdominal hysterectomy, except for catheter and drain management.
2. Clamp the suprapubic catheter on postoperative day 14, and initially measure the residual urine volume every 4 hours, increasing the time interval of clamping as the residual diminishes (see Chapter 3).
3. After radical hysterectomy, patients often have minimal or no bladder sensation, so they must be carefully observed for signs of urinary retention.

4. Actively encourage bowel function with stool softeners, bulk agents, laxatives, enemas, etc., because diminished rectal sensation can lead to fecal impaction.

G. Specific Postoperative Complications
1. Inability to void
   - Teach patients self-catheterization, and remove the suprapubic catheter
     or
   - Leave the catheter in place, and teach the patient the clamping routine (see Chapter 3).
2. Urinary fistula
   - Vesicovaginal or ureteral fistula formation is a recognized complication in 1% to 2% of cases.
   - If urine is draining vaginally, insert 200 mL of water with indigo carmine into the bladder; if colored fluid drains vaginally, the patient has a vesical fistula.
   - If the vaginal fluid remains clear after the above step, give 1 ampule of indigo carmine intravenously (i.v.) to check whether there is a ureteral fistula.
   - After a fistula has been demonstrated at whatever site, intravenous pyelography needs to be performed to exclude ureteral obstruction.
   - If there is no ureteral obstruction and bladder fistula only is present, insert the largest possible size urethral catheter and leave it in place for continuous drainage for 6 weeks.
   - If the vesical fistula does not heal, repair it surgically at 3 months.
   - If ureteral fistula is present or if there is any ureteral obstruction, perform percutaneous nephrostomy and attempt to pass a ureteral stent in an anterograde fashion.
   - If stent passage is successful, leave the stent in place for 6 weeks and remove nephrostomy.
   - If stent passage is unsuccessful, leave nephrostomy for 2 to 3 months, and then perform surgical repair of the fistula.

Note: For other complications, see Chapter 5.

VI. Myomectomy

A. Indications
1. If infertility is thought to be due to uterine fibroids
2. Large, symptomatic, or enlarging fibroids in a young woman who wishes to retain reproductive function

B. Preoperative Investigations
1. Complete blood count
2. Serum chemistry
3. Urinalysis
4. Pap smear
5. Ultrasonographic scan to confirm fibroids
6. Complete infertility investigations when infertility is the main presenting complaint

C. Preoperative Preparation

1. Povidone-iodine douche
2. Abdominal shave
3. Microenema
4. Thromboembolus-deterrant stockings
5. Prophylactic treatment with antibiotics

D. Surgical Technique

1. Perform preliminary dilation and curettage to exclude any pedunculated submucous fibroids. (Hysteroscopy can also be performed.)
2. Insert an indwelling urethral catheter.
3. Make a lower midline incision.
4. Explore the abdomen and pelvis, insert a self-retaining catheter, and pack away intestines.
5. Plan the incision to try to excise all fibroids through a single incision.
6. Insert myomectomy screw into one of the larger fibroids near the fundus, and use this for traction.
7. Place noncrushing clamps or clips across the ovarian and uterine blood supply to diminish blood loss (optional).
8. Injection of a vasoconstricting solution along the incision line and the use of cautery will minimize blood loss.
9. Gently shell out each fibroid by using a combination of sharp and blunt dissection, making use of the false capsule that surrounds fibroids.
10. During the dissection, keep the site of insertion of the fallopian tubes under view at all times to avoid tubal damage, and endeavor to avoid entering the endometrial cavity.
11. Carefully palpate the uterus to be sure all fibroids have been excised.
12. Repair the defect with multiple layers of interrupted 0 synthetic absorbable sutures in a hemostatic fashion, keeping all suture material buried if possible.
13. Apply a sheet of oxidized regenerated cellulose or other adhesive barrier over the incision line to help prevent adhesions.

E. Postoperative Management

The same as for abdominal hysterectomy

F. Specific Postoperative Complications

1. Intraabdominal hemorrhage
   - This is not infrequent, because of the vascularity of a large fibroid uterus.
   - Prevention by meticulous attention to hemostasis at operation is essential.
2. Adhesive bowel obstruction
   - Because of the large incision lines on the uterine surface, the small bowel or omentum can become adherent, causing obstruction.
   - This can occur more easily with incisions on the anterior aspect of the uterus.

VII. Thermal Ablation

A. Indications

1. Dysfunctional uterine bleeding
2. Persistent postmenopausal bleeding due to hormone replacement therapy

B. Preoperative Investigations

1. Pregnancy test when indicated
2. Biopsy to determine whether endometrium is benign.

C. Preoperative Preparation

1. Povidone-iodine douche
2. Microenema

D. Surgical Technique

1. Perform a preliminary dilation and curettage, and measure uterine depth.
2. Inflate the balloon of the ablation device with about 15 to 20 mL of D_5W.
3. Withdraw solution to a negative pressure of -150 to -200 mm Hg to confirm that the balloon has no leaks.
4. Dampen the outside of the balloon with D_5W.
5. Insert probe into the uterine cavity and slowly inflate the balloon with D_5W until a pressure of 160 to 180 mm Hg is maintained for 30 to 45 seconds.
6. Start the heating cycle at 87°C for 8 minutes.
7. Deflate the balloon after allowing it to cool for 30 seconds, and remove the device from the uterus.

VIII. Vaginal Hysterectomy

A. Indications

1. Dysfunctional uterine bleeding
2. Symptomatic fibroids
3. Severe dysmenorrhea and central pelvic pain problems
4. Uterovaginal prolapse
5. Cervical intraepithelial neoplasia
6. Stage IA(1) cervical cancer
7. Atypical adenomatous hyperplasia and in situ endometrial cancer
8. Minimal grade 1 endometrial adenocarcinoma in grossly obese patients

B. Preoperative Investigations

1. Complete blood count
2. Serum chemistry
3. Urinalysis
4. Pap smear
5. Electrocardiography for patients older than 40 years
6. Chest radiography if patient is older than 60 years or if indicated by history
7. Colposcopy with biopsies if cervical intraepithelial neoplasia exists
8. Dilation and curettage if atypical endometrial hyperplasia or adenocarcinoma exist

C. Preoperative Preparation

1. Povidone-iodine douche
2. Perineal shave
3. Microenema
4. Prophylactic treatment with antibiotics

D. Surgical Technique

1. Perform a preliminary dilation and curettage to exclude endometrial or endocervical cancer if patient has a history of abnormal bleeding.
2. Insert a weighted vaginal speculum and three Deaver retractors to expose the cervix.
3. With two tenacula, grasp the cervix on its anterior and posterior lips.
4. Make an elliptical incision around the cervix.
5. With traction downward on the cervix and lifting up the cut edge of the anterior vaginal fornix mucosa with toothed forceps, dissect the bladder off the front of the cervix with Mayo scissors.
6. Push the bladder up digitally until the peritoneal reflection can be felt sliding under the fingertip.
7. Insert a narrow Deaver retractor into this space to retract the bladder.
8. Pick up the peritoneal reflection—identified as a curved white fold—with toothed forceps, and open it with Mayo scissors (Fig. 19).
9. Insert the scissors into the incision in the peritoneum, and open them widely to enable the Deaver retractor to be inserted into the anterior cul-de-sac.
10. Pull the cervix anteriorly with the tenacula, and, while grasping the cut edge of the posterior fornix vaginal mucosa, enter the posterior cul-de-sac with Mayo scissors.

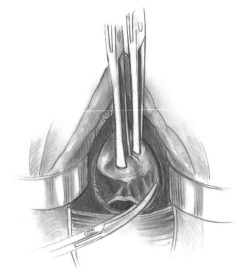

FIG. 20. After the posterior cul-de-sac is opened, the left uterosacral ligament is clamped, divided, and ligated.

11. Insert a finger through the posterior cul-de-sac to palpate the uterus and adnexa and to feel for adhesions, endometriosis, etc.
12. Remove the Deaver retractor on the patient's right side; the assistant on that side retracts the cervix to the patient's right side.
13. Clamp the left uterosacral ligament with curved Heaney clamps, divide, and suture-ligate with a no. 1 synthetic absorbable suture (Fig. 20).
14. Similarly clamp the lower two-thirds of the left cardinal ligament, but before dividing it, palpate the left ureter (Fig. 21).
15. Insert the left index finger into the anterior cul-de-sac, and snap the ureter between this finger and the

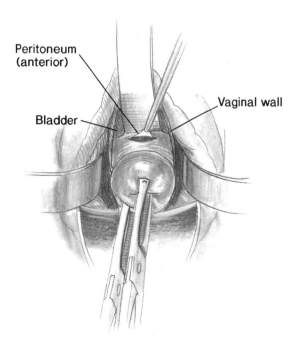

FIG. 19. The bladder is retracted superiorly, and the anterior cul-de-sac peritoneum is opened with scissors.

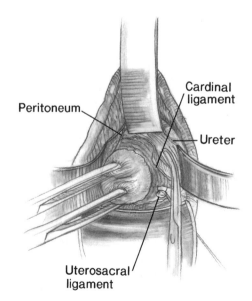

FIG. 21. The lower portion of the cardinal ligament is clamped and divided after the ureter is palpated.

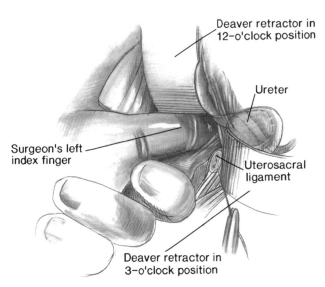

FIG. 22. The ureter is palpated as a cord against the Deaver retractor.

Deaver retractor in the patient's left vaginal fornix (Fig. 22).

16. After determining that the ureter is well clear of the clamp, divide, transfix, and ligate the cardinal ligament.

17. Similarly clamp the upper one-third of the cardinal ligament, which contains the uterine artery. Be sure that the anterior and posterior peritoneal surfaces are approximated in this clamp, and then divide, transfix, and ligate the cardinal ligament.

18. The Deaver retractor in the left vaginal fornix is then moved to the right side, and the cervix is pulled to the left by the assistant on the patient's left side.

19. Perform a similar clamping routine on the right side of the uterus. The ends of all the sutures are left long and tagged for later identification during closure of the vault.

20. The tenaculum from the posterior lip of the cervix is removed, and with the anterior tenaculum being used to pull vertically on the cervix, the posterior fundus comes into view through the posterior cul-de-sac, where it is delivered into the vagina by grasping with a tenaculum.

21. With the left index finger inserted behind the uterus to keep the bowel away, place a Heaney clamp across the remaining supports of the uterus on the right side (tube, ovarian ligament, and round ligament) and transect the pedicle.

22. Place a similar clamp on the left side after rotating the fundus superiorly, and remove the uterus.

23. These last two clamped pedicles are then suture-ligated, and the long ends of the sutures are tagged and placed up on the abdominal wall.

24. Inspect the ovaries and tubes carefully. If they are abnormal or if the patient is menopausal, they can be removed at this point by clamping across their pedicle

with a long curved clamp and doubly ligating the pedicle or by using the endoscopic GIA stapler.

25. Grasp the posterior cul-de-sac peritoneum with an Allis forceps, and dissect the peritoneum back to where it reflects on the front of the rectum.

26. Excise the redundant peritoneum of the cul-de-sac to prevent a future enterocele (Fig. 23).

27. If the posterior fornix mucosa is excessive, resect a narrow wedge to give further support, thus preventing a future enterocele.

28. Grasp the anterior peritoneum with a second Allis forceps, and insert a small pack into the peritoneal cavity to pack away the intestine.

29. Insert a modified McCall stitch of a no. 1 synthetic absorbable suture through the posterior fornix mucosa on the patient's left side, just lateral to the resected wedge, up through the posterior peritoneal edge, picking up the left pararectal tissue posterior to the uterosacral ligament tie. Take multiple bites across the front of the rectum, around the right pararectal tissue, out through the posterior peritoneal edge on the right and then through the patient's right posterior vaginal fornix exactly opposite the insertion of the suture on the left (Fig. 24).

30. When tied, this suture approximates the uterosacral ligaments in the midline and pulls the posterior vaginal fornix posteriorly, thus providing prophylaxis against a future enterocele.

31. Close the pelvic peritoneum with a purse-string stitch of 2-0 synthetic absorbable suture.

32. Place this suture so that the ligament stumps are placed extraperitoneally. By again picking up each uterosacral ligament in the purse string and bringing the ends of this suture (after tying it) through the posterior fornix mucosa, a second McCall suture is created.

33. Suture-ligate the ligament stumps on each side into the corners of the vault.

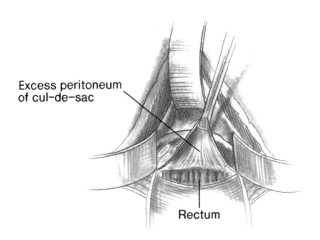

FIG. 23. The cul-de-sac peritoneum is dissected back to its reflection on the rectum, and the excess peritoneum of the potential enterocele is excised.

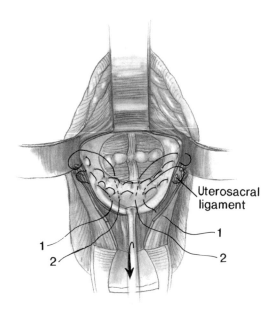

FIG. 24. One or two modified McCall sutures are inserted to approximate the uterosacral ligaments and to obliterate the cul-de-sac after a wedge of posterior vaginal fornix mucosa is excised.

34. Close the vault mucosa with interrupted 2-0 synthetic absorbable sutures.
35. Insert a pack into the vagina and a Foley catheter into the urethra.

E. Special Techniques: Morcellation

1. Use this technique if the uterus is large and cannot be delivered through the posterior vaginal fornix.
2. It is performed after the uterine vessels have been clamped and ligated.
3. Grasp the cervix at the 3 and 9 o'clock positions, and,

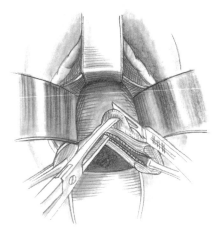

FIG. 26. Wedges of myometrium are removed by morcellation, causing the uterus to collapse in on itself, allowing it to be delivered through the vagina.

with either scissors or a scalpel, split the uterus and cervix vertically as high as possible (Fig. 25).
4. Occasionally, if the uterus is not too large, this maneuver results in the fundus being delivered through the vault.
5. With a larger uterus that will not deliver, resect wedges of myometrium from the middle of the uterine body by using a tenaculum to grasp the uterus and by incising with a scalpel (Fig. 26).
6. Alternately, resect wedges from the front and the back of the uterus, shelling out any fibroids that are present (Fig. 27).
7. The uterus eventually collapses in on itself, and the remaining pedicles can be divided and the uterus removed.
8. It is important to check all the pedicles carefully for hemostasis after removing the uterus by morcellation,

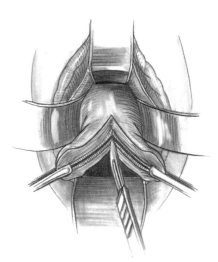

FIG. 25. Before morcellation of the uterus, the uterus is transected in the midline.

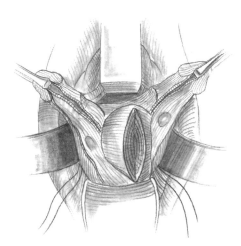

FIG. 27. Often a fibroid can be shelled out of the uterus, thereby decreasing uterine size.

because the forceful traction on the uterus may have loosened some ties.

F. Intraoperative Complications

1. Cystotomy
   * Mark the defect with a suture.
   * Repair it in two overlapping layers with 3-0 synthetic absorbable interrupted sutures after the uterus has been removed.
2. Enterotomy
   Repair as for cystotomy.
3. Bleeding
   * It occurs mainly in the gap between vascular pedicles.
   * Identify by placing ligated pedicles on traction and oversew bleeding points with figure-of-eight 3-0 synthetic absorbable suture.
   * If bleeding is from retracted pedicle, retract with Deaver retractors, pick up bleeding pedicle with toothed forceps, clamp across it with long curved forceps, and oversew with 3-0 synthetic absorbable suture.

G. Postoperative Complications

1. Vault abscess
   * Drain through the center of the vault by probing with sterile curved forceps.
   * Culture and start treatment with antibiotics.
2. Bleeding
   * Remove the vaginal pack and inspect the vault.
   * If obvious bleeding point is visible, oversew to obtain hemostasis.
   * If bleeding is intraabdominal, open abdomen, remove clot, search for bleeding site, and ligate.
   * If no actual bleeding vessel is found, ligate the anterior division of the internal iliac artery on both sides.
3. Ureteral obstruction: see Chapter 5.
4. Urinary fistula: see Chapter 5.

H. Postoperative Management

1. Remove the vaginal pack and catheter the morning after the operation.
2. Mobilize the patient the day after the operation, and start oral fluids.
3. Check the serum levels of hemoglobin, creatinine, and electrolytes on the morning after the operation.

IX. Congenital Anomalies

A. Indications

1. Infertility
2. Dysmenorrhea

B. Preoperative Investigations

Intravenous pyelography should be performed to exclude congenital renal abnormalities.

C. Surgical Technique

1. Septate uterus
   Endoscopic removal of the septum with use of the hysteroscope has now replaced open techniques (see Chapter 25).
2. Bicornuate uterus
   Make a vertical incision in the medial aspect of each horn, and approximate the edges to make a single uterine cavity.

X. Endometrial Biopsy

A. Indications

1. Infertility
2. Screening of patients who receive exogenous estrogens
3. Screening of high-risk patients for endometrial cancer
4. Checking results of hormonal therapy for endometrial hyperplasia

B. Preoperative Investigations

None are necessary.

C. Preoperative Preparation

1. Swab cervix with povidone-iodine.
2. Methods
   * Curette-type instruments (e.g., Novak curette)
   * Suction-type instruments (e.g., Vabra, Pipelle)
   * Brush or spiral sampling technique

D. Surgical Technique

1. Grasp the cervix with a single-toothed tenaculum.
2. Sound the uterus for depth and direction of the cavity.
3. Insert the sampling instrument, and take a sample by scraping or suction, involving all quadrants of the cavity.
4. Remove the instruments, and send the specimen for pathologic examination.

XI. Cesarean Hysterectomy

A. Indications

1. Intractable hemorrhage after a cesarean section
2. In selected cases of placenta percreta or accreta
3. Malignant cervical, uterine, or ovarian tumor in pregnancy

B. Preoperative Investigations

The same as for total abdominal hysterectomy (see section III of this chapter)

C. Preoperative Preparation

1. Abdominal shave
2. Microenema

3. Thromboembolus-deterrent stockings and sequential calf compression device
4. Prophylactic treatment with antibiotics

D. Surgical Technique

The technique is the same as for total abdominal hysterectomy except for the following:

1. The infant may be delivered via a classic or lower segment uterine incision.
2. Close the incision in the uterus for hemostatic purposes with continuous synthetic absorbable suture.
3. Tissue planes are edematous and easily dissected, but veins are large and easily traumatized.
4. The ureters are somewhat dilated in late pregnancy and more difficult to palpate.
5. Multiple clamping may be necessary down the side of the uterus and cervix, rather than the usual single-clamp technique.
6. If the cervix is effaced, it may be difficult to palpate, and care must be taken to ensure that all the cervix is excised.

E. Postoperative Management

The same as for total abdominal hysterectomy

F. Specific Postoperative Complications

Venous thrombosis with embolism is more frequent in pregnant women, and active measures are used to prevent this complication.

Reading List

Pratt JH, Lee MJ Jr, Hasskarl WF Jr, et al. Morbidity after total abdominal hysterectomy. *Am J Obstet Gynecol* 1951;61:407–413.

Counseller VS. Vaginal hysterectomy: indications, advantages, and surgical technic. *Obstet Gynecol* 1953;1:84–93.

Symmonds RE, Counseller VS, Pratt JH. Prolapse of the fallopian tube as a complication of hysterectomy: report of three cases. *Am J Obstet Gynecol* 1957;74:214–217.

Pratt JH. Techniques of vaginal hysterectomy. *Clin Obstet Gynecol* 1959;2:1125–1135.

Pratt JH, Nelson GA, Wilcox CF III, et al. Blood loss during vaginal hysterectomy. *Obstet Gynecol* 1960;15:101–107.

Symmonds RE, Pratt JH, Welch JS. Total abdominal hysterectomy by the Mayo Clinic (Masson-Counseller) technique. *Surg Gynecol Obstet* 1961;113:379–386.

Welch JS, Pratt JH, Symmonds RE. The Wertheim hysterectomy for squamous cell carcinoma of the uterine cervix: thirty years' experience at the Mayo Clinic. *Am J Obstet Gynecol* 1961;81:978–987.

Pratt JH. Operative and postoperative difficulties of vaginal hysterectomy. *Obstet Gynecol* 1963;21:220–226.

Symmonds RE, Pratt JH, Welch JS. Extended Wertheim operation for primary, recurrent, or suspected recurrent carcinoma of the cervix. *Obstet Gynecol* 1964;24:15–24.

Pratt JH, Galloway JR. Vaginal hysterectomy in patients less than 36 or more than 60 years of age. *Am J Obstet Gynecol* 1965;93:812–821.

Symmonds RE. Morbidity and complications of radical hysterectomy with pelvic lymph node dissection. *Am J Obstet Gynecol* 1966;94:663–673.

Brown JM, Malkasian GD Jr, Symmonds RE. Abdominal myomectomy. *Am J Obstet Gynecol* 1967;99:126–129.

Janes DR, Smith RA, Williams TJ. Cesarean hysterectomy. *Minn Med* 1968;51:17–20.

Pratt JH, Gunnlaugsson GH. Vaginal hysterectomy by morcellation. *Mayo Clin Proc* 1970;45:374–387.

Williams TJ. Vaginal hysterectomy. *Dallas Med J* 1974;60:525–534.

Pratt JH. Common complications of vaginal hysterectomy: thoughts regarding their prevention and management. *Clin Obstet Gynecol* 1976;19:645–659.

Webb MJ, Gaffey TA. Outpatient diagnostic aspiration curettage. *Obstet Gynecol* 1976;47:239–242.

Webb MJ, Symmonds RE. Radical hysterectomy: influence of recent conization on morbidity and complications. *Obstet Gynecol* 1979;53:290–292.

Webb MJ, Symmonds RE. Wertheim hysterectomy: a reappraisal. *Obstet Gynecol* 1979;54:140–145.

Webb MJ, Symmonds RE. Site of recurrence of cervical cancer after radical hysterectomy. *Am J Obstet Gynecol* 1980;138:813–817.

Webb MJ. Surgical treatment of cervical cancer. *Postgrad Obstet Gynecol* 1982;2:1–5.

Lee RA. Total abdominal hysterectomy. *OB-GYN Illustrated* 5, 1984.

Symmonds RE, Lee RA. Simple abdominal hysterectomy. *In:* Nyhus LM, Baker RJ, eds. *Mastery of surgery,* vol 2. Boston: Little, Brown, 1984:1171–1182.

Lee RA. Abdominal hysterectomy (simple). *In:* Breen JL, Osofsky HJ, eds. *Current concepts in gynecologic surgery. Vol 3: Advances in clinical obstetrics and gynecology.* Baltimore: Williams & Wilkins, 1987:151–169.

Podratz KC, Symmonds RE. Radical hysterectomy and pelvic lymphadenectomy. *In:* Alberts DA, Surwit EA, eds. *Cervix cancer,* vol 3. The Hague: Martinus Nijhoff, 1987:67–88.

Kinney WK, Egorshin EV, Podratz KC. Wertheim hysterectomy in the geriatric population. *Gynecol Oncol* 1988;31:227–232.

Symmonds RE, Lee RA. Simple abdominal hysterectomy. *In:* Nyhus LM, Baker RJ, eds. *Mastery of surgery,* vol 2, 2nd ed. Boston: Little, Brown, 1992:1497–1509.

Kinney WK, Hodge DO, Egorshin EV, et al. Identification of a low-risk subset of patients with stage Ib invasive squamous cancer of the cervix possibly suited to less radical surgical treatment. *Gynecol Oncol* 1995;57:3–6.

Kinney WK, Hodge DO, Egorshin EV, et al. Surgical treatment of patients with stages Ib and IIa carcinoma of the cervix and palpably positive pelvic lymph. *Gynecol Oncol* 1995;57:145–149.

Lee RA. Radical hysterectomy. *In:* Donohue JH, Van Heerden JA, Monson JRT, eds. *Atlas of surgical oncology.* Cambridge: Blackwell Scientific Publications, 1995:295–302.

Magrina JF, Goodrich MA, Weaver AL, et al. Modified radical hysterectomy: morbidity and mortality. *Gynecol Oncol* 1995;59:277–282.

Moen MD, Webb MJ, Wilson TO, et al. Vaginal hysterectomy in patients with benign uterine enlargement. *J Pelv Surg* 1995;1:197–203.

Kammer-Doak DN, Magrina JF, Weaver A, et al. Vaginal hysterectomy with and without oophorectomy. *J Pelv Surg* 1996;2:304–309.

Webb MJ. Transvaginal oophorectomy using the endoscopic stapler. *J Pelv Surg* 1996;2:128–130.

Cliby WA. Total abdominal hysterectomy. *Baillieres Clin Obstet Gynecol* 1997;11:77–94.

Webb MJ. Radical hysterectomy. *Baillieres Clin Obstet Gynecol* 1997;11:149–166.

CHAPTER 8

Surgery of the Cervix

Timothy O. Wilson, M.D.

I. Laser Vaporization and Cryosurgery

A. Indications
1. Abnormal findings on Pap smear, with colposcopy revealing the entire lesion, and no invasive disease found on adequate biopsy of the lesion.
2. Goal is ablation of all abnormal epithelium of the ecto/endocervix.

B. Preoperative Investigations
1. Pap smear
2. Colposcopy with colposcopically directed biopsy
3. Visualization of the entire lesion, with identification of squamocolumnar junction

C. Preoperative Preparation
1. None
2. It is important to avoid douche or vaginal suppository, which may traumatize the cervix and make visualization difficult.

D. Surgical Technique
1. Laser vaporization
   - Inject 2% lidocaine (Xylocaine) into cervical stroma at the 3 and 9 o'clock positions.
   - Smoke evacuation speculum is mandatory for visualization and for preventing heat buildup.
   - The patient must be relaxed to permit good visualization of the cervix.
   - Sedation is seldom necessary when treating the cervix alone.
   - Use carbon dioxide laser with micromanipulator, and view the cervix with a colposcope.

   - Use a power setting of 10 to 15 W (depends on spot size), and ablate the lesion to a depth of 5 to 7 mm to vaporize endocervical glands that may harbor disease.
   - Control any bleeding with cautery, silver nitrate, Monsel solution, or suture placement.
   - Skin hooks to manipulate the cervix are helpful if disease is on the lateral cervix or fornix.
2. Cryosurgery
   - For cryosurgery, it is mandatory that the entire lesion be seen.
   - Choose a probe tip to conform to the contour of the lesion.
   - Colposcopic identification of the lesion is best just before treatment.
   - The double freeze technique with formation of an adequate ice ball is preferred.

E. Specific Postoperative Management
1. No tampons, douche, or coitus for 1 month
2. A watery discharge is normal for 3 to 4 weeks postoperatively.
3. Analgesics seldom are necessary.

F. Specific Postoperative Complications
1. Bleeding
   - Can occur 7 to 14 days after treatment as eschar loosens
   - Usually will stop, with only observation needed
   - Cautery, silver nitrate, Monsel solution, or a suture may be needed.
2. Cervical stenosis
   - Uncommon unless endocervical canal was treated deeply
   - Causes dysmenorrhea, amenorrhea, or decreased menstrual flow
   - Treated with cervical dilation
3. Infection
   - Seldom a problem
   - Routine treatment with antibiotics is not indicated.

Timothy O. Wilson: Consultant, Departments of Obstetrics and Gynecology and Surgery, Mayo Clinic and Mayo Foundation; Assistant Professor of Obstetrics and Gynecology, Mayo Medical School, Rochester, Minnesota.

II. Cone Biopsy

A. Indications
1. Pap smear shows dysplasia, but colposcopy does not identify either the entire lesion or the squamocolumnar junction.
2. Pap smear or biopsy findings are suggestive of possible invasive disease.
3. Lack of correlation between findings on Pap smear and biopsy
4. Microinvasive disease found on biopsy

B. Preoperative Investigation
1. Pap smear
2. Colposcopy

C. Preoperative Preparation
1. None
2. It is important to avoid douche or vaginal suppository, which may traumatize the cervix.

D. Surgical Technique
1. Laser conization
   - Can be performed in the surgeon's office
   - Inject 2% lidocaine with epinephrine at the 3 and 9 o'clock positions.
   - Use a superpulse or high-oscillating current to outline the area to be removed, and then perform deeper vaporization.
   - Use skin hooks to grasp the cervix.
   - Remove the specimen by sharply cutting the apex of the cone.
   - Use cautery, silver nitrate, Monsel solution, or suture if bleeding occurs.
2. Cold knife conization

   - Needs to be performed in an operating room, with patient under anesthesia
   - Identify the lesion (with colposcopy if necessary or by staining with Lugol solution).
   - Tailor the conization to the size and shape of the lesion and with regard to patient age and fertility considerations.
   - Remove specimen sharply to avoid tissue trauma from cautery (Fig. 1).
   - Place sutures at the 3 and 9 o'clock positions for hemostasis.
   - Cauterize cervix for hemostasis.
   - Perform dilation and curettage after conization.

E. Specific Postoperative Management
1. No tampons, douche, or coitus for 1 month.
2. Discharge is usual for 3 to 4 weeks.
3. Analgesics seldom are necessary.

F. Specific Postoperative Complications
1. Bleeding
   - Can occur 7 to 14 days after conization as eschar loosens
   - Can often be controlled by insertion of a vaginal pack for 12 to 14 hours
   - If bleeding is significant, placement of a suture or pack is usually required.
   - Bleeding can be heavy; if visualization or discomfort is a problem in the office or emergency area, return to the operating room; anesthesia may be necessary.
2. Cervical stenosis
   - Symptoms are amenorrhea, dysmenorrhea, or decreased menstrual flow.
   - Ultrasonography, computed tomography, or magnetic resonance imaging will reveal fluid collection in the uterus.
   - Treated with cervical dilation

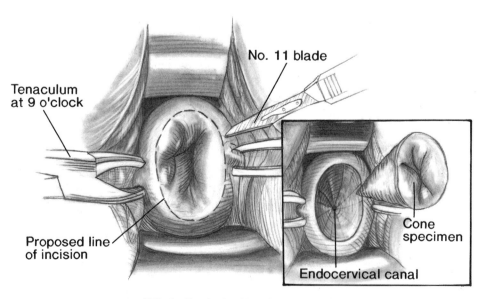

FIG. 1. Cervical cold knife conization.

3. Infection
   • Seldom a problem
   • Routine treatment with antibiotics is not indicated.

III. Trachelectomy/Excision of Cervical Stump

A. Indications
1. Pathologic condition of the cervix warranting removal
2. Either vaginal or abdominal approach, depending on disease process

B. Preoperative Investigation
1. Varies with the surgical indication
2. Pap smear
3. Colposcopy if Pap smear is abnormal
4. Intravenous pyelography, ultrasonography, computed tomography, or magnetic resonance imaging if cervical mass

C. Preoperative Preparation
1. Avoid cervical trauma if trachelectomy is for cervical dysplasia.
2. Prophylactic treatment with antibiotics.

D. Surgical Technique
1. Vaginal approach
   • Grasp cervix with tenaculum.
   • Make a circumferential incision, as in vaginal hysterectomy.
   • Enter the peritoneum anteriorly and posteriorly.
   • Clamp the uterosacral and cardinal ligament pedicles (two bites on each side).
   • Palpation of the ureters is critical because of possible altered position from supracervical hysterectomy.
   • Note bowel or bladder that may be adherent at the apex from supracervical hysterectomy.
   • Perform McCall suture/vaginal vault closure in routine fashion.
2. Abdominal approach
   • Place a vaginal pack and Foley catheter.
   • Identify the cervical stump by palpation.
   • Grasp with two tenacula.
   • Identify the ureters.
   • Dissect the bladder and rectum off the cervix.
   • Clamp and ligate remnants of the cardinal ligaments (Fig. 2).
   • Transect the uterosacral ligaments.
   • Remove the specimen, and close the vaginal vault in the usual fashion, reattaching uterosacral and cardinal ligament pedicles.
   • Again, check the ureters.

E. Specific Postoperative Management
The same as for hysterectomy

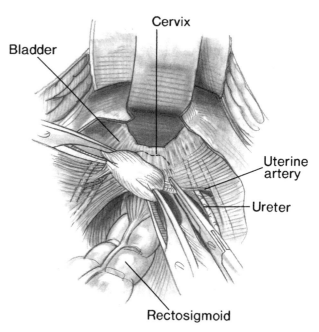

FIG. 2. Excision of cervical stump.

F. Specific Postoperative Complications
The same as for hysterectomy

IV. Radical Excision of Cervical Stump for Cancer

A. Indications
Invasive carcinoma of the cervical stump

B. Preoperative Investigation
1. Biopsy, confirming invasive cancer
2. Computed tomography or magnetic resonance imaging of the pelvis and/or intravenous pyelography

C. Preoperative Preparation
1. Enema
2. Vaginal douche if no active bleeding
3. Prophylactic treatment with antibiotics

D. Surgical Technique and Difficulties Encountered
1. Place a vaginal pack and Foley catheter.
2. A lower midline incision is preferred.
3. Collect peritoneal washings for cytologic examination.
4. Explore the abdomen and pelvis for metastatic disease.
5. Grasp the cervical stump with two tenacula.
6. Clamp, cut, and ligate the remnant of the round ligament.
7. Identify the ureter, and develop the paravesical and pararectal spaces.
8. Remove lymph nodes from the external iliac, common iliac, internal iliac, and obturator areas (see Chapter 24).

9. Ligate the anterior division of the internal iliac artery.
10. Ligate the lateral pelvic web adjacent to the pelvic sidewall between the paravesical and pararectal spaces.
11. Perform the identical procedure on the opposite side.
12. Separate the ureter from its attachment to the medial leaf of the broad ligament.
13. Incise the peritoneum of the medial leaf of the broad ligament to the base of the cul-de-sac.
14. Bluntly dissect the cervical stump and vagina from the rectum.
15. Transect the uterosacral ligaments lateral to the rectum.
16. Dissect the bladder off the cervical stump anteriorly.
17. Ligate the obliterated hypogastric artery anteriorly, adjacent to the bladder.
18. Dissect the ureter out of its tunnel, as described in Radical Hysterectomy (see Chapter 7).
19. Make an incision into the vagina, removing the proximal 3 cm of vagina with the cervical stump and parametrium.
20. Close the vagina, and achieve hemostasis.
21. Deep drains may or may not be placed, depending on the surgeon's preference.
22. Because of bladder denervation, place a suprapubic catheter and bring it out through a separate abdominal stab wound.
23. Close the abdomen.
24. This is technically a more difficult procedure than radical hysterectomy because the supracervical portion of the uterus is absent, and adequate countertraction is difficult to obtain. Also, there is often scarring from the previous supracervical hysterectomy.

E. Specific Postoperative Management
1. If used, deep drains are left in place until the lymphatic output is 50 mL/24 h on 2 consecutive days.
2. Suprapubic catheter clamping is begun 21 days postoperatively; it usually can be removed within 4 weeks.
3. The patient usually is dismissed from the hospital the day the deep drains are removed.

F. Specific Postoperative Complications
1. The incidence of ureteral fistula is approximately 2%.
2. Sensory denervation of the bowel and bladder may occur, with sensation varying from no sensation of an urge for voiding or defecating to normal sensation for both.
3. Long-term development of lymphocyst in the area of the pelvic lymphadenectomy is uncommon (<5%). If it occurs, it may be observed on computed tomographic scan, or if symptomatic, it may be drained through computed tomographically directed aspiration. Reoperation is seldom necessary.
4. Lymphedema of the lower extremity is uncommon (<5%), unless adjuvant radiotherapy is administered.

V. Cerclage

A. Indications
1. Patient has a history of an incompetent cervix.
2. Patient has premature cervical dilation without uterine contractions.
3. Patient has intact membranes.
4. Patient has no uterine bleeding.
5. Patient has no evidence of intraamniotic infection.
6. Fetus would benefit from a longer intrauterine confinement.

B. Preoperative Investigation
Ultrasonographic scan may delineate cervical dilation.

C. Preoperative Preparation
1. Prophylactic treatment with antibiotics
2. Fetal monitoring
3. Uterine monitoring for contractions
4. General anesthesia to relax uterus

D. Surgical Technique
1. Shirodkar
   • Grasp the cervix with ring forceps to minimize trauma.
   • Make an incision anteriorly on the cervix.
   • Mobilize the bladder from the lower uterine segment.
   • Make an incision posteriorly on the cervix.
   • Use a wide braided nylon (Mersilene) tape double armed with large needles, and pass it submucosally from the anterior incision laterally to the posterior incision (Fig. 3).
   • Perform the identical procedure on the opposite side.

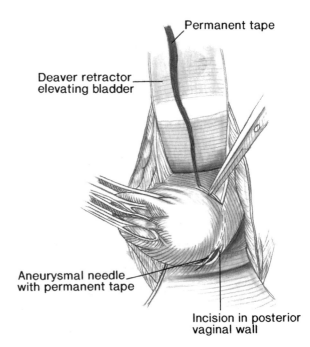

FIG. 3. Insertion of Shirodkar suture.

- Next, tie the tape securely posteriorly, reducing the membranes (if necessary) to their intrauterine position.
- Close the vaginal mucosal incisions or leave the ends of the tape protruding into the posterior vaginal fornix.

2. McDonald
- Grasp the cervix with ring forceps to minimize trauma.
- Without incising the vaginal mucosa, take four to six bites of the vaginal mucosa and underlying cervix in a purse-string fashion.
- Use braided nylon (Mersilene).
- Tie the suture securely anteriorly.

E. Specific Postoperative Management
1. The patient is monitored for fetal heart rate and uterine contractions postoperatively.
2. The suture can be removed at 38 weeks or with the onset of labor; however, with the Shirodkar procedure, this can be difficult. Occasionally, it needs to be performed in the operating room.

F. Specific Postoperative Complications
1. Rupture of membranes intraoperatively or postoperatively.
2. Uterine irritability (contractions) may be produced by the procedure, and tocolytics may be necessary.
3. Infection rarely occurs if antibiotics are used prophylactically.

VI. Excision of Cervical Polyp

A. Indications
In general, a polyp at the cervical os is always removed to prevent bleeding except if the patient is pregnant.

B. Preoperative Investigation
Pap smear

C. Preoperative Preparation
None

D. Surgical Technique
1. Can be performed in the office
2. No anesthetic is needed.
3. Grasp the polyp with a curved clamp, Allis forceps, or ring forceps.
4. Twist and remove the polyp.
5. Sharp dissection is seldom necessary.
6. Apply silver nitrate, Monsel solution, or cautery for hemostasis.

E. Specific Postoperative Management
No tampons, douche, or coitus for 72 hours.

F. Specific Postoperative Complications
Bleeding: is usually managed with silver nitrate, Monsel solution, or cautery; suture placement is rarely required.

VII. Cervical Stenosis/Atresia/Pyometra/Hematometra

A. Indications
1. In premenopausal patients, these conditions result in hematometra with cyclic dysmenorrhea, with or without menstrual blood flow.
2. In menopausal patients, development of hematometra or pyometra is usually asymptomatic.

B. Preoperative Investigation
1. Probe the cervix with a fine silver probe or a uterine sound; if the sound can be readily passed into the uterine cavity, the patient does not have stenosis or hematometra/pyometra.
2. With pyometra or hematometra, ultrasonography reveals a fluid-filled uterine cavity.
3. With cervical atresia, a remnant of cervix may or may not be present; again, ultrasonography will reveal whether a blind uterine cavity with hematometra exists.
4. With cervical atresia, other congenital anomalies of the genitourinary tract are common; therefore, intravenous pyelography or computed tomography should be performed.

C. Preoperative Preparation
Povidone-iodine douche

D. Surgical Technique
1. General anesthesia
2. Grasp the cervix with a tenaculum.
3. Insert a fine probe into the cervical os if possible.
4. If a fine probe cannot be inserted, use a fine curved clamp to probe the cervical canal and break down the scarring.
5. Insert a sound.
6. Progressively dilate the cervix to at least 30 F with Hegar or Pratt dilators (ideally to 40 F).
7. In older patients, sample the endometrium after evacuation of the hematometra/pyometra to exclude carcinoma.
8. With atresia, gently probe the cervix to find the communication with the body of the uterus, and then gently dilate the cervix.

E. Specific Postoperative Management
None

F. Specific Postoperative Complications
1. Uterine perforation secondary to difficulty entering the uterine cavity and also to thinning of the myometrial wall by hematometra/pyometra
2. Recurrence of cervical stenosis is common, and patients need to be observed for recurrence of symptoms.

Reading List

Williams TJ, Johnson TR, Pratt JH. Time interval between cervical conization and hysterectomy. *Am J Obstet Gynecol* 1970;107:790–796.

Pratt JH, Jefferies JA. The retained cervical stump: a 25-year experience. *Obstet Gynecol* 1976;48:711–715.

Magrina JF, Kempers RD, Williams TJ. Cervical cerclage: 20 years' experience at the Mayo Clinic. *Minn Med* 1983;66:599–602.

Noller KL, Stanhope CR. Colposcopic accuracy: comparison of satisfactory examinations with results of conization. *Colp Gynecol Laser Surg* 1984;1:181–184.

Williams TJ. Cerclage for cervical incompetence. *Female Patient* 1985;10:81.

Kinney WK, Egorshin EV, Ballard DJ, et al. Long-term survival and sequelae after surgical management of invasive cervical carcinoma diagnosed at the time of simple hysterectomy. *Gynecol Oncol* 1992;44:24–27.

CHAPTER 9

Surgery of the Fallopian Tubes

Tiffany J. Williams, M.D. and William A. Cliby, M.D.

I. Introduction

Surgery of the fallopian tubes may be divided into two categories, reconstructive and extirpative.

A. Reconstructive Operations
1. These are performed because of disease and infertility.
   • Iatrogenic problems, such as tubal ligation and the desire for restoration of fertility
   • Disease processes, which may be divided into three categories:
      — Adhesive disease: affects ovum pickup and transport because of partial obstruction or compromise of motility
      — Distal tubal obstruction: such as hydrosalpinx, in which ovum pickup cannot occur
      — Proximal tubal obstruction: may occur in salpingitis isthmica nodosa and may be partial or complete
2. Management methods
   • Salpingo-ovariolysis: adhesive disease may be corrected with lysis and excision of adhesions involving the tubes and ovaries. Adhesive disease often accompanies the other tubal occlusions and requires correction, even if it is not the primary problem.
   • Fimbrioplasty is the correction of adhesion or agglutination of the fimbria and partial distal obstruction of the tubes. Obstruction may be complete with hydrosalpinx.
   • Neosalpingostomy is the construction of a patent tubal lumen after there has been complete distal occlusion.

Tiffany J. Williams: Emeritus Member, Departments of Obstetrics and Gynecology and Surgery, Mayo Clinic and Mayo Foundation; Emeritus Professor of Obstetrics and Gynecology, Mayo Medical School, Rochester, Minnesota.

William A. Cliby: Consultant, Department of Obstetrics and Gynecology and Surgery, Mayo Clinic and Mayo Foundation; Assistant Professor of Obstetrics and Gynecology, Mayo Medical School, Rochester, Minnesota.

Agglutination of the fimbria within the hydrosalpinx may require lysis as well.
   • Anastomosis involves the resection of an obstructed portion of the tube and approximation of the adjacent patent lumina, regardless of location of causation.

Note: Reconstructive surgery performed on the fallopian tubes requires the use of optical augmentation to improve not only visualization intraoperatively but also the results of reconstruction.

B. Extirpative Operations
Disease of the tubes requires removal of
1. Tube (salpingectomy)
2. Tube and ovary (salpingo-oophorectomy)
3. Uterus, tubes, and ovaries (hysterectomy and salpingo-oophorectomy)

C. Preoperative Investigations
1. Documentation of the normalcy of other fertility factors
   • Semen analysis
   • Hysterosalpingography
   • Laparoscopy
2. Evidence of ovulation
   • Basal body temperature chart
   • Serum level of progesterone
   • Endometrial biopsy
   • Follicle-stimulating hormone in older women
3. Weight: obesity is a relative contraindication; it may significantly complicate the operation because of compromise of exposure. The patient should be close to her ideal weight for height.

D. Preoperative Preparation
1. Povidone-iodine douche
2. Abdominoperineal shave
3. Enema
4. Prophylactic treatment with antibiotics
5. Perform operation during the *postmenstrual* phase of

the cycle to avoid increased vascularity and possible bleeding from a corpus luteum.

6. Anesthesia should provide adequate relaxation to improve exposure.
7. *Lithotomy* position with vaginal preparation for insertion of intrauterine catheter device to inject dye to confirm subsequent tubal patency
8. Pack the vagina to elevate the uterus and to improve exposure to the adnexa.
9. Insert bladder catheter for drainage.

II. Reconstructive Surgical Techniques

A. Salpingo-ovariolysis

1. Indication
   Infertility in the absence of other factors related to sterility (pain is not an appropriate or logical indication for adhesiolysis for tubal obstructive disease, either partial or complete)
2. Surgical technique
   - Incision
     — A low midline incision has the advantage of speed and adequate visualization.
     — A transverse (Pfannenstiel) incision has more bleeding and may not allow adequate visualization and optimal use of the operating microscope (partially with thicker abdominal walls).
   - Explore the abdomen to evaluate its contents.
   - Pack the intestines away from the operative field, and protect them with plastic sheeting to avoid serosal trauma and to decrease formation of adhesions.
   - Free adhesions to allow packing of the cul-de-sac to elevate the uterus further. This improves visualization and allows delicate tissue management with use of fingers.
   - Lysis of adhesions, which may hold uterus and adnexa posteriorly, may require use of visual magnification together with microelectrocautery or laser (Fig. 1). These have the advantage of speed and hemostasis, compared with sharp dissection.
   - Pack the cul-de-sac with a polymeric silicone (Silastic)-covered pack to avoid peritoneal and serosal trauma and subsequent information of adhesions and to elevate and immobilize the fundus and adnexa.
   - Remove patient from the steep Trendelenburg position to allow better visualization and better access to the adnexal structures.
   - Tilting the patient laterally may facilitate visualization, delicate tissue handling, and ease of operative manipulation.
   - Immobilization of the organs in a flat plane is necessary because of the small depth of field related to the optics of the microscope.
   - The assistant must also keep the area of the operation centered in the field of vision while working only in a two-dimensional setting.

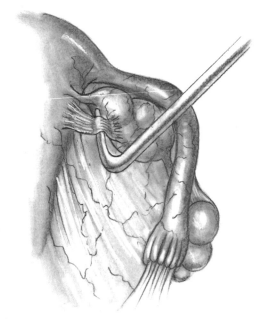

FIG. 1. Freeing adherent adnexa.

- Small movements are required while attending to exposure and traction.
- Continuous lavage improves visualization and requires attention from the assistant for accurate placement.
- Continuous suction removes the fluid and decreases the difficulties caused by surface tension effects.
- Excise adhesions by starting at the ovary and proceeding to free the tube from the ovary along the line of adhesions, avoiding damage to the serosa, peritoneum, or ovarian capsule (Fig. 2).
- Hemostasis with bipolar cautery or microelectrocautery should be exact and meticulous.

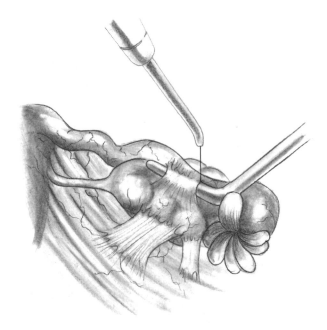

FIG. 2. Freeing ovarian adhesions.

- Cleanse the cornual portion of the uterus and tubo-ovarian hiatus between the tube and the ovary, and then remove adhesions from the surface of the tube, avoiding any peritoneal defects.
- Meticulous hemostasis: thorough flushing with balanced physiologic solution containing 5,000 U of heparin (1 mL heparin/1,000 mL solution).

Note: The entire operation is performed under continuous irrigation to flush away blood and clot as well as to decrease the effects of desiccation from air, heat, and light.

- With extensive cul-de-sac adhesions, consider ovarian suspension.
- Use of an adhesion barrier may be considered if there is a peritoneal defect so as to minimize subsequent adhesion formation.
- Documentation of patency
  — Intrauterine catheter injection
  — Cervical occlusion and direct transmural intrauterine injection (the use of an intracath-type needle is effective for this)
  — Retrograde injection or sounding
  — Documentation is mandatory and is best performed in a way to minimize damage to the tubal endothelium.
  — Attempts at retrograde intraluminal probing should be avoided if possible because of endothelial damage.
- Remove the packs.
- Replace the omentum and the bowel.
- Thoroughly irrigate the pelvis to remove all clots or debris.
- Close the abdomen.
- Remove the intrauterine catheter immediately postoperatively.
- Remove the bladder catheter either immediately postoperatively or on the morning after the operation.
3. Intraoperative complications
- Bleeding: immaculate hemostasis is required.
- Damage to peritoneum from dissection:
  — Subsequent reconstruction
  — Consideration of use of adhesion barriers
- Bowel damage and bladder damage, as with any operative procedure: appropriate management should be with minimally reactive sutures.
4. Specific postoperative management
  The same postoperative management routine as for all abdominal procedures
5. Specific postoperative complications
- Infection or even low-grade inflammation:
  — Continuation of antibiotic coverage
  — Pelvic examination is needed to document tenderness, guarding, or rebound.
  — Cervical, vaginal, and blood cultures are indicated.
- Bleeding: vaginal bleeding is not uncommon because of the intrauterine manipulations and, unless profuse, requires no specific management.

B. Fimbriolysis
1. Indication
  Infertility in the absence of other factors related to sterility (correctable factors should be identified so they can be managed postoperatively)
2. Surgical technique
- Make a low midline incision.
- Explore the abdomen to evaluate the contents.
- Pack the intestines away from the operative field, and protect them with plastic sheeting.
- Adhesions are likely to be encountered; use the same technique as for salpingo-ovariolysis.
- Excise adhesions by starting at the ovary and proceed to free the tube from the ovary along the line of adhesions, avoiding damage to the serosa, peritoneum, or ovarian capsule.
- Hemostasis is achieved with bipolar cautery or microelectrocautery and should be exact and meticulous.
- The fimbria and the areas of scarring must be visualized.
- Microdissection with microelectrocautery (or laser) may excise the scarred areas, allowing the fimbria to open. This should be accomplished to allow as normal-appearing a position as possible.
- High magnification may be necessary to determine the lines of dissection.
- Because reocclusion is a common cause of failure, use a fine, permanent suture (8–0 nylon [Ethilon]). Suture the fimbria open in as normal-appearing a position as possible.
- First, complete one side and allow it to remain in that position.
- Manage the second side in a similar fashion before returning to the first side.
- At this time and before placing the sutures, evaluate the maintenance of the dissection.
- If the appearance and position are not normal, additional dissection is indicated before suture placement.
- Suture placement is recommended, first at the region of the ovary (6 o'clock), and then at 12 o'clock, then adding whatever number of sutures seems appropriate.
- Document patency as in salpingo-ovariolysis.
- Remove the packs, irrigate, and close as described above.
3. Intraoperative complications
- The same as for salpingo-ovariolysis
- Damage to the blood supply of the tube or ovary during the dissection:
  — If viability of the tissue is questionable, excision of the compromised area is recommended.
4. Specific postoperative management
  Hydrotubation: enzyme, antibiotic, steroid solution
- Cervicovaginal cleansing
- Sterile technique

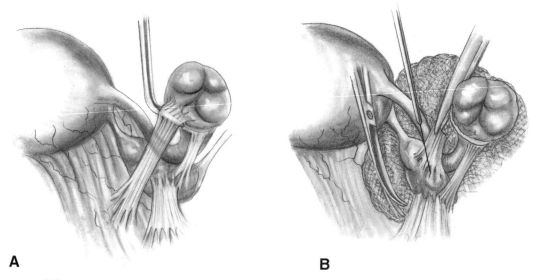

FIG. 3. A: Freeing ovarian adhesions. **B:** Lines of adherence of fimbria at hydrosalpinx.

- Contraindicated by bleeding or discharge or clinical evidence of infection
- Instilled on three to four occasions at 3- to 4-day intervals
- The risk of infection is 3%.
5. Specific postoperative complications
   The same as for salpingo-ovariolysis

C. Neosalpingostomy
1. Indication
   Infertility in the absence of other factors related to sterility
2. Surgical technique
- Make a low midline incision.
- Explore the abdomen to evaluate its contents.
- Pack the intestines away from the operative field, and protect with plastic sheeting.
- Adhesions are likely to be encountered; use the same technique as for salpingo-ovariolysis.
- Pack the cul-de-sac with polymeric silicone-covered packs.
- Excise adhesions by starting at the ovary and proceeding to free the tube from the ovary along the line of adhesions, avoiding damage to the serosa, peritoneum, or ovarian capsule (Fig. 3).
- With optical magnification, visualize the scar lines and make an incision into the hydrosalpinx.
- Fill the tube with dye to distend it and to make the sites for dissection more obvious.
- Continue the incision along the scarred areas until the fimbria flowers open (Fig. 4).
- Fimbrial agglutination may be encountered:
  — The fimbria and the areas of scarring must be visualized.
  — Microdissection with microelectrocautery (or laser)

may excise the scarred areas, allowing the fimbria to open. This should be accomplished to allow as normal-appearing a position as possible.
- Because reocclusion is a common cause of failure, the use of a fine, permanent suture (8-0 nylon) is recommended; suture the fimbria open in as normal-appearing a position as possible, as for fimbrioplasty (Fig. 5).
- Manage the second side in a similar fashion before returning to the first side.
- At this time and before placing the sutures, evaluate the maintenance of the dissection.

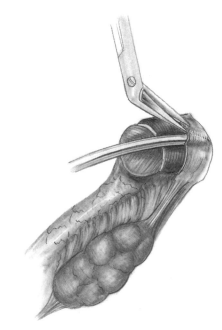

FIG. 4. Fimbria flowering open.

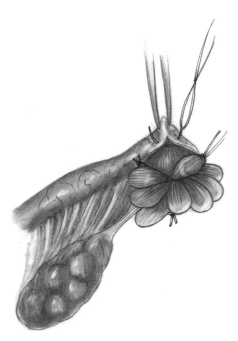

FIG. 5. Suturing to maintain patency.

- If the appearance and position are not normal, additional dissection is indicated before suture placement, as for fimbrioplasty.
- Document patency as described above.
- Attempts at retrograde intramural probing should be avoided because of possible endothelial damage.
- Remove the packs, replace the omentum and bowel, irrigate the pelvis, and close the incision.
3. Intraoperative complications
   The same as for fimbriolysis
4. Specific postoperative management
   Hydrotubation: enzyme, antibiotic, steroid solution, as for fimbriolysis
5. Specific postoperative complications
   The same as for fimbriolysis

D. Anastomosis
1. Indication
   Infertility in the absence of other factors related to sterility (correctable factors should be identified so they can be managed postoperatively)
2. Surgical technique
   - Adhesions are likely to be encountered; use the same technique as for salpingo-ovariolysis.
   - Identify the obstructed portion of the tubes; the operation is facilitated by optical magnification so that minimal tubal resection is possible.

Note: The resection must excise scarred and abnormal tissue until normal endothelium and muscularis are observed.

- Pick up the obstructed portion with a fine-needle 5-0 or 6-0 synthetic absorbable suture.
- Score the area of planned incision with microelectrocautery.

- With sharp dissection, excise the obstructed portion with either fine scissors or a scalpel.
- Identify the normal-appearing tube and then document patency.
  — Document distal patency by using no. 90 polymeric silicone tubing attached to a 30-gauge needle attached to a syringe filled with methylene blue. (Because of the bacteriostatic properties of methylene blue, it is preferred to indigo carmine.)
  — Document proximal patency with the intrauterine device. If this is not satisfactory, cervical occlusion and intrauterine injection are required.
  — For retrograde injection, polymeric silicone tubing may be helpful.
  — Lacrimal duct probes and Garcia probes may be used to document patency if dye flow is not satisfactory.
  — Choose the method that causes the least endosalpingeal irritation and damage.
- After documenting patency proximally and distally, approximate the mesosalpinx with 5-0 or 6-0 suture. (Permanent suture is recommended.) Avoid undue traction.
- Close the mesosalpingeal defect by using the same or an additional suture, which may be absorbable.
- Place a horizontal muscular suture at the 6 o'clock position, generally by using 7-0 synthetic absorbable suture (Fig. 6).
- Insert mucomuscular sutures of 8-0 synthetic absorbable suture:
  — A minimum of four sutures is used in the lower proximal portion of the tube where the lumen is narrow.
  — More distal approximations may require more sutures for meticulous and adequate approximation.

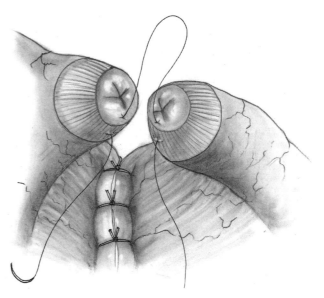

FIG. 6. Mucomuscular suture.

- Polymeric silicone tubing placed in the lumen is helpful when there is difficulty visualizing the placement of the sutures and the position of the muscularis and lumen (Fig. 7). The tubing is removed as the final sutures are placed.
- Place the sutures individually, and tie at the completion of each suture placement.
- Accurate placement is required. Avoid any endothelium or peritoneum between the approximated muscular walls.
- Next, place musculoserosal sutures, interdigitating them with the previously placed sutures.
- Document patency. Watertight anastomosis should be anticipated.
- Cut the internal sutures on the knot having four throws (square knots).
- Cut the external sutures with the scissor blade above the knot.
- Interstitial anastomosis may require placement of all internal sutures before they are tied individually.
- In most instances, shaving through the cornual area will allow interstitial anastomosis, which is preferable to implantation.
- Achieve meticulous hemostasis.
- Document patency as described above.
- Remove the packs, replace the omentum and bowel, irrigate the pelvis, and close the incision.

3. Intraoperative complications
   Failure to demonstrate patency suggests inadequate anastomosis. Patency must be achieved, even if the sutures have to be removed and the anastomosis redone.
4. Postoperative management
   The same as for salpingo-ovariolysis
5. Postoperative complications
   The same as for salpingo-ovariolysis

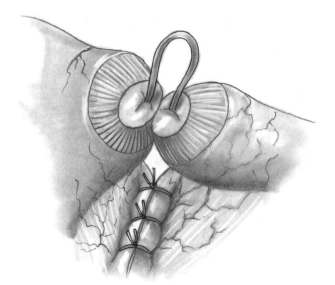

FIG. 7. Identifying lumen.

III. Extirpative Surgical Techniques

A. Salpingectomy
1. Indications
   - Tubal disease: symptomatic and recurrent inflammatory disease
   - Damage such that normal tubal function may not be expected, e.g., ectopic pregnancy
2. Preoperative investigations
   - Complete blood count
   - Documentation of the normalcy of other fertility factors if future pregnancy is planned
3. Preoperative preparation
   - Povidone-iodine douche
   - Abdominoperineal shave
   - Enema
   - Prophylactic treatment with antibiotics
4. Surgical technique
   - Make a low midline incision.
   - Explore the abdomen to evaluate its contents.
   - Pack the intestines away from the operative field and protect with plastic sheeting.
   - Perform adhesiolysis starting with the ovary and the centripetal surrounding structures if indicated.
   - Clamp, cut, and tie the mesosalpinx with minimally reactive sutures (2-0 synthetic absorbable).
   - Take separate bites until reaching the uterine cornu.
   - The tube may be cross-clamped, cut, and tied. Alternatively, a wedge at the base of the tube may be resected from the uterus and the defect closed with a figure-of-eight suture.
   - In either instance, the area may be covered by the round ligament by using a modified Coffey suspension.
   - Check for hemostasis.
   - Remove the packs, replace the omentum and bowel, irrigate the pelvis, and close the incision.
   - This procedure may be performed endoscopically (see Chapter 26).
5. Intraoperative complications
   - Bleeding from the mesosalpinx: control under direct vision and suture-ligate bleeding sites
   - Blood supply of the ovary damaged during the dissection
6. Specific postoperative management
   The same as for salpingo-ovariolysis
7. Specific postoperative complications
   The same as for salpingo-ovariolysis

B. Salpingo-oophorectomy
1. Indications
   - Diseased tube and ovary, such that tubal or ovarian preservation is not possible with adequate blood supply

- Benign neoplasm of ovary
- Ovarian malignancy
- Inflammatory tubo-ovarian mass
- Repeated infections (this may have socioeconomic implications, such as loss of work time)

2. Preoperative investigation
   Complete blood count

3. Preoperative preparation
   - Povidone-iodine douche
   - Abdominoperineal shave
   - Enema
   - Prophylactic treatment with antibiotics

4. Surgical technique
   - Make a low midline incision.
   - Explore the abdomen to evaluate its contents.
   - Pack the intestines away from the operative field.
   - Perform adhesiolysis as indicated.
   - Open the broad ligament.
   - Isolate the infundibulopelvic ligament.
   - Check by visualization and palpation to be sure that the ureter is clear.
   - Clamp, cut, and tie the infundibulopelvic ligament with synthetic absorbable suture.
   - Clamp, cut, and tie the utero-ovarian ligament and tube.
   - Separate anatomical clamping is preferred to a single-clamp technique that includes all structures.
   - Reperitonealization is not necessary.
   - Laparoscopic salpingo-ophorectomy is an alternative technique.

5. Intraoperative complications
   - Bleeding from the infundibulopelvic ligament
   - Bleeding from the utero-ovarian ligament: should be controlled under direct vision with clamping and tying, being sure of the position of the ureter

6. Specific postoperative management
   Routine postoperative management

7. Postoperative complications
   The same as for salpingo-ovariolysis

C. Tubal Sterilization

1. Indications
   Requested by patient

2. Preoperative investigation
   Pregnancy test if menses are delayed

3. Preoperative preparation
   - Povidone-iodine douche
   - Abdominoperineal shave
   - Emptying the bladder
   - Prophylactic treatment with antibiotics

4. Surgical technique
   - Laparoscopic
     — Patient in modified lithotomy position (ski position)
     — Insert uterine elevator into the uterus.

— Insert orogastric tube to decompress stomach.
— Insert Veres needle through a small subumbilical incision, and establish pneumoperitoneum.
— Place patient in the Trendelenburg position.
— Insert a trocar through the umbilical incision, and insert laparoscope.
— Insert a second, smaller trocar suprapubically.
— Insert forceps through the suprapubic trocar, and inspect pelvic and abdominal organs.
— Elevate the uterus toward the abdominal wall and to one side, and grasp the midpoint of the tube with forceps.
— Examine the entire tube, including the fimbria.
— Coagulate a segment at least 1.5 cm long in the midisthmus portion of the tube and divide with scissors.
— Repeat a similar procedure on the contralateral side.
— Inspect the pelvis for hemostasis.
— Expel gas from the peritoneal cavity.
— Close the incisions with no. 0 absorbable sutures on the fascia and close skin with subcuticular 3-0 synthetic absorbable sutures.

- Minilaparotomy
  — Place patient in modified lithotomy position.
  — Insert uterine elevator into the uterus.
  — Make a small vertical or transverse incision two fingerbreadths above the symphysis.
  — Place patient in the Trendelenburg position.
  — Retract the edges of the incision with four goiter retractors.
  — Elevate the uterus toward the incision, and deliver one tube.
  — Identify the distal end of the tube, and inspect the ovary.
  — Perform tubal ligation by incising a 1-cm segment of the tube, ligating each end, and cauterizing the stump.
  — Perform a similar procedure on the opposite side.
  — Check for hemostasis.
  — Close the wound in layers with synthetic absorbable sutures.

- Transvaginal
  — Place patient in lithotomy position.
  — Grasp the posterior lip of the cervix with a tenaculum.
  — With Mayo scissors, make a transverse incision in the posterior vaginal fornix to open into the cul-de-sac.
  — With a vein retractor, hook around the fallopian tube on one side and deliver its distal end through the incision.
  — Excise the distal half of the tube, and doubly ligate the stump.
  — Repeat the procedure on the opposite side.
  — Check for hemostasis.

— Close the incision in the vaginal wall with multiple interrupted 2-0 synthetic absorbable sutures.

5. Specific postoperative management
- No coitus allowed for 6 weeks after the transvaginal approach.
- All procedures may be performed on an outpatient basis.

6. Specific postoperative complications
- Perforation of viscus or major vessel with laparoscopic technique
- Bleeding from tubal mesentery

Reading List

Starkey TA, Williams TJ. Plastic operations on the fallopian tubes. *Minn Med* 1969;52:903–908.

Smith RA, Symmonds RE. Vaginal salpingectomy (fimbrectomy) for sterilization. *Obstet Gynecol* 1971;38:400–402.

Thorsteinsson VT, Pratt JH. Gynecologic operations for sterilization. *Minn Med* 1972;55:204–210.

Thie JL, Williams TJ, Coulam CB. Repeat tuboplasty compared with primary microsurgery for postinflammatory tubal disease. *Fertil Steril* 1986;45:784–787.

Patton PE, Williams TJ, Coulam CB. Microsurgical reconstruction of the proximal oviduct. *Fertil Steril* 1987;47:35–39.

Patton PE, Williams TJ, Coulam CB. Results of microsurgical reconstruction in patients with combined proximal and distal tubal occlusion: double obstruction. *Fertil Steril* 1987;48:670–674.

Williams TJ. Surgical procedures for inflammatory tubal disease. *Obstet Gynecol Clin North Am* 1987;14:1037–1048.

Williams TJ. Tubal microsurgery for pelvic inflammatory disease. *Postgrad Obstet Gynecol* 1987;4:1–8.

Jacobs LA, Thie J, Patton PE, et al. Primary microsurgery for postinflammatory tubal infertility. *Fertil Steril* 1988;50:855–859.

Williams TJ. Reoperation of the tubes and ovaries. *In:* Nichol DH, ed. *Reoperative gynecologic surgery.* St. Louis, MO: Mosby Year Book, 1991:123–132.

CHAPTER 10

Surgery of the Ovaries

Maurice J. Webb, M.D. and Timothy O. Wilson, M.D.

I. Ovarian Cystectomy

A. Indications
1. Persistent simple ovarian cyst
2. Simple cyst >6 cm in diameter
3. Symptomatic cyst
4. Complex cyst that appears benign

B. Preoperative Investigations
1. Complete blood count
2. Urinalysis
3. Ultrasonography usually is performed to help decide whether to observe the patient or to operate.
4. Pregnancy test if indicated

C. Preoperative Preparation
1. Abdominal shave
2. Empty patient's bladder.

D. Surgical Technique
1. Make a midline lower abdominal incision. A transverse incision may be used if there is convincinge vidence that the cyst is benign and small (e.g., dermoid).
2. Laparoscopic removal is possible with small benign cysts.
3. Inspect the abdominal contents.
4. Collect peritoneal washings for cytologic examination.

Maurice J. Webb: Chairman, Division of Gynecologic Surgery and Consultant, Department of Surgery, Mayo Clinic and Mayo Foundation; Professor of Obstetrics and Gynecology, Mayo Medical School, Rochester, Minnesota.
Timothy O. Wilson: Consultant, Departments of Obstetrics and Gynecology and Surgery, Mayo Clinic and Mayo Foundation; Assistant Professor of Obstetrics and Gynecology, Mayo Medical School, Rochester, Minnesota.

5. Inspect the uterus, tubes, and ovaries, and determine whether cyst appears benign and is suitable for cystectomy with conservation of ovarian tissue.
6. If there is doubt about whether the cyst is benign or malignant, oophorectomy may be preferable to avoid rupturing a malignant tumor.
7. Grasp the utero-ovarian ligament and infundibulopelvic ligament with Allis forceps to stabilize the ovary.
8. Pack off the peritoneal cavity to avoid contamination if the cyst ruptures.
9. Inspect the ovary containing the cyst, and plan an appropriate incision in the ovarian stromal capsule that conserves as much normal ovarian tissue as feasible.
10. With a scalpel, cut the stroma superficially around the base of the cyst circumferentially.
11. Use Metzenbaum scissors and toothed Adson forceps to tunnel between the cyst wall and the stromal capsule, and cut along the previously demarcated incision line.
12. After completing the incision, peel the cyst out of the ovary, and achieve hemostasis with cautery and 3-0 synthetic absorbable sutures.
13. Send the ovarian cyst for frozen section analysis.
14. Reconstruct the ovary in layers with 3-0 or 4-0 synthetic absorbable sutures.
15. Place a small piece of adhesion barrier over the suture line, and close the incision.
16. Alternatively, the ovary may not be reconstructed.

E. Specific Postoperative Management
Remove the urethral catheter on the morning after the operation.

F. Specific Postoperative Complications
Bleeding from the cystectomy site produces ovarian hematoma or hemoperitoneum.

II. Oophorectomy

A. Indications

1. Large benign ovarian cyst in which partial ovarian conservation and reconstruction are not feasible
2. Stage IA ovarian cancer in which preservation of ovarian function is desired
3. Torsion of ovary with infarction
4. Residual ovary syndrome
5. Unilateral pelvic pain
6. Tubo-ovarian abscess
7. Ovarian pregnancy
8. In association with hysterectomy

B. Preoperative Investigations

Depends on presumed diagnosis but may include
1. Ultrasonography
2. Assay for human chorionic gonadotropin
3. Complete blood count
4. Diagnostic laparoscopy

C. Preoperative Preparation

The same as for ovarian cystectomy

D. Surgical Technique

1. Make a midline lower abdominal incision.
2. Explore the abdominal contents.
3. Collect peritoneal washings for cytologic examination if indicated.
4. Inspect the opposite ovary and the uterus if present.
5. If the ovary is adherent to the medial leaf of the broad ligament peritoneum, do not dissect it free; remove the peritoneum attached to the ovary, thereby preventing ovarian remnant syndrome.
6. Open the broad ligament by incising the peritoneum lateral and parallel to the infundibulopelvic ligament.
7. Retract the ovary medially, and identify the ureter.
8. Perforate the broad ligament peritoneum beneath the ovary. Clamp and divide the ovarian vessels between the two straight Kocher clamps, and ligate the pedicle.
9. Divide the peritoneum beneath the ovary up toward the uterus.
10. Clamp, divide, and ligate the tube and ovarian ligament flush with the uterus if present.
11. Irrigate the pelvis, and close the abdominal incision.
12. Laparoscopic oophorectomy is feasible in many cases; however, the principle of opening the broad ligament to identify the ureter before stapling the ovarian vessels with the endo-GIA instrument is important.
13. This may be best accomplished by first dividing the tube and ovarian ligament with the stapler and incising the broad ligament peritoneum with endoscopic scissors, thus opening the broad ligament to display the ureter. Finally, staple across the ovarian vessels.

E. Specific Postoperative Management

Remove the uretheral catheter on the morning after the operation.

F. Specific Postoperative Complications

1. Bleeding from loose pedicle
2. Ovarian remnant syndrome, wherein some ovarian stroma is left attached to the ovarian pedicle or pelvic sidewall peritoneum and becomes symptomatic

III. Ovarian Transposition

A. Indication

Patient is to receive pelvic irradiation and there is a desire to preserve ovarian function, e.g., at the time of radical hysterectomy for cervical cancer.

B. Preoperative Investigations

Depends on the indications for the operation

C. Preoperative Preparation

The same as for the primary operation

D. Surgical Technique

1. Divide the peritoneum on each side of the ovarian vessels high above the pelvic brim.
2. Place a metallic hemostatic clip on each end of the ovary that is to be transposed for purposes of later radiographic localization.
3. On the right side, bring the ovarian vessels beneath the ascending colon, and tack the ovary to the parietal peritoneum up high in the right paracolic gutter.
4. On the left side, bring the ovarian vessels out beneath the descending colon and attach the ovary to the left paracolic gutter peritoneum at a high level.
5. Avoid twisting the ovarian pedicle and causing torsion.
6. An intraoperative radiograph may be made to confirm that the ovaries are placed outside the planned field of radiation.

E. Specific Postoperative Management

Depends on the primary operation

F. Specific Postoperative Complications

1. Cystic change in transposed ovaries is not uncommon.
2. Not all transposed ovaries have normal hormonal function.
3. Cyclic pain may develop in the region of the transposed ovary.
4. Rarely, metastasis can occur to the transposed ovary.

IV. Ovarian Cancer Staging

A. Indication
Known or suspected ovarian cancer

B. Preoperative Investigations
1. Complete blood count
2. Serum chemistry
3. Serum CA-125
4. Chest radiography
5. Urinalysis
6. Ultrasonography, computed tomography, or magnetic resonance image if indicated

C. Preoperative Preparation
1. Polyethylene glycol-electrolyte solution (GoLYTELY) or standard bowel preparation
2. Prophylactic treatment with antibiotics
3. Place transurethral Foley catheter

D. Surgical Technique
1. The principle is to determine the pathologic diagnosis; after ovarian carcinoma has been confirmed, it is mandatory to assess the entire peritoneal cavity and retroperitoneal lymph nodes to determine pathologically whether there is any evidence of metastasis.
2. A lower midline incision is mandatory for known or suspected ovarian cancer staging.
3. On opening the peritoneal cavity, promptly obtain peritoneal cytologic specimens.
4. Carefully explore the abdominal cavity to assess the peritoneal surfaces for evidence of spread of disease, especially the right hemidiaphragm. Palpate and examine all intraabdominal and retroperitoneal organs to look for evidence of metastatic disease.
5. Perform a unilateral or bilateral salpingo-oophorectomy in the customary fashion, as described above. If the patient has completed childbearing, perform a total abdominal hysterectomy and bilateral salpingo-oophorectomy. If the patient wishes preservation of childbearing potential and has a low-grade lesion confined to one ovary, perform a similar staging procedure, but with preservation of the uterus and normal remaining tube and ovary.
6. Submit the ovary suspected to have cancer to pathology for frozen section evaluation to confirm the diagnosis of ovarian carcinoma.
7. Next, perform a formal staging procedure, consisting of 11 pairs of peritoneal biopsies, complete omenectomy, and pelvic and aortic lymphadenectomy.
8. Complete the pelvic portion of the operation first. Next, extend the incision above the umbilicus, and complete the upper abdominal portion of the procedure.
9. Obtain two biopsy samples from each of the following sites: bladder peritoneum, right and left pelvic sidewalls, cul-de-sac, right and left colic gutters, ileal mesentery and serosa, sigmoid mesentery and serosa, and right hemidiaphragm. Note any other suspicious lesion and excise it and submit it for pathologic examination.
10. Perform a bilateral pelvic lymphadenectomy, removing the lymph nodes from the external iliac, common iliac, internal iliac, and obturator areas. This may be a unilateral lymphadenectomy if the patient has disease confined to one ovary only.
11. Extend the incision above the umbilicus.
12. Dissect the omentum from its attachment to the transverse colon, and ligate it at its origin from the stomach. Anesthesia personnel should place a nasogastric tube in the stomach.
13. On the right side, extend the retroperitoneal defect in the broad ligament cephalad, identifying the ureter and ovarian vessels as well as the inferior vena cava and the aorta. Complete an aortic lymphadenectomy, removing the lymph nodes to the level of the right renal vessels. Ligate the ovarian vessels where they enter the vena cava and aorta. Excise these vessels, and submit them for pathologic assessment.
14. On the left side, reflect the sigmoid to the right, and extend the broad ligament incision, revealing the ureter and left side of the aorta. Excise the lymph nodes to the level of the renal vessels, and, again, ligate the ovarian vessels where they enter the aorta and left renal vein, and submit them to pathology.
15. Perform a routine appendectomy, especially if the ovarian malignancy has mucinous histologic features.
16. If the retroperitoneal spaces are closed, place drains in the lymphatic spaces. If the lymphatic spaces are left open, then drains are not placed.
17. Irrigate the abdomen, and close the incision, leaving a subcutaneous suction drain.

E. Specific Postoperative Management
1. Remove the nasogastric tube the morning after surgery if the patient is not nauseated and the output is minimal.
2. Remove the urethral catheter on the second morning postoperatively.
3. Oral intake resumes 1 to 2 days postoperatively.

F. Specific Postoperative Complications
1. Same as for hysterectomy
2. Ileus is common, especially with paraaortic dissection.
3. Lymphocyst formation is uncommon and may be treated, if large and symptomatic, with radiologically guided aspiration. Operation is seldom necessary.

V. Ovarian Cancer Debulking

A. Indication
Metastatic ovarian cancer

B. Preoperative Investigations
1. Complete blood count
2. Serum chemistry
3. Serum CA-125
4. Chest radiography
5. Urinalysis
6. Colon radiography if indicated
7. Ultrasonography, computed tomography, or magnetic resonance imaging, if indicated

C. Preoperative Preparation
1. Polyethylene glycol-electrolyte solution (GoLYTELY) or standard bowel preparation
2. Prophylactic treatment with antibiotics
3. Parenteral nutrition if weight loss is significant

D Surgical Technique
1. The principle is to remove the uterus, both tubes and ovaries, the omentum, all visible intraperitoneal disease, and the pelvic and aortic lymph nodes.
2. In practice, no two operations are identical because of the large variation with metastases.
3. With extensive pelvic peritoneal disease, en bloc retroperitoneal hysterectomy, bilateral salpingo-oophorectomy, anterior resection of the rectosigmoid, and removal of all the pelvic peritoneum are necessary for pelvic clearance. The essential steps of this operation are as follows:
4. Grasp the uterus with straight Kocher forceps, as in a hysterectomy.
5. Open the broad ligament peritoneum, and identify the ureters.
6. Develop the pararectal and paravaginal spaces.
7. Clamp, divide, and ligate the infundibulopelvic ligaments.
8. Clamp, divide, and ligate bilaterally the anterior division of the internal iliac artery.
9. Dissect the bladder peritoneum away from the back of the bladder downward to expose the cervix (Fig. 1).
10. Dissect the bladder away from the front of the cervix and vagina, and open the vagina at the 12 o'clock position.
11. Place a Henrontin tenaculum on the outer edge of the vagina and on the cervix, and proceed with the hysterectomy in a retrograde fashion.
12. Continue the incision around the vaginal cuff.
13. Dissect the rectum away from the back of the vagina below the peritoneal reflection.
14. Place the right hand in the presacral space, and mobilize the rectosigmoid from the front of the sacrum.
15. Clamp and ligate the middle rectal vessels, and skeletonize, clamp, and transect the rectum at the appropriate level below the peritoneal reflection.
16. Lift up the uterus, tubes and ovaries, rectosigmoid, and pelvic peritoneum out of the pelvis and cover them with sponges (Fig. 2).

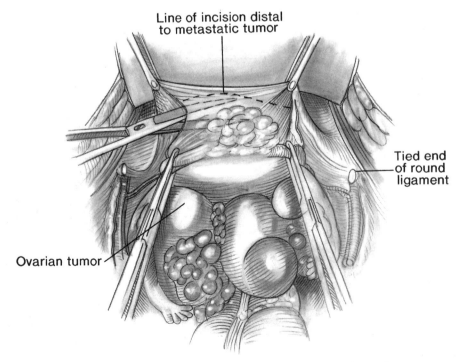

FIG. 1. Dissection of bladder peritoneum involved with metastatic ovarian cancer.

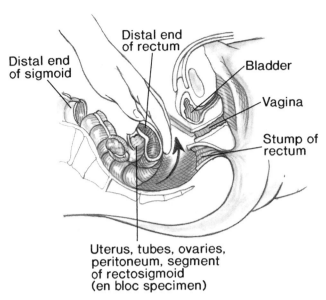

FIG. 2. En bloc resection of the uterus, tubes, ovaries, and rectosigmoid.

Labels in figure:
Distal end of sigmoid
Distal end of rectum
Bladder
Vagina
Stump of rectum
Uterus, tubes, ovaries, peritoneum, segment of rectosigmoid (en bloc specimen)

21. The ultrasonic surgical aspirator or argon beam coagulator is useful for removing peritoneal deposits, especially subdiaphragmatic ones.
22. Leave two Jackson-Pratt drains down in the pelvis on either side of the colorectal anastomosis, and bring them out through the anterior abdominal wall.
23. Irrigate the peritoneal cavity thoroughly, and close the incision, leaving a subcutaneous suction drain.

E. Specific Postoperative Management
1. Remove the urethral catheter on the second morning postoperatively.
2. Remove one pelvic drain when drainage is < 50 mL / 24 h.
3. Remove the second pelvic drain when intestinal function returns.
4. Parenteral nutrition may be required postoperatively.

F. Specific Postoperative Complications
1. Prolonged ileus is not uncommon.
2. Intestinal anastomotic leak: colostomy is required.

VI. Second-Look Laparotomy

A. Indication
1. Patient with epithelial ovarian carcinoma who responded postoperatively to chemotherapy and is clinically free of disease

B. Preoperative Investigations
1. Complete blood count
2. Urinalysis

17. Clamp and divide the mesentery of the sigmoid at an appropriate level above the pelvic tumor, and transect the sigmoid.
18. Remove the specimen, and send it for pathologic examination.
19. Reanastomose the descending colon to the rectal stump in two layers with running 3-0 synthetic absorbable suture supported by interrupted 3-0 silk sutures or by using the intraluminal stapler (Fig. 3).
20. Perform the total omentectomy and pelvic and aortic lymphadenectomy.

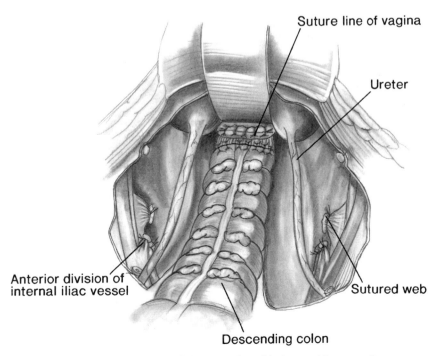

Labels in figure:
Suture line of vagina
Ureter
Sutured web
Descending colon
Anterior division of internal iliac vessel

FIG. 3. Reanastomosis of the rectosigmoid after en bloc resection.

3. Chest radiography
4. Computed tomography of abdomen and pelvis
5. Serum CA-125

C. Preoperative Preparation

1. Polyethylene glycol-electrolyte solution (GoLYTELY) bowel preparation
2. Abdominal shave

D. Surgical Technique

1. Make a midline incision.
2. Free all peritoneal adhesions.
3. Collect washings from the pelvis, right and left paracolic gutters, and right diaphragmatic region for cytologic examination.
4. Inspect the entire peritoneal cavity, including all parietal and visceral peritoneal surfaces.
5. Perform biopsy of any suspicious areas.
6. In addition to samples from specific biopsy sites, take random biopsy samples from the cul-de-sac peritoneum, bladder peritoneum, pelvic sidewall peritoneum, ovarian pedicles, both paracolic gutters, the undersurface of the right leaf of the diaphragm, the omental remnant, the mesentery and serosa of the sigmoid, and the mesentery and serosa of the ileum.
7. If lymphadenectomy was not performed at primary operation, proceed to perform pelvic and aortic lymphadenectomy up to the level of the renal vessels.
8. Irrigate the abdomen, and close the incision.
9. If macroscopic residual disease is detected and it is potentially resectable to no visible residual disease, then proceed with secondary debulking.
10. If gross macroscopic disease is present but is not completely resectable, secondary debulking is not beneficial except in grade 1 or low malignant-potential disease.

Reading List

Pratt JH. Surgery of endometriosis. *J Okla State Med Assoc* 1961;54:586–591.

Malkasian GD Jr, Pratt JH, Dockerty MB. Primary ovarian pregnancy: report of two cases. *Obstet Gynecol* 1963;21:632–635.

Malkasian GD Jr, Symmonds RE. Treatment of unilateral encapsulated dysgerminoma. *Am J Obstet Gynecol* 1964;90:379–382.

Thompson JP, Dockerty MB, Symmonds RE, et al. Ovarian and paraovarian tumors in infants and children. *Am J Obstet Gynecol* 1967;97:1059–1065.

Puga FJ, Gibbs CP, Williams TJ. Castrating operations associated with metastatic lesions of the breast. *Obstet Gynecol* 1973;41:713–719.

Webb MJ, Decker DG, Mussey E, et al. Factors influencing survival in stage I ovarian cancer. *Am J Obstet Gynecol* 1973;116:222–228.

Williams TJ. Management of malignant, premalignant, and minimally invasive ovarian lesions. *Prog Clin Cancer* 1973;5:183–186.

Williams TJ, Symmonds RE, Litwak O. Management of unilateral and encapsulated ovarian cancer in young women. *Gynecol Oncol* 1973;1:143–148.

Hill LM, Johnson CE, Lee RA. Ovarian surgery in pregnancy. *Am J Obstet Gynecol* 1975;122:565–569.

Lee RA, Kazmier FJ. Ovarian hematoma complicating anticoagulant therapy. *Mayo Clin Proc* 1977;52:19–23.

Webb MJ, Snyder JA Jr, Williams TJ, et al. Second-look laparotomy in ovarian cancer. *Gynecol Oncol* 1982;14:185–293.

Buskirk SJ, Schray MF, Podratz KC, et al. Ovarian dysgerminoma: a retrospective analysis of results of treatment, sites of treatment failure, and radiosensitivity. *Mayo Clin Proc* 1987;62:1149–1157.

Lee RA. Ovarian remnant syndrome. *In:* Nichols DH, ed. *Clinical problems, injuries, and complications of gynecologic surgery,* 2nd ed. Baltimore: Williams & Wilkins, 1988:16–19.

Podratz KC, Malkasian GD Jr, Wieand HS, et al. Recurrent disease after negative second-look laparotomy in stages III and IV ovarian carcinoma. *Gynecol Oncol* 1988;29:274–282.

Podratz KC, Schray MF, Wieand HS, et al. Evaluation of treatment and survival after positive second-look laparotomy. *Gynecol Oncol* 1988;31:9–21.

Webb MJ. Cytoreduction in ovarian cancer: achievability and results. *Baillieres Clin Obstet Gynaecol* 1989;3:83–94.

Webb MJ. Ovarian remnant syndrome. *Aust NZ J Obstet Gynaecol* 1989;29:433–435.

Moen MD, Cliby WA, Wilson TO. Stage III papillary serous cystadenocarcinoma of the ovary in a 15-year-old female. *Gynecol Oncol* 1994;53:274–276.

van Winter JT, Simmons PS, Podratz KC. Surgically treated adnexal masses in infancy, childhood, and adolescence. *Am J Obstet Gynecol* 1994;170:1780–1786.

Zanetta G, Keeney GL, Cha SS, et al. Flow-cytometric analysis of deoxyribonucleic acid content in advanced ovarian carcinoma: its importance in long-term survival. *Am J Obstet Gynecol* 1996;175:1217–1225

CHAPTER 11

Surgery of the Vagina

Maurice J. Webb, M.D.

I. Cystocele Repair

A. Indications
1. Symptomatic prolapse
2. Urinary stress incontinence associated with prolapse

B. Principles
1. Cystocele repair usually is performed as part of a vaginal hysterectomy and repair for prolapse or repair of a posthysterectomy vaginal vault prolapse.
2. Repair of cystocele alone is an uncommon operation, because an anterior vaginal wall prolapse is usually associated with uterine or vault descensus and rectocele.

C. Preoperative Investigations
1. Complete blood count
2. Urinalysis with culture if indicated
3. Serum chemistry
4. Electrocardiography if older than 40 years
5. Chest radiography if older than 60 years or if indicated by history
6. Cystoscopy and urodynamics if indicated by history of mixed incontinence or other bladder symptoms

D. Preoperative Preparation
1. Povidone-iodine douche
2. Perineal shave
3. Microenema
4. Suprapubic catheter inserted

E. Surgical Technique
1. Usually, vaginal hysterectomy (see Chapter 7) or repair of the enterocele of a vaginal vault prolapse (see section II below) will have been performed just before the cystocele repair.

Maurice J. Webb: Chairman, Division of Gynecologic Surgery and Consultant, Department of Surgery, Mayo Clinic and Mayo Foundation; Professor of Obstetrics and Gynecology, Mayo Medical School, Rochester, Minnesota.

2. Grasp the cut anterior edge of the vaginal vault transverse incision with straight Kocher forceps at either edge of the wedge of the vaginal wall to be excised.
3. Grasp the suburethral vaginal mucosa with a third Kocher forceps.
4. Tunnel beneath the vaginal mucosa in the midline vertically, and divide the mucosa with Metzenbaum scissors, creating a vertical linear incision (Fig. 1).
5. Grasp the cut edge of the mucosa on each side with two Allis forceps, retracting the mucosa by putting traction on the Allis and Kocher forceps.
6. Dissect the pubocervical fascia and bladder off the mucosa with Metzenbaum scissors on the patient's left side.
7. Repeat the dissection on the right vaginal wall flap, with the first assistant grasping the bladder fascia with long Russian forceps to maintain traction during the dissection.
8. Imbricate the bladder fascia (pubocervical) from the vaginal vault upward to the urethral meatus with multiple 2-0 synthetic absorbable interrupted sutures.
9. Make a special effort to reconstruct the urethrovesical angle by plicating the pubocervical fascia beneath the urethra and bladder neck.
10. Remove the Allis and Kocher forceps from each vaginal cut edge of the mucosa, assess the amount of redundant mucosa to be excised, and remove it bilaterally with scissors (Fig. 2).
11. Approximate the vaginal mucosal edges starting at the urethral meatus and working inferiorly, using multiple interrupted 2-0 synthetic absorbable sutures.
12. Inspect for hemostasis, and insert a vaginal pack or proceed to rectocele repair if indicated.

F. Specific Postoperative Management
1. The vaginal pack is removed the morning after the operation.
2. Suprapubic catheter clamping is commenced on the third day postoperatively.

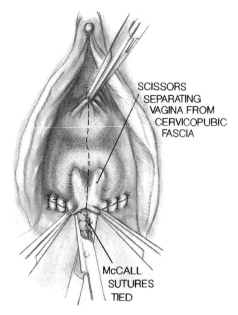

FIG. 1. Tunneling beneath the vaginal mucosa during repair of cystocele. (Redrawn from Lee RA. *Atlas of gynecologic surgery.* Philadelphia: WB Saunders, 1992:142, with permission.)

G. Specific Postoperative Complications

1. Hemorrhage: usually due to dissection in the wrong plane when developing vaginal mucosal flaps
   - Hemostasis must be secured before inserting the pack. Do not rely on the pack to maintain hemostasis.
   - If bleeding occurs, inspect carefully and insert mucosal sutures if bleeding is from the edge.
   - If there is hematoma, open the mucosal incision, evacuate the hematoma, secure hemostasis, and reapproximate the incision.

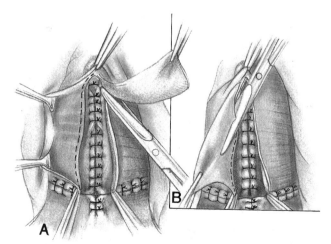

FIG. 2. A and **B:** Excision of redundant anterior vaginal wall mucosa. (Redrawn from Lee RA. *Atlas of gynecologic surgery.* Philadelphia: WB Saunders, 1992:146, with permission.)

2. Inability to void: rarely is a prolonged problem; patience usually corrects the difficulty.
   - Self-catheterization may be preferable to prolonged suprapubic catheterization if voiding difficulties persist.
   - Avoid removal of sutures, dilation of the urethra, etc., because the problem will almost always resolve with time.
3. Urinary fistula: due to unrecognized trauma to the bladder or urethra
   - Insert a large-bore urethral catheter, and leave to drain freely for at least 4 weeks.
   - Perform intravenous pyelography to check that there has been no damage to the ureters.
   - If the fistula persists, do not attempt repair until 3 months postoperatively.
4. Ureteral obstruction: due to fascial plication sutures being placed too deeply
   - Obstruction is recognized by a slight increase in the serum level of creatinine 2 days postoperatively and confirmed by intravenous pyelography or ultrasonography.
   - Place an anterograde or retrograde ureteral stent (see Chapter 5) if possible.
5. Vaginal stenosis: due to excessive excision of vaginal mucosa
   - Always assess the functional diameter and the depth of the vagina carefully before excising mucosa.
   - Surgical correction may be required (see section IV below).

II. Enterocele Repair

A. Prophylaxis

1. Prophylaxis at the time of abdominal or vaginal hysterectomy may prevent subsequent enterocele formation.
2. Abdominal prophylaxis
   - Excise deep cul-de-sac peritoneum.
   - Excise a wedge of posterior fornix vaginal mucosa.
   - Suture plication of the uterosacral ligaments in the midline.
   - High closure of cul-de-sac peritoneum (Moscowitz- or Halban-type procedure)
   - Prophylaxis of enterocele is especially important if abdominal hysterectomy is being combined with a retropubic suspension, because enterocele is common after this operation.
3. Vaginal prophylaxis
   - This is performed at the time of vaginal hysterectomy.
   - Modified McCall-type sutures are inserted at every vaginal hysterectomy, possibly combined with excision of a wedge of posterior fornix vaginal mucosa (see Chapter 7).
   - The redundant cul-de-sac peritoneum of a potential enterocele is also excised at this time.

B. Indications

1. Symptomatic prolapse
2. Enterocele is usually associated with a cystocele and rectocele except occasionally after a previous vaginal repair, when an enterocele may protrude but the anterior and posterior vaginal walls remain well supported.

C. Preoperative Investigations

1. The same as for cystocele repair
2. Intravenous pyelography may be indicated to assess ureters in patients with recurrent enterocele.

D. Preoperative Preparation

The same as for cystocele repair

E. Surgical Technique: Vaginal Approach

1. Grasp the vaginal vault scar with two or three Kocher forceps.
2. Make an elliptical incision around the vault to excise the scar (Fig. 3).
3. Partially reflect the bladder off the vault anteriorly.
4. Enter the enterocele sac posteriorly behind the scar.
5. With a finger in the enterocele sac, dissect the bladder away from the anterior peritoneum, and open the anterior peritoneum (Fig. 4).
6. Clamp the uterosacral/cardinal ligament tissue on either side with Heaney clamps, and then divide, transfix, and ligate it after palpating the ureter with the index finger against the Deaver retractor in the lateral vaginal fornix (see Chapter 7), thus excising the vault scar.
7. Dissect the redundant cul-de-sac peritoneum (enterocele sac) back to its reflection on the rectum, and excise it (Fig. 5).
8. Occasionally, the enterocele is of a sliding type, with the contents being sigmoid colon.

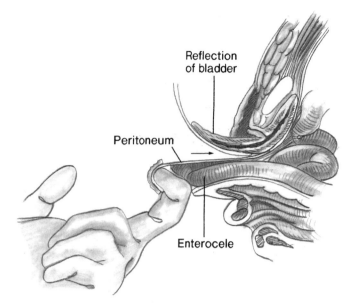

FIG. 4. Dissection of the enterocele sac for excision.

9. Remove a wedge from the posterior fornix vaginal mucosa; the width of the wedge determines the subsequent diameter of the vagina.
10. Grasp the anterior and posterior peritoneal reflections with Allis forceps, and insert a pack into the pelvic cavity.
11. Insert a number of modified McCall sutures using no. 1 synthetic absorbable suture (see Chapter 7) to approximate the uterosacral ligaments and to obliterate the cul-de-sac.
12. Close the pelvic peritoneum at a high level with a purse string of 2-0 synthetic absorbable sutures.
13. Bring the ends of this suture out through the posterior fornix mucosa and tie.

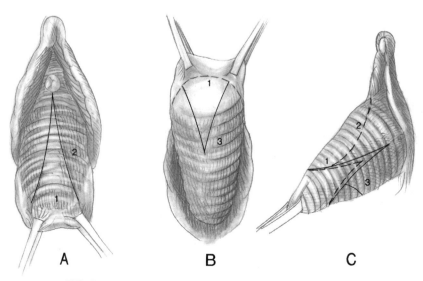

FIG. 3. Incisions used in vaginal repair of vault prolapse.

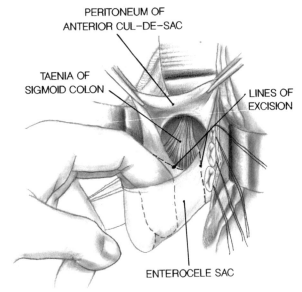

PERITONEUM OF
ANTERIOR CUL-DE-SAC

TAENIA OF
SIGMOID COLON

LINES OF
EXCISION

ENTEROCELE SAC

FIG. 5. Preparing the enterocele sac for excision. (Redrawn from Lee RA. *Atlas of gynecologic surgery.* Philadelphia: WB Saunders, 1992:138, with permission.)

14. Tie the McCall sutures.
15. Close the vaginal vault with interrupted 2-0 synthetic absorbable sutures.
16. Perform anterior and posterior vaginal repairs (Fig. 6).
17. Place a pack in the vagina.

F. Specific Postoperative Management

1. Remove the pack the next morning.

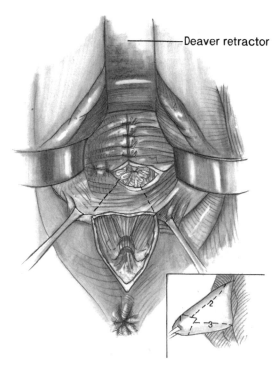

Deaver retractor

FIG. 6. Posterior vaginal wall incisions used in repair of rectocele.

2. If cystocele repair was performed, clamp the suprapubic catheter on postoperative day 3.
3. If there was no anterior repair, remove the urethral catheter the morning after the operation.

G. Specific Postoperative Complications

Ureteral obstruction

1. This may occur because McCall sutures were placed too high or too anteriorly.
2. These sutures should always be inserted posteriorly and lateral to the rectum and well behind the 3 o'clock and 9 o'clock positions at the vault.

H. Surgical Technique: Abdominal Approach

Used for patients in whom further vaginal surgery would severely compromise vaginal dimensions and for whom continued vaginal function is required.

1. Treat prophylactically with antibiotics perioperatively.
2. Distend the vagina with a gauze pack or plastic mold.
3. Insert an indwelling urethral catheter.
4. Make a midline lower abdominal incision.
5. Incise the peritoneum between the bladder and the distended vaginal vault transversely.
6. Carefully dissect the bladder from the front of the vagina, approximately 4 cm.
7. Make a vertical incision in the peritoneum on the right side of the sigmoid mesentery, from the sacral promontory down to the vaginal vault.
8. Reflect the rectosigmoid to the patient's left side, and expose the front of the upper sacrum.
9. Take care to avoid traumatizing the presacral veins.
10. Excise the redundant peritoneum of the cul-de-sac enterocele sac.
11. Select and trim a piece of polytef (Teflon) or expanded polytef (Gore-Tex) mesh so that it easily reaches from the vagina to the sacrum.
12. Suture the mesh to the anterior aspect of the upper 3 cm of the vagina with multiple nonabsorbable sutures [e.g., 3-0 silk, monofilament (Prolene)].
13. Take care to prevent the sutures from entering the vaginal lumen.
14. Suture the upper end of the mesh strip to the front of vertebra S2 periosteum so that the mesh is not under tension (Fig. 7).
15. Secure meticulous hemostasis.
16. Close the pelvic peritoneum over the mesh sling so that it lies retroperitoneally, thereby obliterating the cul-de-sac.
17. Close the incision, and remove the vaginal pack or mold.

I. Specific Postoperative Management

1. Remove the urethral catheter on the second postoperative morning.
2. Have the patient avoid lifting or straining for 6 to 8 weeks.

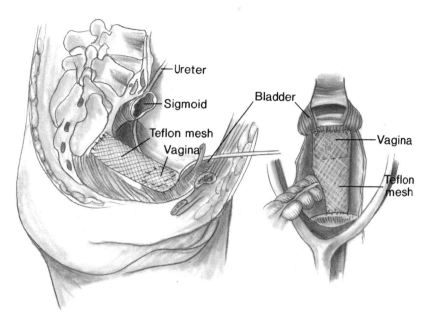

FIG. 7. Insertion of mesh to support the prolapsed vaginal vault.

J. Specific Postoperative Complications

1. Ureteric obstruction caused by kinking of the ureter during closure of the cul-de-sac peritoneum
2. Sepsis related to the presence of foreign material in the pelvis
3. Vesicovaginal fistula related to unrecognized bladder trauma
4. Urinary stress incontinence occurs in a significant number of patients, possibly because of flattening of the urethrovesical angle with traction on the vaginal vault.
5. Later, ulceration of the vaginal mucosa with exposure of the mesh. This may require removal of the mesh.

III. Rectocele Repair

A. Indications

1. Symptomatic protrusion of the posterior vaginal wall
2. Digital splinting of the posterior vaginal wall required to expel feces from the rectum
3. Usually, this operation is performed in association with vaginal hysterectomy and repair or with vault prolapse repair.

B. Preoperative Investigations

1. The same as for cystocele repair
2. Proctoscopy, manometry, and colonoscopy if indicated by symptoms

C. Preoperative Preparation

1. Povidone-iodine douche
2. Perineal shave
3. Microenema

D. Surgical Technique

1. Place patient in the lithotomy position.
2. Grasp the forchette with tenacula at approximately the 5 o'clock and 7 o'clock positions.
3. Take a V-shaped wedge from the forchette and perineum as determined by the anatomical defect (a wide shallow wedge if deficient perineum and large rectocele or a narrow deeper wedge if minimal buildup of the perineum is necessary).
4. Grasp the midline vaginal mucosa with straight Kocher forceps.

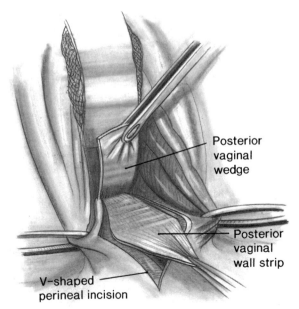

FIG. 8. Wedge of posterior vaginal wall mucosa excised in repair of rectocele.

5. Excise a wedge of the posterior vaginal wall with Mayo scissors (Fig. 8).
6. Extend the incision line up to the vaginal vault.
7. The width of the posterior vaginal wall to be excised is determined by the size of the rectocele and the required postoperative diameter of the vagina.
8. Approximate the posterior vaginal mucosa with a running locked 2-0 synthetic absorbable suture.
9. Undermine the distal 2 cm of the vaginal wall, and approximate the levator muscles in the midline with one or two no. 1 synthetic absorbable sutures.
10. Approximate the perineal skin with continuous subcuticular 3-0 synthetic absorbable suture.
11. Insert a vaginal pack and urethral catheter.

E. Specific Postoperative Management
The vaginal pack and catheter may be removed the morning after the operation.

F. Specific Postoperative Complications
1. Hemorrhage: bleeding is more common from the posterior than the anterior vaginal wall and usually is easily controlled with sutures.
2. Vaginal stenosis: due to too much excision of vaginal mucosa
3. Transverse ridge or bar across the posterior vaginal wall: the levator muscles have been approximated too high, creating a ridge that can cause dyspareunia.
4. Rectovaginal fistula: sutures were placed in the rectal lumen at the time of the repair of the rectocele.

IV. Vaginal Stenosis and Introital Stenosis

A. Indications
1. Narrowing of the vagina causing dyspareunia or apareunia
2. May be caused by obstetric trauma, surgery, or radiation therapy
3. May be of various degrees, from a tight band in one section of the vagina to narrowing of the full length of the vagina

B. Preoperative Investigations
The same as for repair of cystocele and rectocele

C. Preoperative Preparation
The same as for rectocele repair

D. Surgical Technique
1. Individualization of techniques must occur, dependent on the site and the degree of stenosis.
2. For a simple introital stenosis, narrow vaginal band, or ring stenosis, vertical division of the stenotic band with transverse closure of the single or multiple incisions may suffice.
3. For more severe degrees of stenosis, a Z-plasty with rotation of Z-shaped flaps will provide additional diameter (see Chapter 23).

4. Additional diameter may be obtained by swinging a single or multiple perineal or vulval skin flaps into the vagina after laying open the stenotic segment.
5. Skin flaps are usually routine in the management of postradiation stenosis.

E. Specific Postoperative Management
The same as for repair of cystocele and rectocele

F. Specific Postoperative Complications
1. Restenosis: regular coitus or the wearing of a mold may be necessary to prevent restenosis.
2. Fistula: more likely to occur in postirradiated patients

V. Imperforate Hymen

A. Indications
Hematocolpos in menstruating female or before menarche if diagnosed

B. Preoperative Investigations
1. No specific tests required
2. May be confirmed with pelvic ultrasonography

C. Preoperative Preparation
1. Microenema
2. Prophylactic treatment with antibiotics

D. Surgical Technique
1. Place patient in the lithotomy position.
2. Make a cruciate incision in the imperforate hymen, allowing hematocolpos to drain.
3. Excise excess hymenal skin, and secure hemostasis with small 3-0 synthetic absorbable sutures.
4. Do not irrigate or insert anything into the vagina because of the risk of ascending infection.

E. Specific Postoperative Management
Nothing allowed in the vagina for 4 to 6 weeks

F. Specific Postoperative Complications
1. Ascending uterotubal infection
2. Infertility due to uterotubal damage caused by infection, hematometra, or hematosalpinx

VI. Vaginal Agenesis: The McIndoe Procedure

A. Indication
Vaginal reconstruction in the presence of congenital absence of the vagina

B. Preoperative Investigations
1. Intravenous pyelography is mandatory because associated renal abnormalities are common.

2. Pelvic ultrasonography, laparoscopy, and chromosomal analysis may provide information about the rest of the genital tract.

C. Preoperative Preparation
1. Microenema
2. Prophylactic treatment with antibiotics

D. Surgical Technique
1. The patient lies on her side with knees flexed.
2. Collect a split-skin graft from the buttock/hip region.
3. Apply plastic occlusive dressing to the donor site.
4. Reposition the patient to the lithotomy position.
5. Fashion a mold out of plastic foam and cover with a condom.
6. Tie the open end of the condom with heavy silk thread, and leave the ends long.
7. Suture the split-skin graft over the mold with continuous 3-0 synthetic absorbable suture; avoid placing sutures in the condom (Fig. 9).
8. Make a transverse incision across the center of the dimple of the vaginal remnant.
9. With a combination of blunt and sharp dissection and the use of two Deaver retractors, dissect in the avascular plane up to the cul-de-sac peritoneal reflection.
10. Secure meticulous hemostasis with cautery and fine sutures.
11. Insert skin-graft-covered mold into the vaginal space, and suture the introitus together to hold the mold in place.
12. Pass a urethral catheter into the bladder and leave it to drain freely.

E. Specific Postoperative Management
1. With the patient under general anesthesia, remove the mold on postoperative day 7.
2. Inspect the graft to see whether it has taken, and gently irrigate the vagina.

3. Suture the skin of the graft to the skin of the introitus with multiple interrupted 3-0 synthetic absorbable sutures.
4. Insert a plastic obturator into the vagina, and remove the catheter.
5. The obturator is worn continuously for 8 weeks and is removed daily for cleansing.
6. The obturator, then, is worn regularly at night until the patient is coitally active.
7. Leave the donor site alone until the adhesive dressing falls off.

F. Specific Postoperative Complications
1. If the graft does not take: may cause localized stenosis or granulation
2. Vesicovaginal, urethrovaginal, or rectovaginal fistula: may be due to dissection in the wrong plane or to pressure from the mold
3. Vaginal stenosis: caused by poor take of the graft or failure to wear the mold.

Note: Repair of a fistula or stenosis often results in a vaginal cavity that is less than satisfactory.

VII. Vaginal Septa

A. Types
1. Transverse
   - Develops at the junction of the müllerian and ectodermal components of the embryonic vagina
   - Usually presents with coital problems or with difficulty inserting a tampon
2. Longitudinal
   - Develops because of failure of fusion of the two müllerian ducts
   - May be complete, giving two vaginas or a partial septum extending partway down the vagina
   - May be associated with duplication of the cervix or uterus
   - May be associated with renal abnormalities

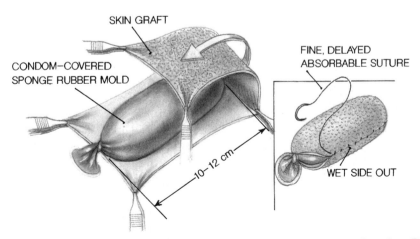

FIG. 9. Split-skin graft being sutured over the condom-covered mold. (Redrawn from Lee RA. *Atlas of gynecologic surgery.* Philadelphia: WB Saunders, 1992:26, with permission.)

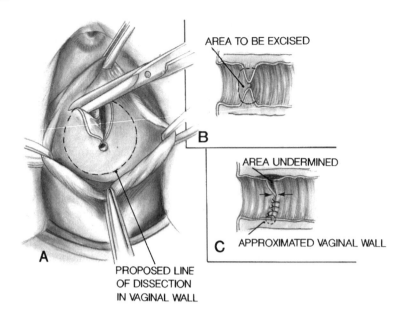

AREA TO BE EXCISED

B

AREA UNDERMINED

C APPROXIMATED VAGINAL WALL

A

PROPOSED LINE
OF DISSECTION
IN VAGINAL WALL

FIG. 10. A–C: Excision of transverse septum. (Redrawn from Lee RA. *Atlas of gynecologic surgery.* Philadelphia: WB Saunders, 1992:35, with permission.)

B. Preoperative Investigations

1. Perform urography if there is a longitudinal septum.
2. Ultrasonography and laparoscopy may give further information about the uterus and adnexa.

C. Preoperative Preparation

1. Povidone-iodine douche
2. Microenema

D. Surgical Technique

1. Transverse septum
  - Make a cruciate incision in the septum.
  - Excise each of the four quadrants of the septum individually (Fig. 10).
  - Take care not to remove underlying vaginal mucosa.
  - Suture the vaginal mucosal edges together with interrupted 3-0 synthetic absorbable sutures.
2. Longitudinal septum
  - With scissors, incise the middle of the septum from the introitus up to the cervix.
  - With traction on the septum, excise the anterior and posterior segments.
  - Take care not to remove the adjacent vaginal mucosa.
  - Approximate the vaginal mucosal edges with interrupted 3-0 synthetic absorbable suture.
  - Insert a vaginal pack and urethral catheter.

E. Specific Postoperative Management

1. Remove the catheter and vaginal pack the next morning.
2. Patient may resume coitus when healed, approximately 4 to 6 weeks.

F. Specific Postoperative Complications

Vaginal stenosis: due to removal of some of the vaginal wall mucosa along with the septum

VIII. Vaginal Reconstruction (Postoperatively)

A. Indications

1. The most common indication for vaginal reconstruction postoperatively is after pelvic exenteration.
2. Skin grafting with the McIndoe technique may be indicated immediately after vaginectomy, either complete or partial, to maintain vaginal function.
3. Vaginal lengthening procedures may be necessary after partial vaginal resection, e.g., Wertheim hysterectomy with upper vaginectomy.

B. Preoperative Investigations

Routine laboratory tests

C. Preoperative Preparation

Depends on the technique to be used, e.g., bowel preparation for sigmoid neovagina

D. Surgical Technique

1. McIndoe technique
  - The technique described in section VI above may be used after vaginectomy by the vaginal route (e.g., for vaginal intraepithelial neoplasia) by placing the graft-covered mold in the vaginal cavity after mucosal resection (partial or complete).
  - Stenosis may develop at the junction of the graft and the normal vaginal mucosa after partial vaginectomy.
  - After pelvic exenteration, the graft-covered mold may be wrapped in an omental pedicle and placed in the pelvis to create a neovagina.
  - Prolapse of the neovagina is not uncommon with the latter technique.

2. Sigmoid neovagina
   - At exenteration, isolate a segment of sigmoid colon as a conduit.
   - Rotate the conduit through 180 degrees, and suture it to the introitus.
   - Close the proximal end (Fig. 11).
3. Cecal neovagina
   - Isolate the cecum, terminal ileum, and part of the ascending colon on ileocolic vessels.
   - Rotate the segment through 180 degrees, and anastomose the open end of the ascending colon to the introitus.
   - Perform ileoascending anastomosis to restore bowel continuity.
4. Gracilis neovagina
   - Develop myocutaneous flaps based on the gracilis muscle from the medial aspect of each thigh.
   - Make the flap approximately 20 cm long × 6 cm wide.
   - The vascular pedicle of the gracilis muscle arises approximately 7 cm from the pubic tubercle.
   - Loosely suture the muscle to the overlying skin to prevent skin separation.
   - Tunnel the flaps beneath the skin lateral to the introitus and let lie in approximation.
   - Construct a pouch by suturing one flap to the other with continuous 2-0 synthetic absorbable suture.
   - Rotate the pouch of the neovagina through 90 degrees, and place it in the pelvic cavity.
   - Suture the neovagina to the presacral area to keep it in place.
   - Suture the distal edge of the pouch to the introitus with interrupted 2-0 synthetic absorbable sutures.
   - Reapproximate the thigh wounds over suction drains with subcuticular 3-0 synthetic absorbable sutures.
5. Rectus abdominus flaps
   - Similar indications and technique as for gracilis flaps, but the myocutaneous flap is based on the rectus abdominus muscle and the underlying deep epigastric vessels.
   - Develop a large unilateral skin flap, and roll it into a cylinder to construct the neovagina.
   - Close the abdominal wound over suction drains.
6. Pudendal thigh fasciocutaneous flaps
   - Develop a fasciocutaneous flap from each groin based on the pudendal artery.
   - Make the flaps approximately 15 × 6 cm, and base them posteriorly (Fig. 12).
   - Construct a pouch as before, insert it into the pelvic cavity, and suture it to the presacral area.
   - Close the groin defects over suction drains.
   - The major advantage of this technique is that the scars are all hidden, and the viability of the flaps is not a problem.
7. Williams operation
   - It is useful as a vaginal lengthening technique rather than for reconstruction.
   - Make a V-shaped incision around the introitus.
   - Suture the mucosal cut edge side to side across the introitus with interrupted 2–0 synthetic absorbable sutures.
   - Similarly, reapproximate the outer skin layer edges, thereby constructing a somewhat vertical pouch that adds vaginal length.

E. Specific Postoperative Management
1. All drains can be removed when the output is <20 mL/24 h.

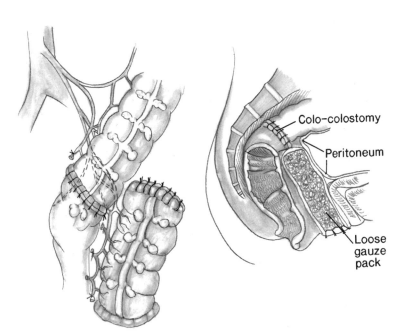

FIG. 11. Construction of a sigmoid neovagina.

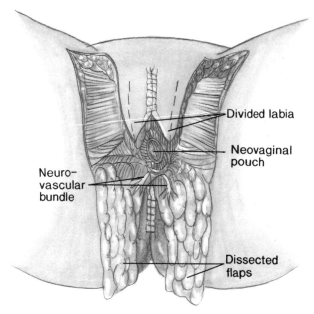

FIG. 12. Neovaginal construction using pudendal thigh fasciocutaneous flaps.

2. Patients with myocutaneous flaps are kept at bed rest for 2 to 3 days to prevent tension on the vascular pedicle.

F. Specific Postoperative Complications

1. Flap necrosis is not uncommon with gracilis and less common with rectus myocutaneous flaps.
2. Prolapse of the neovagina can occur with all techniques but is especially common with sigmoid neovagina or McIndoe technique with omental pedicle wrap.
3. Intestinal fistula may develop in relation to intestinal anastomosis.
4. Vaginal stricture occurs if McIndoe or sigmoid graft is attached to normal lower vagina. (It is best to excise the vagina completely.)
5. Splitting of the forchette skin occurs with coitus with the Williams operation.
6. If flap necrosis occurs, a split-skin graft may be applied after the infection has subsided and granulation tissue develops.
7. If prolapse occurs, the vagina may be reattached abdominally or, in the case of the sigmoid or cecum, the prolapsed portion of the bowel is amputated vaginally and the cut edge reapproximated to the introitus.

Reading List

Symmonds RE, Pratt JH, Ellis FH Jr. Ruptured enterocele. *Am J Obstet Gynecol* 1957;74:1150–1153.

Pratt JH. Vaginal relaxations. *Mississippi Doctor* 1959;37:107–110.

Kempers RD, Smith RA, Pratt JH. Descensus uteri and prolapse of the vaginal vault and enterocele: clinical and surgical considerations. *Minn Med* 1960;43:543–547.

Symmonds RE, Pratt JH. Vaginal prolapse following hysterectomy. *Am J Obstet Gynecol* 1960;79:899–908.

Pratt JH. The colon in vaginal reconstructions. *Proc Staff Meet Mayo Clin* 1961;36:34–40.

Pratt JH. Sigmoidvaginostomy: a new method of obtaining satisfactory vaginal depth. *Am J Obstet Gynecol* 1961;81:535–544.

Symmonds RE. Genital and rectal prolapse. *Gynecol Obstet Guide* 1963;721–745;761–763.

Symmonds RE. Uterovaginal prolapse. *Northwest Med* 1965;64:114–119.

Symmonds RE, Sheldon RS. Vaginal prolapse after hysterectomy. *Obstet Gynecol* 1965;25:61–67.

Pratt JH. Surgical repair of pelvic relaxations. *Chicago Med* 1966;69:1057–1062.

Pratt JH, Smith GR. Vaginal reconstruction with a sigmoid loop. *Am J Obstet Gynecol* 1966;96:31–40.

Cali RW, Pratt JH. Congenital absence of the vagina: long-term results of vaginal reconstruction in 175 cases. *Am J Obstet Gynecol* 1968;100:752–763.

Pratt JH. Vaginal atresia corrected by use of small and large bowel. *Clin Obstet Gynecol* 1972;15:639–649.

Pratt JH. Surgical repair of rectocele and perineal lacerations. *Clin Obstet Gynecol* 1972;15:1160–1172.

Lee RA. The vaginal approach to anterior vaginal relaxation. *Clin Obstet Gynecol* 1972;15:1098–1106.

Lee RA, Symmonds RE. Surgical repair of posthysterectomy vault prolapse. *Am J Obstet Gynecol* 1972;112:953–956.

Day TG Jr, Stanhope R. Vulvovaginoplasty in gynecologic oncology. *Obstet Gynecol* 1977;50:361–364.

Pratt JH, Field CS, Symmonds RE. Congenital absence of the vagina. *Excerpta Medica Int Congress Ser* 1977;412:343–348.

Symmonds RE. Relaxation of pelvic supports. *In:* Benson RC, ed. *Current obstetric & gynecologic diagnosis & treatment.* Los Altos: California, Lange Medical Publications, 1980:245–263.

Symmonds RE, Williams TJ, Lee RA, et al. Posthysterectomy enterocele and vaginal vault prolapse. *Am J Obstet Gynecol* 1981;140:852–859.

Pratt JH. Incarcerated procidentia. *In:* Nichols DH, Anderson GW, eds. *Clinical problems, injuries, and complications of gynecologic surgery,* 2nd ed. Baltimore: Williams & Wilkins, 1988:92–94.

Buss JG, Lee RA. McIndoe procedure for vaginal agenesis: results and complications. *Mayo Clin Proc* 1989;64:758–761.

Cliby WA, Dodson MK, Podratz KC. Uterine prolapse complicated by endometrial cancer. *Am J Obstet Gynecol* 1995;172:1675–1680.

Cliby WA, Podratz KC. Procidentia with adenocarcinoma of the endometrium. *In:* Nichols DH, DeLancey JOL, eds. *Clinical problems, injuries, and complications of gynecologic and obstetric surgery,* 3rd ed. Baltimore: Williams & Wilkins, 1995:170–173.

Lee RA. Pelvic organ prolapse. *ACOG Tech Bull* 1995;214.

Podratz KC, Ferguson LK, Hoverman VR, et al. Abdominal sacral colpopexy for posthysterectomy vaginal vault descensus. *J Pelv Surg* 1995;1:18–23.

Polasek PM, Erickson LD, Stanhope CR. Transverse vaginal septum associated with tubal atresia. *Mayo Clin Proc* 1995;70:965–968.

Webb MJ. Resection of the vagina, vaginal reconstruction, and dealing with the empty pelvis. *Magyar Noorvosok Lapja* 1995;58[Suppl 2] Evfolyam Kulonsyam:1–94.

Kammer-Doak DN, Magrina JF, Weaver A, et al. Vaginal hysterectomy with and without oophorectomy. *J Pelv Surg* 1996;2:304–309.

Webb MJ. Mayo culdoplasty in the treatment of vaginal vault prolapse. *In:* Gershenson DM, ed. *Operative techniques in gynecologic surgery.* Philadelphia: WB Saunders, 1996:104–110.

Webb MJ, Kinney WK. Radical vaginectomy and parametrectomy after inadvertent simple hysterectomy in cervical cancer. *In:* Panici PB, Scambia E, Maneochi F, Sevin BU, Mancuso S, eds. *Wertheims radical hysterectomy.* Rome Societa Editrice Universo, 1996:27–33.

Lee RA. Vaginal hysterectomy with repair of enterocele, cystocele, and rectocele. *In:* Rock JA, Thompson JD, eds. *Te Linde's operative gynecology,* 8th ed. Philadelphia: Lippincott-Raven, 1997:1059–1076.

Zanetta G, Welter VE, Lee RA. An unusual complication after a McIndoe procedure for vaginal agenesis. *J Pelv Surg* 1997;3:221–223.

Webb MJ, Aronson MP, Ferguson LK, et al. Posthysterectomy vaginal vault prolapse: primary repair in 693 patients. *Obstet Gynecol* 1998;92:281–285.

CHAPTER 12

Surgery of the Vulva

Maurice J. Webb, M.D.

I. Bartholin Duct Cyst/Abscess

A. Indications
1. Cystic enlargement of the Bartholin duct
2. Abscess formation in a cyst of the Bartholin duct

B. Preoperative Investigation
Culture the cervix and urethra if a gonococcal infection is suspected.

C. Preoperative Preparation
Povidone-iodine douche and perineal wash

D. Surgical Technique
1. Principles
   - Options involve:
     — Incision and drainage
     — Word catheter
     — Marsupialization
     — Excision
   - Recurrences are least likely with excision and most common with incision and drainage.
2. Incision and drainage
   - These usually are performed in association with acute abscess formation.
   - Infiltrate the skin with local anesthetic, and incise the abscess with a scalpel.
   - Take a sample of contents for culture.
   - A small gauze wick may be inserted into the cavity.
   - Recurrences are common.
3. Word catheter
   - This usually is performed with abscess formation.
   - Infiltrate the skin with local anesthetic.
   - Make a small incision over the abscess; drain the contents and culture.

- Insert a Word catheter, and inflate the bulb.
- Remove the catheter in about 5 to 7 days, after the sinus tract has had time to epithelialize.
4. Marsupialization
   - It can be used to treat abscess or cyst formation.
   - Infiltrate the skin with local anesthetic or use general anesthesia.
   - Excise an ellipse of skin over the cyst at the approximate location of the duct orifice.
   - Culture the contents.
   - Approximate the mucosal lining of the cyst wall to the vulval skin with multiple interrupted 3-0 synthetic absorbable sutures (Fig. 1).
5. Excision
   - Excision can be used if the site is not infected. If abscess formation is present, incise and drain first, and excise later when healed.
   - The advantage is that the gland and duct are excised, so that recurrences are rare.
   - Excision needs to be performed with the patient under general anesthesia.
   - Make an elliptical incision over the cyst, and retract the skin edges with Allis forceps.
   - Continue the dissection deep into the labia, and use cautery to maintain hemostasis.
   - Excise the duct and gland, and examine them histologically.
   - Secure hemostasis, and close the incision in layers with 3-0 synthetic absorbable sutures.

E. Specific Postoperative Management
1. Apply an ice pack to the vulva in the initial postoperative period.
2. Prescribe frequent sitz baths or perineal washes until healed.

F. Specific Postoperative Complications
1. Hematoma formation is not uncommon with excision of the Bartholin duct and gland; thus, hemostasis must be meticulous.

Maurice J. Webb: Chairman, Division of Gynecologic Surgery and Consultant, Department of Surgery, Mayo Clinic and Mayo Foundation; Professor of Obstetrics and Gynecology, Mayo Medical School, Rochester, Minnesota.

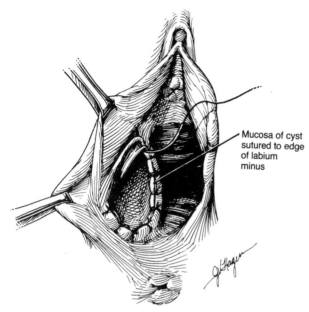

Mucosa of cyst
sutured to edge
of labium
minus

FIG. 1. Marsupialized Bartholin duct cyst. (From Lee RA. *Atlas of gynecologic surgery.* Philadelphia: WB Saunders, 1992:3, with permission.)

2. Recurrence of cyst/abscess is relatively common with incision and drainage and occasionally after Word catheter insertion or marsupialization.

II. Vulval Biopsy

A. Indications

Biopsy should be performed on any lesion on the vulva and the specimen examined histologically before treatment is initiated.

B. Surgical Technique
1. Infiltrate the lesion with local anesthetic.
2. Drill out a disk of representative tissue with a Key punch.
3. Cauterize the base or insert a single absorbable suture for hemostasis.

III. Hemivulvectomy

A. Indications
1. Unilateral invasive squamous cell carcinoma of the vulva in a lateral position which can be widely excised with good margins, especially in a young patient (the rest of the vulva should be normal)
2. Localized vulval melanoma
3. Localized Paget disease of the vulva
4. Localized vulval sarcoma
5. Unilateral Bartholin gland adenocarcinoma

Note: Inguinofemoral lymphadenectomy is indicated for squamous cell carcinoma or adenocarcinoma and possibly for melanoma with invasion >1 mm.

B. Preoperative Investigations
1. Chest radiography to exclude metastasis
2. Complete blood count
3. Computed tomography of the abdomen and pelvis if nodal metastases are suspected
4. Colposcopy as indicated

C. Preoperative Preparation
1. Vulval/perineal shave
2. Povidone-iodine douche and perineal wash
3. Prophylactic treatment with antibiotics
4. Mini-dose of heparin given subcutaneously if indicated

D. Surgical Technique
1. Grasp the skin of the vulva on the side of the lesion superiorly, inferiorly, medially, and laterally with Allis forceps.
2. Make an elliptical incision that extends at least 2 cm beyond the lesion in all directions, and dissect down below the superficial fascia to the fascia of the perineal musculature of the urogenital diaphragm. Use cautery to obtain hemostasis.
3. Check histologically that all margins are free of tumor.
4. Reapproximate the vulval tissue in layers with interrupted 3–0 synthetic absorbable sutures, obliterating all dead space.
5. Insert a small suction drain if indicated.

E. Specific Postoperative Management
1. Apply ice pack to the vulva in the initial postoperative period.
2. Prescribe frequent sitz baths or perineal washes until healed.

F. Specific Postoperative Complications
1. Infection
2. Hematoma formation
3. Separation of the skin incision

IV. Simple Vulvectomy

A. Indications
1. Extensive, superficially invasive squamous cell carcinoma
2. Intractable, severely symptomatic vulval dystrophy
3. Extensive Paget disease of the vulva

B. Preoperative Investigations
1. Routine laboratory tests depending on age and medical status
2. Colposcopy of the vulva if indicated

C. Preoperative Preparations
The same as for hemivulvectomy

D. Surgical Technique

1. Map out the line of incision depending on the nature of the lesion and the results of the colposcopic examination (Fig. 2).
2. Make incisions that extend from the midpoint of the mons above the clitoris downward in a curved fashion lateral to the labia majora.
3. The lowermost point of the lateral incisions is just lateral to the anterior aspect of the anus.
4. The perineal incision curves up and around the anus in a reversed U-shaped fashion.
5. This "butterfly-shaped" perineal incision prevents "dog ears" when the skin flaps are approximated.
6. With straight Kocher clamps on vulval skin edges and rakes to retract the lateral skin flaps, dissect down to the superficial fascia on each side of the vulva, using cautery.
7. Free the superior aspect of the vulva from the underlying symphysis pubis.
8. With traction on the vulval skin, dissect the posterior aspect of the vulva in a curved fashion, identifying the transverse perineal muscles and dissecting anteriorly to them.
9. Continue the perineal incision superiorly until it reaches the posterior vaginal fourchette.
10. Continue the lateral incisions medially until they reach the vaginal mucosa at the hymenal region.
11. Cut through into the vagina at the posterior fourchette, and carry the incision anteriorly on the vaginal wall up to the level of the urethral meatus.

12. Bring the incisions together above the urethral meatus in a reversed V-shape; this enables the meatus to be fixed in the midline to prevent spraying of urine.
13. The vulva is now attached only by the crura of the clitoris.
14. Clamp across the base of the clitoris, and then divide and ligate the clitoral stump.
15. Secure hemostasis and undermine the lateral skin flaps if necessary to allow tissue approximation.
16. Undermine the posterior vaginal wall a little to allow approximation of the vaginal mucosa to the perineal skin.
17. Close the incisions with interrupted vertical mattress 2–0 synthetic absorbable sutures in two layers.
18. Pay particular attention to the area around the urethral meatus to be sure that it is central and not pulled to one side. Also, do not allow it to retract into the vagina.
19. This is achieved by fixing the apex of the tissue above the urethra to the fascia over the symphysis pubis.

E. Specific Postoperative Management

1. The same as for hemivulvectomy
2. Indwelling catheter for 2 to 3 days

F. Specific Postoperative Complications

The same as for hemivulvectomy

V. Radical Vulvectomy

A. Indications

1. Invasive squamous cell carcinoma or adenocarcinoma of the vulva: cases in which the size or location of the lesion, the age of the patient, or the presence of widespread dystrophy make hemivulvectomy or wide local excision not feasible.
2. In young patients with widespread dystrophy or vulval intraepithelial neoplasia but with a locally resectable lesion, it is best to resect the cancer widely and treat the vulval intraepithelial neoplasia with laser therapy rather than remove the whole vulva.

B. Preoperative Investigations and Preparation

The same as for hemivulvectomy

C. Surgical Technique

1. The technique is similar to that for simple vulvectomy, except that the incision extends to the crural folds laterally.
2. Continue the dissection down to the periosteum of the symphysis, the deep fascia overlying the adductor muscle laterally, and the urogenital diaphragm centrally.

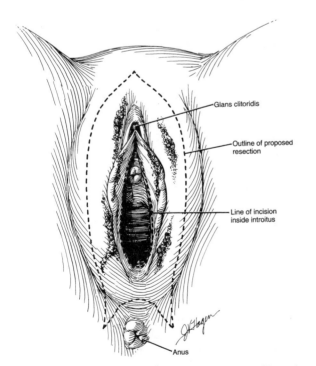

FIG. 2. Lines of excision for simple vulvectomy. (From Lee RA. *Atlas of gynecologic surgery.* Philadelphia: WB Saunders, 1992:6, with permission.)

Glans clitoridis

Outline of proposed resection

Line of incision inside introitus

Anus

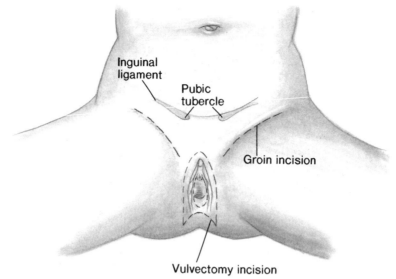

FIG. 3. Radical vulvectomy and groin node dissection through separate incisions.

3. It may be necessary to resect a segment of the distal urethra or a portion of the distal vaginal wall to get adequate clearance.
4. Surgical margins should be a minimum of 1 cm.
5. The procedure should be as radical as necessary to achieve clearance, because the resulting defect can be closed by the use of skin flaps (see Chapter 23).
6. Radical vulvectomy is normally performed in conjunction with inguinofemoral lymphadenectomy.
7. Inguinofemoral lymphadenectomy may be performed through separate incisions (Fig. 3; see Chapter 24) or as an en bloc procedure in conjunction with radical vulvectomy (see section VI below).

D. Specific Postoperative Management
The same as for simple vulvectomy

E. Specific Postoperative Complications
1. The same as for hemivulvectomy
2. Lymphadenectomy places the patient at risk for deep vein thrombosis and lymphocyst formation.
3. Use of mini-dose of heparin may predispose patient to lymphocyst formation or to excessive lymphatic drainage.

VI. Basset Operation: En Bloc Radical Vulvectomy with Bilateral Inguinofemoral Lymphadenectomy

A. Indications
1. Centrally located malignancy involving the clitoris or mons
2. Large anterior vulval lesion, even if lateral
3. Skin lymphatic metastases between the groin and the vulva

B. Preoperative Investigations and Preparation
The same as for hemivulvectomy

C. Surgical Technique
1. Place the patient in a modified lithotomy position: the ski position.
2. Make a downward curved incision that extends from one anterior superior iliac spine to the other and that reaches a point approximately 2 cm above the symphysis in the midline.
3. Continue the incision down to the anterior rectus muscle fascia, using cautery.
4. Undermine the abdominal wall skin flap about 3 to 4 cm to allow approximation of the skin edges later.
5. Continue the inferior incision inferiorly and medially in the groin skin creases, down to the crural skin folds lateral to the vulva.
6. Undermine the lower flap just below the superficial fascia down to the apex of the femoral triangle (Fig. 4).
7. Perform groin node dissection with a technique similar to the separate groin incision technique (see Chapter 24), leaving the nodes attached to the strip of excised groin skin (Fig. 5).
8. W-shaped lateral end of groin incisions may help prevent "dog ears."
9. Perform a similar groin dissection on the contralateral side.
10. Extend the incisions down to the vulva, and perform en bloc radical vulvectomy, leaving the nodes attached to vulval tissue in a "butterfly-shaped" specimen.
11. Reapproximate the vulval skin in two layers with interrupted 2–0 synthetic absorbable sutures.
12. Close the groin incisions in two layers with absorbable deep sutures and nonabsorbable interrupted skin sutures or clips over a suction drain.

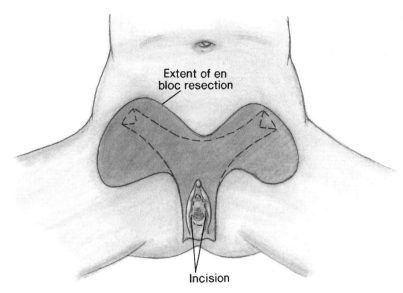

FIG. 4. Basset en bloc radical vulvectomy and groin node dissection showing extent of subcutaneous dissection.

D. Specific Postoperative Management

1. The same as for radical vulvectomy
2. Remove the groin suction drains when <50 mL of fluid is collected per 24 hours over a 2-day period or when wound breakdown allows drainage of lymphatic fluid.
3. Thromboembolus-deterrent stockings, sequential calf compression devices, and subcutaneous heparin should be considered for deep vein thrombosis prophylaxis.

E. Specific Postoperative Complications

1. The same as for radical vulvectomy and inguinofemoral lymphadenectomy

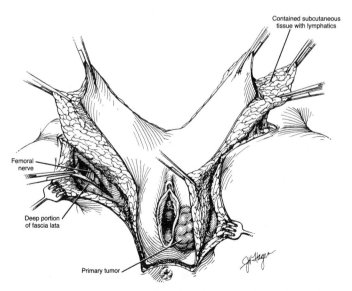

FIG. 5. En bloc radical vulvectomy and bilateral inguinofemoral lymphadenectomy for left vulval carcinoma. (From Lee RA. *Atlas of gynecologic surgery.* Philadelphia: WB Saunders, 1992:17, with permission.)

2. Wound breakdown is common; treatment includes debridement, grafting, packing, and skin flaps.
3. Femoral artery rupture is rare and associated with necrosis of the groin flaps.
4. If a large defect is present after resection, coverage with skin flaps (see Chapter 23) is preferable to closure with excessive tension.

VII. Skinning Vulvectomy

A. Indications

1. Extensive vulval intraepithelial neoplasia
2. Laser vaporization has less morbidity and is preferable to skinning vulvectomy.

B. Preoperative Investigations

Colposcopy and biopsy to define the lesion

C. Preoperative Preparation

1. Vulvoperineal shave
2. Povidone-iodine douche and perineal wash
3. Prophylactic treatment with antibiotics

D. Surgical Technique

1. With a colposcope, map out the area of vulval skin to be excised.
2. Incise the skin around the lesion with a scalpel, down to the subcutaneous fat.
3. Grasp the skin edges, and dissect the skin off the vulva, using scalpel, scissors, or cautery and continuously applying traction.
4. Secure meticulous hemostasis.
5. Apply the previously harvested split-skin graft to the denuded area and suture in place, using multiple interrupted 3-0 synthetic absorbable sutures.
6. Leave a number of the sutures long to tie over the dressing.

7. Perforate the skin graft in a number of places to allow serum to escape from beneath the graft.
8. Apply xeroform gauze and then fluffed gauze dressings over the graft and tie in place, using long sutures tied across the dressing.
9. Apply occlusive plastic dressing to the skin donor site.

E. Specific Postoperative Management

1. Keep the wound dry.
2. Remove the dressing from the graft site in 7 days.
3. Leave the donor-site dressing until it separates and falls off.

F. Specific Postoperative Complications

Loss of the skin graft may result in scarring and contracture, with less than desirable cosmetic results.

VIII. Laser Vaporization

A. Indications

1. Vulval condylomata
2. Vulval intraepithelial neoplasia
3. Vulval dystrophy

B. Preoperative Investigations and Preparation

1. Apply 3% acetic acid.
2. Perform colposcopy, and perform biopsy on the lesion.
3. Povidone-iodine douche and perineal wash

C. Surgical Technique

1. Identify the abnormal epithelium with colposcopy.
2. Map out the area to be vaporized with multiple short bursts of laser beam, going 3 to 5 mm beyond the lesion.
3. Systematically vaporize the abnormal skin in a constant painting type of motion to a depth of 3 mm.
4. Remove the carbonized debris with a moist sponge.

D. Specific Postoperative Management

1. Frequent sitz baths
2. Dry vulva with a hair dryer.
3. Apply povidone-iodine washes or antiseptic cream after each bath.
4. Analgesics as necessary

E. Specific Postoperative Complications

1. Secondary infection
2. Excessive scarring from extensive laser vaporization

Reading List

Dockerty MB, Pratt JH. Extramammary Paget's disease: a report of four cases in which certain features of histogenesis were exhibited. *Cancer* 1952;5:1161–1169.

Pratt JH, Watson JR. Carcinoma of the vulva: a new incision for one-stage radical vulvectomy and bilateral nodal dissection. *Proc Staff Meet Mayo Clin* 1955;30:23–31.

Pratt JH. Carcinoma of the vulva and its treatment. *Proc Natl Cancer Conf* 1960;363–370.

Symmonds RE, Pratt JH, Dockerty MB. Melanoma of the vulva. *Obstet Gynecol* 1960;15:543–553.

Kempers RD, Symmonds RE. Invasive carcinoma of the vulva and pregnancy: report of 2 cases. *Obstet Gynecol* 1965;26:749–751.

Pratt JH. Carcinoma of the vulva. *Curr Ther* 1969;841–842.

Yackel DB, Symmonds RE, Kempers RD. Melanoma of the vulva. *Obstet Gynecol* 1970;35:625–631.

Williams TJ. The role of surgery in the management of endometriosis. *Mayo Clin Proc* 1975;50:198–203.

Magrina JF, Webb MJ, Gaffey TA, et al. Stage I squamous cell carcinoma of the vulva. *Am J Obstet Gynecol* 1979;134:453–459.

Lee RA, Dahlin DC. Paget's disease of the vulva with extension into the urethra, bladder, and ureters: a case report. *Am J Obstet Gynecol* 1981; 140:834–836.

Podratz KC, Symmonds RE, Taylor WF. Carcinoma of the vulva: analysis of treatment failures. *Am J Obstet Gynecol* 1982;143:340–351.

Webb MJ. Complications of vulval and vaginal surgery. *In:* Delgado G, Smith JP, eds. *Management of complications in gynecologic oncology.* New York: John Wiley & Sons, 1982:213–228.

Podratz KC, Gaffey TA, Symmonds RE, et al. Melanoma of the vulva: an update. *Gynecol Oncol* 1983;16:153–168.

Podratz KC, Symmonds RE, Taylor WF, et al. Carcinoma of the vulva: analysis of treatment and survival. *Obstet Gynecol* 1983;61:63–74.

Podratz KC. Melanoma of the vulva. *Postgrad Obstet Gynecol* 1984;4:1–6.

Cliby WA, Dodson MK, Podratz KC. Cervical cancer complicated by pregnancy: episiotomy site recurrences following vaginal delivery. *Obstet Gynecol* 1994;84:179–182.

Magrina JF, Gonzalez-Bosquet J, Weaver AL, et al. Primary squamous cell cancer of the vulva: radical versus modified radical vulvar surgery. *Gynecol Oncol* 1998;71:116–121.

CHAPTER 13

Surgery of the Anus and Rectum

C. Robert Stanhope, M.D.

Repair of Fourth-Degree Perineal Tear and Anal Incontinence

A. Indications
1. Anal incontinence: uncontrolled and unacceptable loss of gas, liquid, or solid stool
2. Sexual dysfunction due to vaginal laxity
3. Recurrent urinary tract infections due to soilage

B. Preoperative Investigations
1. Anorectal manometry with compliance
   - Anal canal resting pressure
   - Anal canal squeeze pressure
   - Rectal anal sphincter inhibitory response
   - Rectal capacity and sensory status
2. Electromyographic study: to demonstrate
   - Denervation
   - Pudendal nerve terminal motor latency (PNTML) (surgical success is unlikely in presence of pudendal neuropathy)
   - Endoanal ultrasonography for concentric anal sphincter mapping
3. Proctoscopy or flexible sigmoidoscopy: to rule out
   - Inflammatory bowel disease
   - Neoplasm
   - Fistula
4. Complete blood count
5. Midstream urine culture

C. Preoperative Preparation
1. Mechanical bowel preparation [buffered oral saline laxative (Phospho-Soda)]
2. Perioperative treatment with broad-spectrum antibiotics

3. Povidone-iodine vaginal douche
4. Perineal shave, excluding mons pubis

D. Surgical Technique
1. General or regional anesthesia
2. Place patient in lithotomy position.
3. Povidone-iodine vaginal and perineal skin preparation
4. Carefully excise introital scar tissue if present.
5. Widely mobilize the distal vagina (posterior vaginal wall) off the anterior rectal wall.
6. Expose the levator ani, external anal sphincter, and internal anal sphincter muscles (Fig. 1).
7. Identify the separated ends of the external anal sphincter and the puborectalis muscles by using a peripheral nerve stimulator (optional).
8. Use interrupted no. 0 monofilament synthetic delayed absorbable sutures, inserting all sutures through the identified internal sphincter muscles and incorporating the internal sphincter by including the intervening wall of the rectum without entering the lumen.
9. Plicate the sphincter muscles so that the diameter of the lumen of the anal canal is decreased approximately 50% (it usually will feel snug around a small finger).
10. Approximate the external sphincter muscles over the entire length of the anal canal (approximately 4 cm).
11. Plicate the medial aspect of the puborectalis muscles (avoid developing a band of tissue that may cause vaginal stricture).
12. Achieve hemostasis as each suture is placed.
13. Reconstruct the perineal body.

E. Specific Postoperative Management
1. Apply an ice pack to the perineum for the first 12 hours postoperatively to decrease edema.
2. Use Foley catheter drainage for 24 hours or as needed.
3. Allow a low-residue diet when tolerated.
4. Encourage the use of stool softeners for at least 6 weeks: docusate sodium (Colace), 100 mg twice daily, or psyllium (Metamucil), twice daily.

C. Robert Stanhope: Consultant, Departments of Obstetrics and Gynecology and Surgery and Section of Medical Information Resources, Mayo Clinic and Mayo Foundation; Professor of Obstetrics and Gynecology, Mayo Medical School, Rochester, Minnesota.

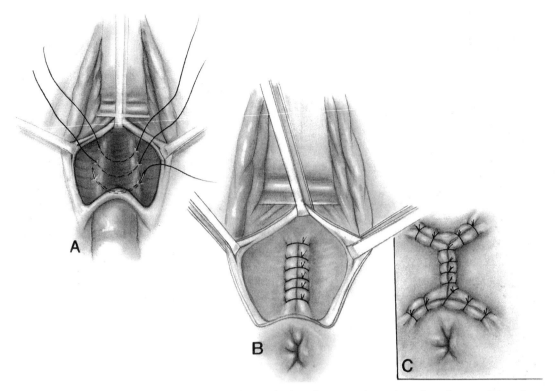

FIG. 1. A: Rectum dissected off the posterior vaginal wall, separating external anal musculature from internal anal sphincter; internal sphincter muscle plicated with interrupted sutures over the entire length of the anal canal. **B:** External sphincter muscle approximated, decreasing the lumen of the anal canal approximately 50%. **C:** Vulvovaginal and cutaneous margins approximated without tension.

5. Avoid the use of suppositories, laxatives, or enemas in the immediate postoperative period.
6. No coitus allowed for at least 6 weeks.

F. Specific Postoperative Complications
1. Hematoma
   Drain only if infected, expanding, or causing incapacitating pain.
2. Infection
   Use broad-spectrum antibiotics with good coverage for *Pseudomonas*.
3. Wound disruption
   • Close primarily if wound is not infected and disrupted less than 24 hours.
   • If infected, do not close until all inflammation resolves.

4. Persistent fecal incontinence
   • Repeat anal manometry.
   • If muscles are intact, use biofeedback.

Reading List

Manning PC Jr, Pratt JH. Fecal incontinence caused by lacerations of the perineum. Delayed repair. *Arch Surg* 1964;88:569–576.

Pezim ME, Spencer RJ, Stanhope CR, et al. Sphincter repair for fecal incontinence after obstetrical or iatrogenic injury. *Dis Colon Rectum* 1987;30:521–525.

Aronson MP, Lee RA, Berquist TH. Anatomy of anal sphincters and related structures in continent women studied with magnetic resonance imaging. *Obstet Gynecol* 1990;76:846–851.

Moen MD, Lee RA. Anorectal function in women: effects of episiotomy and repair. *J Pelv Surg* 1995;1:161–166.

Lee RA, Moen MD. Anal sphincteroplasty in operative techniques in gynecologic surgery. *Gynecol Surg* 1996;1:118–122.

CHAPTER 14

Surgery of the Urethra

Raymond A. Lee, M.D.

I. Diverticulum of the Female Urethra

A. Indications
1. Most of the patients experience urgency, frequency, and dyspareunia.
2. A history of recurrent urinary tract infections is usually present.
3. If symptomatic and identified, the diverticulum should be excised and the urethra repaired.
4. If it is an incidental finding and is asymptomatic, it may not require operation.

B. Preoperative Investigations
1. A palpable suburethral mass is found in 60% of the patients.
2. The diagnosis is confirmed by cystoscopic examination and voiding pressure cystourethrography.
3. Double-balloon urethrograms are helpful in demonstrating diverticula.
4. Diverticula may also be seen on ultrasonography of the urethra and noted with urodynamic studies.

C. Preoperative Preparation
1. Povidone-iodine douche
2. Prophylactic treatment with antibiotics

D. Surgical Technique
1. Make a vertical incision in the anterior vaginal wall.
2. Mobilize the vaginal mucosa laterally, as in a Kelly-Kennedy type anterior colporrhaphy.
3. Incise the pubocervical fascia in a similar fashion and mobilize laterally, exposing the underlying muscular coat of the urethra and the diverticulum.
4. The identification of the diverticulum may be enhanced by the cystoscopic placement of a ureteral catheter within the diverticulum.

Raymond A. Lee: Consultant, Departments of Obstetrics and Gynecology and Surgery, Mayo Clinic and Mayo Foundation; Professor of Obstetrics and Gynecology, Mayo Medical School, Rochester, Minnesota.

5. Others have suggested filling the diverticulum with latex material.
6. In most patients, the diverticulum can be identified without anything within the cavity itself.
7. Do not evacuate the diverticulum, because this may make identification difficult.
8. Dissection must be sharp, accurate, and meticulous.
9. Occasionally, the wall of the diverticulum is in immediate apposition to the pubocervical fascia and is entered as the fascia is mobilized.
10. If this is the case, an index finger may be inserted into the diverticulum and the diverticulum dissected until flush with its entrance into the urethra.
11. Resect the diverticulum, leaving a small remnant of the neck of the diverticulum at its entrance to the urethral mucosa.
12. The surgeon will be aware of the location of the ostium of the diverticulum from the cystoscopic examination and will also know whether more than one ostium is present.
13. Close the urethra in a linear direction over a 10 to 14 F polymeric silicone (Silastic) catheter with interrupted 4-0 synthetic absorbable sutures in an extramucosal fashion.
14. Rarely, the ostium of the diverticulum is repaired more appropriately in a transverse fashion.
15. After the urethral defect has been repaired, imbricate the pubocervical fascia in a side-to-side (vest-over-pants) fashion with interrupted 3-0 synthetic absorbable sutures.
16. Providing these additional layers and avoiding overlying suture lines reduce the potential for fistula formation.
17. Perfect hemostasis must be accomplished, after which the vaginal wall is approximated with interrupted 2-0 sutures.
18. The urethral catheter generally is left in place for 7 days.
19. In selected patients, a suprapubic catheter may be preferable, and occasionally both are indicated.

E. Specific Postoperative Management

1. The catheter is left connected to drainage for at least 1 week, after which the urethral catheter is removed or the suprapubic catheter is clamped and the patient is permitted to void transurethrally.
2. Avoid recatheterizing the patient transurethrally.

F. Postoperative Complications

1. Persistent pain, dysuria, and urinary tract infections may occur.
2. Recurrence of the diverticulum or reoccurrence in another location may occur.
3. Urethrovaginal fistula occurred in 1 of 85 patients in our series.
4. Urethral syndrome occurred in two patients.

G. Alternative Surgical Techniques

1. Perform a transurethral marsupialization by resection of the roof of the diverticulum with the use of a transurethral knife electrode.
2. Where the diverticulum is located in the distal urethra, use scissors to simply incise the urethra with one blade in the vagina, resulting in a vaginal marsupialization or distal urethrovaginal fistula.

II. Slough of the Floor of the Urethra

A. Indication

1. Major slough of the floor of the urethra, resulting in significant urinary incontinence
2. Can be one of the most difficult types of urinary incontinence to correct

B. Preoperative Investigation

Cystourethroscopic examination

C. Preoperative Preparation

1. Povidone-iodine douche
2. Prophylactic treatment with antibiotics

D. Surgical Technique

1. Make a midline incision in the anterior vaginal wall.
2. Extend this up and around the margins of the urethral defect as a U-shaped incision (Fig. 1).
3. Continue the dissection laterally, as for an anterior colporrhaphy.
4. Mobilize the remaining urethral margins only enough to provide a tension-free, accurate approximation of the urethral epithelium.
5. To obtain sufficient relaxation with larger defects that involve loss of the bladder neck and much of the trigone, it is essential to dissect up into the retropubic space as well as posteriorly and laterally.
6. Occasionally, the second row of sutures is placed initially in the supporting tissue before the urethral

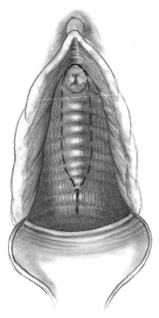

FIG. 1. U-shaped incision made on the side of the deficient urethra.

tube is constructed; this allows checking to be sure that there is no intraluminal placement of the sutures.
7. Next, reconstruct the urethral tube with interrupted 3-0 synthetic absorbable sutures in an accurate, tension-free hemostatic fashion (Fig. 2).
8. Tie the initially placed second row of sutures, and close the vaginal mucosa as a final layer.
9. In patients who have lost a significant portion of the anterior vaginal wall, use a pedicled, Martius-type bulbocavernosus muscle flap to substitute for the defect in the anterior vaginal wall (Fig. 3).
10. Suture this in place with interrupted synthetic absorbable 3-0 sutures (Fig. 4).

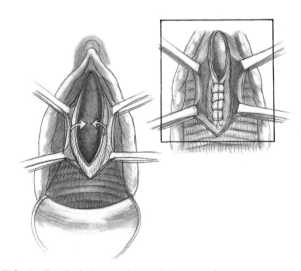

FIG. 2. Roof of the urethra rolled up to form a new narrow urethral tube.

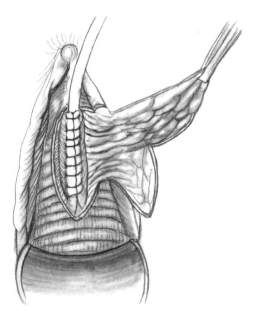

FIG. 3. Vulval skin flap mobilized to correct a vaginal mucosal defect.

E. Postoperative Management

1. A urethral catheter may be required for approximately 7 days; in selected patients, a suprapubic catheter may be placed either as an alternative to or in addition to the urethral catheter.
2. The urethral catheter is removed in approximately 1 week, and the patient is permitted to try to void.
3. Repeat urethral catheterization should be avoided if possible.
4. No attempt should be made to dilate the urethra.

F. Postoperative Complications

1. Urinary stress incontinence: may need retropubic suspension in 6 to 12 months.
2. Urethrovaginal fistula
3. Urinary tract infection
4. Disruption of vaginal incision
5. Prolonged urinary retention

III. Traumatic Disruption of Urethra

A. Indication

Trauma is an infrequent cause of severe injury to the urethra. When it occurs, surgical repair can usually be undertaken after the patient's condition has been stabilized. In the case shown in Figure 5, the urethra was traumatically disrupted from the bladder during operative vacuum extraction delivery.

B. Preoperative Investigations

1. Pelvic examination
2. Cystourethroscopic examination

C. Preoperative Preparation

1. Antibiotics if area is contaminated.
2. Povidone-iodine preparation of the vulva and vagina. Prepare for immediate reanastomosis if the patient's condition is stable.
3. When catheterization is attempted, the catheter will pass through the intact urethral meatus up the distal urethra, where it escapes into the vagina. After the disrupted site has been identified, the catheter should be passed through the bladder neck into the bladder.

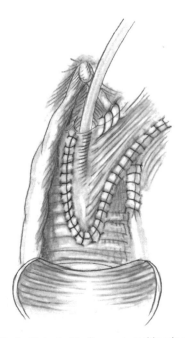

FIG. 4. Vulval skin flap sutured in place.

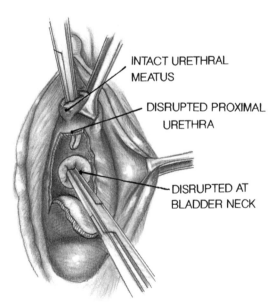

INTACT URETHRAL MEATUS

DISRUPTED PROXIMAL URETHRA

DISRUPTED AT BLADDER NECK

FIG. 5. Segment of proximal urethra disrupted from the bladder neck.

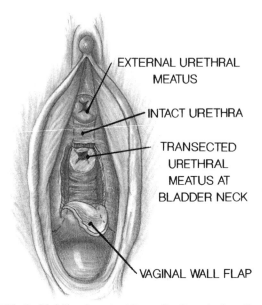

FIG. 6. Mobilized vaginal flap with disrupted urethra.

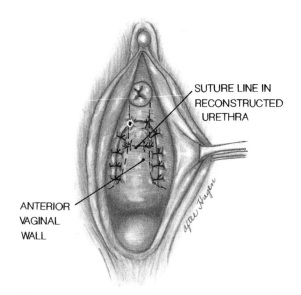

FIG. 8. Reconstructed urethra with closed vaginal flap.

D. Surgical Technique

1. Begin reconstruction by developing a flap of vaginal wall, hinged posteriorly (Fig. 6).
2. Begin reconstruction of the urethra by reanastomosing the disrupted urethra to the bladder neck; place the initial suture in the 12 o'clock position.
3. Place each fine delayed absorbable suture in an extramucosal position, reanastomosing the urethra to the bladder neck (Fig. 7).
4. After the urethra has been firmly attached with the sutures, place the vaginal flap in such a way that it avoids overlying suture lines (Fig. 8).

5. A small urethral catheter (10 F) is left in place for 5 to 7 days, after which it is removed, and spontaneous voiding occurs.
6. Four of these injuries have been repaired by us, and no urinary tract fistulas have developed. Excellent urinary continence has been maintained.

E. Postoperative Management

1. A suprapubic catheter may be used, and the urethral catheter may be removed if the injury to the urethra dictates this. The potential intraluminal placement of sutures could lead to development of a urethrovaginal fistula or slough of the floor of the urethra.

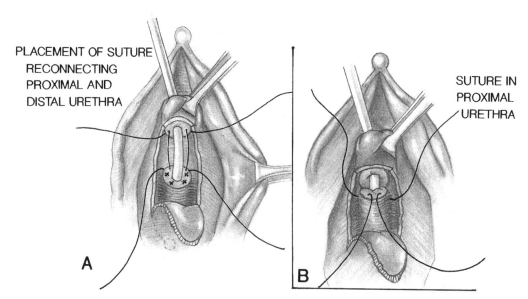

FIG. 7. A: First suture in place at the 12 o'clock position. **B:** Additional suture approximating urethra.

2. Leave the urethral catheter in place for 5 to 7 days, after which it may be removed. If a suprapubic catheter has been placed, it may be clamped on day 5 to 7 to permit voiding.

3. No coitus or vaginal examination allowed for 8 weeks.

F. Postoperative Complications

1. Infection: culture of urine or vaginal suture line as indicated
2. Bleeding from the mucosal edges
3. Development of a urethrovaginal fistula or stress urinary incontinence
4. Delayed voiding because of the snug closure of the urethra

Reading List

Symmonds RE. Loss of the urethral floor with total urinary incontinence: a technique for urethral reconstruction. *Am J Obstet Gynecol* 1969;103: 665–678.

Williams TJ. Reconstruction of the urethra and anterior vaginal wall. *Clin Obstet Gynecol* 1972;15:1122–1132.

Williams TJ, Symmonds RE. Urethral destruction and its management. *Dallas Med J* 1975;61:114–123.

Symmonds RE, Hill LM. Loss of the urethra: a report on 50 patients. *Am J Obstet Gynecol* 1978;130:130–138.

Lee RA. Diverticulum of the female urethra: postoperative complications and results. *Obstet Gynecol* 1983;61:52–58.

Lee RA. Diverticulum of the urethra: clinical presentation, diagnosis, and management. *Clin Obstet Gynecol* 1984;27:490–498.

Cornella JL, Larson TR, Lee RA, et al. Leiomyoma of the female urethra and bladder: report of twenty-three patients and review of the literature. *Am J Obstet Gynecol* 1997;176:1278–1285.

Kim KJ, Jurnalov CD, Lightner DJ, et al. Principles of urodynamics pressure measurement and its implication to female continence function. *J Biomech* 1998;31:861–865

CHAPTER 15

Urinary Fistula

Raymond A. Lee, M.D.

I. Urethrovaginal Fistula

A. Indication
Defect in the floor of the urethra causing urinary leakage

B. Preoperative Investigations
1. Cystoscopic examination
2. Urine culture

C. Preoperative Preparation
1. Antibiotics if infection is present
2. Povidone-iodine preparation of vulva and vagina
3. Do not attempt to repair until 8 to 12 weeks after previous operation.

D. Surgical Technique
1. Place patient in lithotomy position.
2. Perform a bimanual vaginal examination to assess the pelvis and mobility of the anterior vaginal wall.
3. Grasp the anterior vaginal mucosa with a Kocher clamp just proximal to the external urethral meatus.
4. Place Kocher clamps at each corner of the anterior vaginal wall cephalad to the base of the bladder.
5. Make a midline incision to separate the anterior vaginal wall from pubocervical fascia.
6. The incision should encircle the urethrovaginal fistula, leaving a small rim of the edge of vaginal mucosa attached to the edge of the fistula.
7. Mobilization of the anterior vaginal wall laterally is accomplished as with a modified Kelly-Kennedy anterior colporrhaphy (see Chapter 11).
8. Excise the fistula tract to freshen the edges of the urethra to aid approximation.
9. Place the appropriate number of interrupted 3–0 synthetic absorbable sutures in an extramucosal fashion, approximating the edges of the mucosa and submucosa of the urethra.
10. Insert a second inverting suture line of the same material, approximating the fascia and inverting the initial suture line.
11. The second layer of sutures is placed one suture past the proximal and distal ends of the original suture line.
12. If there is sufficient fascia, the second suture line may be closed in a "vest-over-pants" type of technique, overlapping the fascial layers.
13. This gives an additional layer to the repair, because the second suture line does not overlie the original suture line.
14. Leave a urethral catheter, size 12 to 14 F, in place in the urethra.
15. Otherwise, a large suprapubic catheter may be used.

E. Intraoperative Complications
1. Perforation of the base of the bladder
2. Overzealous repair of the fistula, producing slough of the floor of the urethra
3. Intraluminal placement of the sutures, leading to recurrence of the fistula and/or slough of the floor of the urethra

F. Postoperative Management
1. Clamping or removal of the catheter is dictated by the size of the urethral fistula, its location, previous number of repairs, and the surgeon's satisfaction with the closure.
2. No coitus or vaginal examinations for 6 weeks

G. Postoperative Complications
1. Infection: culture of urine and/or vaginal suture line
2. Bleeding from mucosal edges
3. Recurrence of the urethrovaginal fistula: if this occurs, try to divert the urine stream with replacement of the urethral catheter or suprapubic catheter or both.

Raymond A. Lee: Consultant, Departments of Obstetrics and Gynecology and Surgery, Mayo Clinic and Mayo Foundation; Professor of Obstetrics and Gynecology, Mayo Medical School, Rochester, Minnesota.

4. Delayed voiding because of snug closure of the urethra: maintain suprapubic catheter drainage and allow additional time for voiding.

II. Vesicovaginal Fistula

A. Indications

Vesicovaginal fistula that fails to heal after 4 weeks of bladder drainage with a catheter

B. Preoperative Investigations

1. Review of operative or other procedures responsible for fistula formation: any complications associated with the operation or postoperative recovery that would explain the fistula.
2. Cystoscopic examination for determination of the status of the ureters and the site of the defect in relation to ureteric orifices
3. Intravenous pyelography to assess the status of the ureters
4. Retrograde pyelography if indicated
5. Urine culture and sensitivities

C. Preoperative Preparation

1. Avoid operation until approximately 3 months after injury.
2. Vaginal preparation with povidone-iodine douche
3. Treatment of urinary infection if present
4. Prophylactic treatment with antibiotics
5. Ureteric catheterization if the ureters are close to fistula site, to aid in identification at operation

D. Surgical Technique: Vaginal Repair

1. Place patient in lithotomy position.
2. General anesthesia
3. Perform a bimanual vaginal examination to assess the pelvis.
4. Place straight Kocher clamps across the apex of the vagina to expose the fistula.
5. The fistula generally is found just anterior to the hysterectomy vault scar to one side of the midline.
6. Make an incision through the vaginal mucosa about the fistulous tract, and separate the vagina from the endopelvic fascia sufficiently to permit reapproximation of the walls free of tension (Fig. 1).
7. After adequately mobilizing the fistula, grasp the small rim of the vagina that circles the fistula, and excise the fistulous tract.
8. This enlarges the fistula but converts it to a fresh injury.
9. Closure of the fistulous tract, depending on its location, is usually accomplished in a transverse fashion.
10. Place the first layer of sutures, interrupted 3–0 synthetic absorbable sutures, in an extramucosal

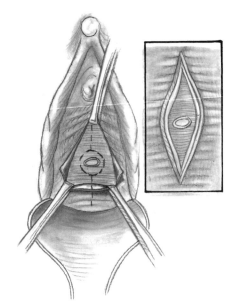

FIG. 1. An incision is made in the vaginal wall around the fistula, and the bladder and vaginal wall are widely mobilized.

fashion to approximate the edges of the mucosa (Fig. 2).
11. Place a second suture line with the suture at the lateral margins, just beyond the most distal sutures of the original suture line.
12. The cul-de-sac is usually entered, and the peritoneum from the back of the bladder is brought down and sutured to cover the suture line of the closed fistula.
13. This peritoneum gives an additional layer of closure.
14. Close the peritoneal cavity with running synthetic absorbable suture.

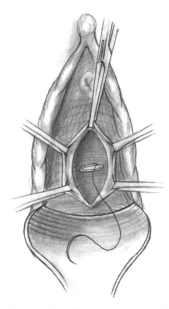

FIG. 2. After excision of the fistula track, the bladder mucosa is closed in the first layer of sutures.

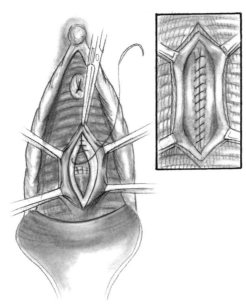

FIG. 3. The bladder muscularis is closed as a second layer, if possible in a direction at right angles to the first suture line.

15. The vagina generally is closed in a vertical fashion but may be closed transversely, depending on the size and location of the fistula (Fig. 3).
16. Care must be taken to ensure that placement of the sutures to close the fistula does not encroach on the ureter.
17. Insert a suprapubic or urethral catheter into the bladder.

E. Surgical Technique: Abdominal Repair

1. Introduction
   - 80% of vesicovaginal fistula repairs are performed vaginally.

- Types of abdominal approach
  — Transperitoneal
  — Transvaginal
- Preferred approach: transperitoneal, because it permits accurate mobilization of the base of the bladder and ureters
2. Indications for abdominal approach
- Large fistula
- Complex fistula (involving ureter and/or bowel)
- Proximity to ureters
- Inadequate exposure transvaginally
3. Technique
- Make a lower midline incision.
- Open the dome of the bladder in the midline.
- Place ureteral stents through the opened bladder.
- Sharply dissect the base of the bladder from the front wall of the vagina (Fig. 4).
- Place the fingers in the bladder and apply traction, with countertraction on the vaginal vault.
- Elevate the base of the bladder, and excise the rim of the fistulous tract in the bladder and vagina.
- Close the vaginal mucosa with running 3-0 synthetic absorbable suture (Fig. 5).
- Insert this layer with a second layer of similar suture material commencing at and extending 0.5 cm beyond the original fistulous opening.
- Occasionally, this defect may best be closed vertically—it is important that it be free of tension and achieve excellent hemostasis and that the second suture line invert the first.
- Submucosal closure of the first layer of the bladder wall accurately approximates the mucosal edges and allows direct inspection and palpation of the ureters (Fig. 6).

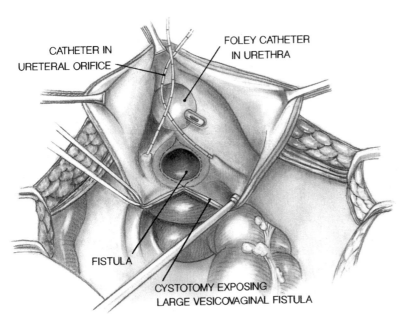

CATHETER IN
URETERAL ORIFICE

FOLEY CATHETER
IN URETHRA

FISTULA

CYSTOTOMY EXPOSING
LARGE VESICOVAGINAL FISTULA

FIG. 4. Opened bladder enabling separation of the bladder wall from the anterior wall of the vagina. (Redrawn from Lee RA. *Atlas of gynecologic surgery.* Philadelphia: WB Saunders, 1992:286, with permission.)

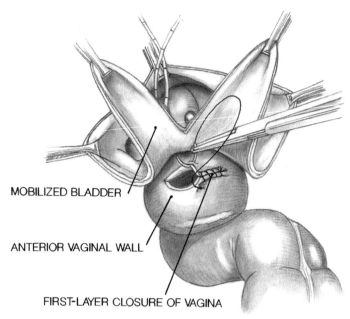

MOBILIZED BLADDER

ANTERIOR VAGINAL WALL

FIRST-LAYER CLOSURE OF VAGINA

FIG. 5. Two-layered closure of vaginal defect after mobilization of the bladder off the vagina. (Redrawn from Lee RA. *Atlas of gynecologic surgery.* Philadelphia: WB Saunders, 1992:287, with permission.)

- The second layer of bladder closure begins and ends 1 cm beyond the original suture line, again inverting it.
- The peritoneum of the back of the bladder may be pulled down over the two suture lines on the posterior bladder wall.
- This flap of peritoneum, or an interposed omental pedicle, helps to separate the bladder from the vaginal suture line (Fig. 7).

- Suture the omental pedicle to the anterior wall of the vagina.
- An omental pedicle is particularly useful in larger, more complex fistula repairs and for radiation-induced fistulas, in which an additional blood supply is brought in via the omental pedicle.
- Close the cystotomy incision in two layers with continuous 3-0 synthetic absorbable suture, leaving a urethral or suprapubic Foley catheter in place.
- If the ureters are close to the incision lines, the ureteral stents may be left in place for 7 days to allow edema to subside; otherwise they are removed before closing the cystotomy.

F. Intraoperative Complications
1. Bleeding
2. Inadvertent cystotomy
3. Ligation of a ureter

G. Postoperative Complications
1. Urinary tract infection
2. Bleeding (must obtain perfect hemostasis at the time of operation)
3. Obstruction of a ureter: locate the level of obstruction and pass a ureteral catheter in an anterograde or retrograde fashion.

H. Postoperative Management
1. Catheter drainage for 1 week (6 weeks, if previous pelvic irradiation)
2. Close monitoring of urine output postoperatively to avoid bladder distention
3. No coitus or vaginal examinations for 6 weeks

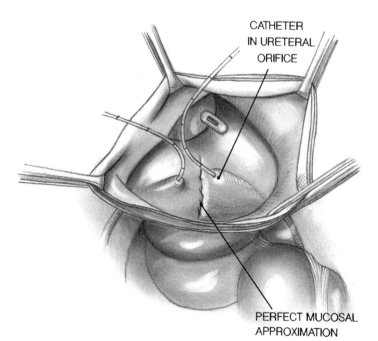

CATHETER IN URETERAL ORIFICE

PERFECT MUCOSAL APPROXIMATION

FIG. 6. Careful closure of the bladder wall with ureteral stents in place. (Redrawn from Lee RA. *Atlas of gynecologic surgery.* Philadelphia: WB Saunders, 1992:287, with permission.)

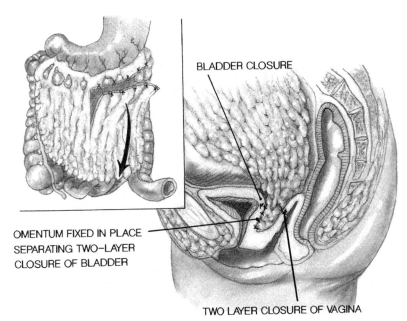

BLADDER CLOSURE

OMENTUM FIXED IN PLACE
SEPARATING TWO-LAYER
CLOSURE OF BLADDER

TWO LAYER CLOSURE OF VAGINA

FIG. 7. Omental pedicle interposed between vaginal and vesical suture lines. (Redrawn from Lee RA. *Atlas of gynecologic surgery.* Philadelphia: WB Saunders, 1992: 289, with permission.)

III. Ureterovaginal Fistula

A. Indications
Ureterovaginal fistula that fails to heal after ureteral stenting or where a stent cannot be passed

B. Preoperative Investigations
1. Cystoscopic examination
2. Intravenous pyelography or retrograde pyelography to exclude obstruction

C. Preoperative Preparation
1. Avoid operation until approximately 3 months postoperatively unless performed within the first 48 hours after injury.
2. Attempt passage of stent; if not possible and any obstruction is present, percutaneous nephrostomy is necessary to protect the kidney.
3. Treat urinary infection if present.
4. Prophylactic treatment with antibiotics

D. Surgical Technique
1. Attempt placement of a ureteral catheter in either a retrograde fashion or anterograde via a percutaneous nephrostomy past the fistula.
2. If this completely corrects the urinary leakage, leave the catheter in place for 4 weeks, then remove it, and perform intravenous pyelography.
3. If normal, repeat pyelography in 3 months to be sure that stenosis has not occurred.
4. If leakage persists and the fistulous opening is close to the bladder, perform an abdominal

ureteroneocystostomy with full-thickness interrupted 4-0 synthetic absorbable sutures, approximating the ureter to the mucosa of the bladder (see Chapter 4).
5. A second layer of sutures approximating the peritoneum of the ureter to the serosa of the bladder is accomplished with interrupted 4-0 sutures, relieving any tension on the anastomosis.
6. A no. 5 double J-catheter is inserted up the ureter, with the distal end in the bladder, and left in place for 2 weeks (6 to 8 weeks, if previous irradiation was given).

E. Specific Postoperative Management
1. The anastomosis is drained in an extraperitoneal fashion with a small suction catheter.
2. After 2 weeks, the ureteral catheter is removed, and intravenous pyelography is performed and repeated in 3 months.

F. Intraoperative Complications
1. Devascularization of segment of ureter
2. Bleeding from dissection near the internal iliac artery and vein
3. Potential trauma to the sigmoid if ureter is adherent to it

G. Postoperative Complications
1. Leakage of anastomosis
2. Stricture of anastomosis

IV. Vesicouterine and Ureterouterine Fistulas

A. Indications
Leakage of urine through the cervix

B. Cause

1. Usually occur after cesarean section
2. Occur when the bladder is traumatized (vesicouterine) or ureter is caught in a suture at the lateral end of a transverse lower segment incision (ureterouterine)
3. Rarely occur in association with uterine malignancy
4. Occasionally occur after difficult instrumental vaginal delivery

C. Preoperative Investigations

1. Intravenous pyelography to exclude ureteral obstruction
2. Cystoscopic examination with retrograde studies if indicated
3. Urine culture

D. Preoperative Preparation

1. Avoid repair for 12 weeks after causative operation, unless performed within 48 hours after injury.
2. If it is a ureteral fistula, attempt passage of an anterograde or retrograde stent.
3. If stenting is not possible and ureteral obstruction is present, it is necessary to perform percutaneous nephrostomy to protect the kidney.

E. Surgical Technique

1. Make a lower abdominal midline incision.
2. Open the vesicouterine fold of peritoneum.
3. Dissect the bladder off the anterior aspect of the cervix and uterus.
4. For vesicouterine fistula, close the defect in the bladder, after freshening edges, with two layers of 2-0 synthetic absorbable sutures.
5. Close the defect in the uterine wall with 2-0 synthetic absorbable sutures.
6. If the patient does not wish to preserve reproductive function, perform hysterectomy.
7. Bring down an omental pedicle and interpose it between the bladder and the uterus if the uterus is present, or between the bladder and the vagina vault if hysterectomy is performed.
8. Drain the pelvis with a suction drain.
9. If ureterouterine fistula is present, open the peritoneum of the broad ligament lateral to the ovarian vessels and identify the ureter.
10. Dissect the ureter distally until reaching the fistula site.
11. Transect the ureter just above this point, and ligate the distal ureteral stump.
12. Perform ureteroneocystostomy, implanting the ureter into the bladder, as described previously, over a stent.
13. Drain the pelvis with a suction drain.
14. Insert a urethral catheter.

F. Specific Postoperative Management

1. Remove the pelvic suction drain in approximately 5 days.
2. Remove the urethral catheter in 7 days.

3. Remove the stent in 2 weeks, if ureterouterine fistula, and perform intravenous pyelography.
4. Repeat pyelography in 3 months to check for stenosis.

G. Specific Postoperative Complications

1. Stricture of ureteric anastomosis
2. Leakage of ureteric anastomosis or bladder repair

V. Ectopic Ureter

A. Principles

1. Ectopic ureter must always be considered in patients with a long history of incontinence.
2. The patients are continuously wet, although variations related to positional changes may occur.
3. The ureter may drain into the vagina, the urethra, or the vaginal introitus.

B. Investigation

Investigation, including cystoscopy, is aided by intravenous injections of methylene blue or indigo carmine dye.

C. Treatment

Treatment is by reimplantation into the bladder or the ipsilateral ureter.

VI. Urinary Fistulas in the Irradiated Patient

Principles of Management

1. Perform biopsy to rule out recurrent malignancy as the cause.
2. Delay any surgical repair until any radionecrosis is nonprogressive.
3. Treat prophylactically with antibiotics.

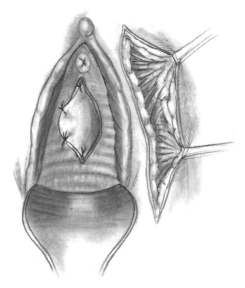

FIG. 8. With a large defect, a Martius myocutaneous flap can be developed from the vulva and sutured into the vaginal defect.

4. Never anastomose irradiated tissue to irradiated tissue.
5. Stent the ureter and/or drain the bladder for at least 6 weeks.
6. Bring in a new blood supply as a vascular pedicle (e.g., omentum, gracilis flap, bulbocavernous flap) (Fig. 8).

Reading List

Symmonds RE, Pratt JH. Prevention of fistulas and lymphocysts in radical hysterectomy: preliminary report of a new technic. *Obstet Gynecol* 1961;17:57–64.

Massee JS, Welch JS, Pratt JH, et al. Management of urinary-vaginal fistula: ten-year survey. *JAMA* 1964;190:902–906.

Pratt JH. Ureteral injuries in pelvic surgery for benign lesions. *Minn Med* 1964;47:389–393.

Hache L, Pratt JH, Cook EN. Vesicouterine fistula. *Mayo Clin Proc* 1966; 41:150–158.

Lee RA, Symmonds RE. Ureterovaginal fistula. *Am J Obstet Gynecol* 1971; 109:1032–1035.

Symmonds RE. Urologic injuries: ureter. *In:* Schaefer G, Graber EA, eds. *Complications in obstetric and gynecologic surgery: prevention, diagnosis, and treatment.* Hagerstown, MD: Harper & Row, 1981:412–430.

Podratz KC, Angerman NS, Symmonds RE. Complications of ureteral surgery in the nonirradiated patient. *In:* Gregorio D, Smith JP, eds. *Management of complications in gynecologic oncology.* New York: John Wiley & Sons, 1982:113–149.

Podratz KC, Symmonds RE, Hagen JV. Vesicovaginal fistula. *Baillieres Clin Obstet Gynaecol* 1987;1:414–445.

Podratz KC. Vesicovaginal fistula. *In:* Monoghan JM, ed. *Rob & Smith's Operative Surgery. Vol 9: Gynaecology and obstetrics,* 4th ed. London: Butterworths, 1987:127–142.

Lee RA, Symmonds RE, Williams TJ. Current status of genitourinary fistula. *Obstet Gynecol* 1988;72:313–319.

Webb MJ. Prevention and management of intraoperative complications in pelvic surgery. *Postgrad Obstet Gynecol* 1990;10:1–5.

Lee RA. Vesicovaginal and ureterovaginal fistulae. *In:* Ostergard DR, Bent AE, eds. *Urogynecology and urodynamics: theory and practice,* 4th ed. Baltimore: Williams & Wilkins, 1996:375–386.

CHAPTER 16

Intestinal Fistula

C. Robert Stanhope, M.D.

I. Introduction

A. Principles of Management for Small-Bowel Fistulas
1. Establishment of intestinal decompression with nasogastric or long intestinal tube
2. Control of vaginal or skin irritation or erosions caused by small intestinal contents
3. Maintenance of nutritional status
4. Decrease intestinal secretions
   Drug: Somatostatin, 150 to 500 μg three times daily

B. Spontaneous Closure
1. Can occur in some intestinal fistulas, making surgical intervention unnecessary
2. Factors conducive to spontaneous closure include
   • Low volume output
   • Narrow tract
   • Absence of foreign body
   • No previous irradiation or inflammatory bowel disease
   • Parenteral nutrition
3. Cancer involving fistula tract or distal obstruction prevents spontaneous closure.

C. Causes of Small-Bowel Fistula Postoperatively
1. Surgical injury
2. Anastomotic leak
3. Postoperative small-bowel obstruction
4. Retained foreign body
5. Previous irradiation
6. Inflammatory bowel disease
7. Any combination of the above

D. Causes of Small-Bowel Fistula in Nonsurgical Cases
1. Small-bowel erosion from pelvic abscess or malignancy

2. Crohn regional enteritis
3. Postirradiation necrosis with sloughing of the intestinal wall

II. Ileovaginal, Ileoperineal, and Ileoabdominal Fistulas

A. Indications for Surgical Treatment
1. Passage of small intestinal contents through the vagina, perineum, or abdominal wall
2. Persistent fistula after adequate trial of conservative nonoperative management

B. Preoperative Investigations
1. Complete blood count
2. Electrolytes and albumin
3. Liver and renal function studies
4. Baseline electrocardiogram
5. Chest radiography
6. Arterial blood gases if indicated by status of patient
7. Radiographic study with contrast media to demonstrate fistula (i.e., small-bowel follow-through or fistulogram)
8. Radiographic study with contrast media to exclude distal bowel obstruction or large bowel involvement
9. Excretory urography or computed tomography with intravenous contrast media to evaluate renal function and the distal genitourinary tract

C. Preoperative Preparation
1. Nasogastric or long intestinal tube drainage
2. Parenteral nutritional support: establish anabolic state preoperatively
3. Perioperative treatment with broad-spectrum antibiotics

D. Surgical Technique
1. Patient in supine position
2. Povidone-iodine skin preparation

C. Robert Stanhope: Consultant, Departments of Obstetrics and Gynecology and Surgery and Section of Medical Information Resources, Mayo Clinic and Mayo Foundation; Professor of Obstetrics and Gynecology, Mayo Medical School, Rochester, Minnesota.

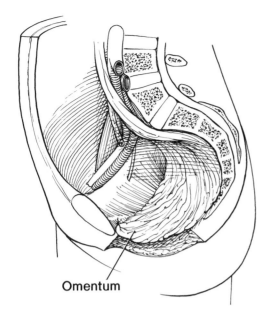

FIG. 1. Omental pedicle graft covering the pelvic floor.

3. Make a midline abdominal incision; if the fistula is located in a previous abdominal incision, excise the entire tract in the abdominal wall.
4. Isolate the involved segment of small bowel.
5. Resect the fistula with the involved small bowel.
6. Anastomose the afferent and efferent bowel segments.
7. Use either hand sewn or stapling techniques.
8. If unable to resect the involved bowel, completely exclude the fistula with a bypass procedure and mucus fistula.

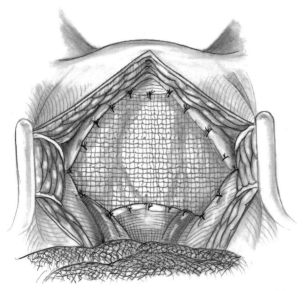

FIG. 2. Synthetic absorbable mesh covering the pelvic floor.

9. Protect the anastomosis with omentum or by placing barriers to prevent its adherence to the previous fistula site if possible (Fig. 1). Absorbable mesh may be used to keep small bowel from adhering deep in the pelvis (Fig. 2).

E. Specific Postoperative Management
1. Intestinal tube drainage until patient passes flatus
2. Hourly urine output measured in the immediate postoperative period
3. Maintenance of fluid and electrolyte balance
4. Hemodynamic monitoring, with replacement of blood products as indicated
5. Treatment with broad-spectrum antibiotics

F. Specific Postoperative Complications
1. Anastomotic leak
   - Signs
     — Fever
     — Leukocytosis
     — Ileus
     — Free air
     — Abscesses
     — New fistula
   - Management
     — Intestinal decompression
     — Treatment with broad-spectrum antibiotics
     — Reoperation if necessary
2. Sepsis
   - Associated with
     — Intraabdominal abscess
     — Pneumonia
     — Pyelonephritis
     — Central catheter infection
   - Management
     After receiving culture results, treat appropriately with antibiotics or central catheter removal.
3. Ileus
   - Causes
     — Anastomotic leak
     — Sepsis
     — Trauma during surgical procedure
   - Management
     — Intestinal decompression
     — Avoid oral intake
4. Malabsorption syndrome, short-bowel syndrome
   - Directly related to length and function of remaining bowel or presence of terminal ileum and cecum and their ability to absorb bile salts
   - Use enteral or parenteral nutrition and monitor
     — Glucose metabolism
     — Amino acid metabolism
     — Electrolytes
     — Liver function
   - May need cholestyramine to bind bile salts or medium-chain triglycerides

III. Rectovaginal Fistula

A. Indications for Surgical Treatment
Unacceptable passage of gas, liquid, or solid stool through the vagina

B. Causes
1. Obstetric injury
2. Perineal laceration
3. Operative injury after hysterectomy, posterior colporrhaphy, or anal surgery
4. Perirectal abscess or chronic fissure
5. Pelvic irradiation (most commonly after brachytherapy)
6. Malignancy

C. Preoperative Investigations
1. Flexible sigmoidoscopy
2. Biopsy of the fistula tract if cancer or chronic inflammatory bowel disease is suspected
3. Complete blood count
4. Midstream urinalysis and culture

D. Preoperative Preparation
1. Mechanical bowel preparation or sodium phosphates (Phospho-Soda) preparation
2. Perioperative treatment with broad-spectrum antibiotics
3. Povidone-iodine vaginal douche

E. Surgical Technique: Vaginal Approach
1. Excise scar tissue and entire fistula tract: the size of the fistula, the viability of tissue, or previous irradiation determines the method of closure and repair.
2. Widely mobilize the anus off the posterior rectal wall.
3. Identify the anal canal musculature.
4. Layered approximation of anal mucosa, anal submucosa, external anal sphincter, and levator and perineal musculature with synthetic absorbable sutures
5. Consider colostomy in previously irradiated patients, patients with chronic inflammatory bowel disease, or patients with large fistulas at the vaginal vault.
6. Because of the size of the fistula or previous irradiation, it may be necessary to mobilize pedicles or flaps of well-vascularized tissue to improve the likelihood of healing (bulbocavernosus, gracilis myocutaneous, omental, etc.).

F. Surgical Technique: Abdominal Approach
1. The abdominal approach may be indicated for very high fistulas where, because of lack of exposure, a safe closure is not possible.
2. Isolate the segment of involved rectum from the vagina, and resect the involved segment and/or establish a diverting colostomy.
3. Reestablish bowel continuity with an end-to-end circularly stapled anastomosis or hand-sewn anastomosis, and separate it from the vagina with omentum or other fat pad if possible. (If patient previously received irradiation, it may be advisable to use a temporary diverting colostomy.)
4. When it is not possible to reestablish bowel continuity, perform the Hartmann procedure or simply divert with a double-barrel or loop colostomy.

G. Specific Postoperative Management
1. Place ice pack to the perineum for the first 12 hours to reduce swelling and to ease discomfort after the vaginal approach.
2. Use stool softeners for 6 weeks or longer: docusate sodium (Colace), 100 mg twice daily, or psyllium (Metamucil), twice daily.
3. Avoid suppositories, enemas, and laxatives.
4. No coitus for 6 weeks or longer.
5. Allow low-residue diet when tolerated.
6. Prescribe nonconstipating analgesics if possible.

H. Specific Postoperative Complications
1. Hematoma: drain only if it is expanding or infected.
2. Infection: use therapeutic doses of broad-spectrum antibiotics and drain only if there is abscess formation.
3. Wound disruption: delay attempts to close until all inflammation has resolved, and consider colostomy before repeating fistula repair.

IV. Sigmoidovaginal/Sigmoidovesical Fistulas

A. Causes
1. Usually, sigmoid diverticulitis with perforation gives rise to abscess formation, producing fistula.
2. Occasionally, gynecologic or colonic malignancy produces fistulas.
3. Rarely, inflammatory bowel disease (Crohn or ulcerative colitis) produces fistulas.
4. Sigmoidovaginal fistula may occur in patients after hysterectomy.

B. Symptoms
Passage of gas and/or stool through the vagina or urethra

C. Preoperative Investigations
1. Complete blood count
2. Midstream urinalysis and culture
3. Colon radiography
4. Intravenous pyelography if vesical fistula
5. Cystoscopy if vesical fistula
6. Sigmoidoscopy
7. Biopsy of fistula tract or bowel if cancer or inflammatory bowel disease is suspected

D. Preoperative Preparation
1. Mechanical bowel preparation or sodium phosphates (Phospho-Soda) preparation
2. Perioperative treatment with broad-spectrum antibiotics
3. Povidone-iodine douche

E. Surgical Technique

1. Make a midline lower abdominal incision.
2. Mobilize the adherent sigmoid from the back of the bladder or vagina.
3. Resect the involved segment of sigmoid colon, and reanastomose the bowel.
4. Oversew the hole in the vaginal vault or bladder with interrupted 2-0 synthetic absorbable suture.
5. Drain the bowel anastomosis site with a Jackson-Pratt suction drain.

F. Specific Postoperative Management

1. If it is a vesical fistula, drain the bladder with a catheter for 7 days or longer if indicated.
2. No enemas or laxatives
3. No coitus for 6 weeks or longer if indicated

G. Specific Postoperative Complications

1. Intestinal anastomosis leak

- Perform proximal diverting colostomy.
- Recheck for healing of leak in 8 weeks, and then close colostomy if healed.

2. Urinary tract infection: from fecal contamination of the bladder

Reading List

Pratt JH, Wychulis AR. Sigmoidovaginal fistulas. *West Surg Assoc Trans* 1996;73:88–92.

Lescher TC, Pratt JH. Vaginal repair of the simple rectovaginal fistula. *Surg Gynecol Obstet* 1967;124:1317–1321.

Schnur PL, Symmonds RE, Williams TJ. Intestinal disorders masquerading as gynecologic problems. *Surg Gynecol Obstet* 969;128:1016–1020.

Raventos JM, Symmonds RE. Surgical management of acute diverticulitis in women. *Obstet Gynecol* 1981;58:557–565.

Schmitt EH III, Symmonds RE. Surgical treatment of radiation induced injuries of the intestine. *Surg Gynecol Obstet* 1981;153:896–900.

Pratt JH: Acute posthysterectomy rectovaginal fistula. *In:* Nichols DH, ed. *Clinical problems, injuries, and complications of gynecologic surgery.* Baltimore: Williams & Wilkins, 1983:62–63.

CHAPTER 17

Pelvic Exenteration

C. Robert Stanhope, M.D.

A. Indications
1. Nondisseminated recurrent cervical, vaginal, endometrial, or vulvar cancer
2. Recurrent bladder or anorectal cancer
3. Recurrent pelvic sarcoma
4. Primary stage IVA cervical cancer
5. Primary stage I or II (large volume) vaginal cancer
6. Primary vulvar cancer with bladder or bowel involvement
7. Incapacitating pelvic pain caused by radiation necrosis or multiple fistulas

B. Types of Exenteration
1. Anterior: removal of pelvic viscera, anterior vagina, bladder, and urethra
2. Posterior: removal of pelvic viscera, posterior vagina, and rectosigmoid colon
3. Total: removal of pelvic viscera, bladder, and rectosigmoid colon

C. Extent of Resection in the Pelvis
1. Supralevator: not necessary to resect levator muscle for clearance
2. Infralevator: necessary to resect some levator muscle for clearance
3. Infralevator with vulvectomy: large lesion requiring resection of some levator muscle and vulva to obtain clearance

D. Preoperative Investigations
1. Histologic evidence of cancer
2. Complete blood count, serum chemistry, hematologic studies, and coagulation panel
3. Chest radiography
4. Medical and psychologic assessment
5. Computed tomography of abdomen and pelvis with intravenous and oral contrast agents to exclude distant metastases and to evaluate renal excretion
6. Scalene lymph node biopsy if paraaortic nodal involvement is suspected
7. Electrocardiography
8. Arterial blood gases for baseline and pulmonary function tests if indicated

E. Preoperative Preparation
1. Mechanical and antibiotic preparation (see Chapter 1)
2. Discussion with and instruction by stomal therapist
3. Stoma site(s) marking
4. Typing and cross-matching of 4 to 6 U of packed erythrocytes
5. Pulmonary preparation if indicated
6. Povidone-iodine douche
7. Treatment with broad-spectrum antibiotics
8. Discussion and planning for possible vaginal reconstruction
9. Insertion of central venous access line
10. Parenteral nutrition if indicated

F. Surgical Techniques: Exploration, Tumor Resection, and Reconstruction
1. Exploration to consider resectability
- Examination under anesthesia
  — Determine mobility or fixation to the pelvic wall or bone.
  — Assess possible preservation of the anal canal and primary sigmoidorectostomy.
- Abdominal exploration through long midline incision
  — Examine the abdomen for possible intraabdominal spread of disease.
  — Perform a gross examination of the pelvic and paraaortic nodal regions.
  — Perform a biopsy on any suspicious areas, and examine frozen sections.

C. Robert Stanhope: Consultant, Departments of Obstetrics and Gynecology and Surgery and Section of Medical Information Resources, Mayo Clinic and Mayo Foundation; Professor of Obstetrics and Gynecology, Mayo Medical School, Rochester, Minnesota.

- Operative assessment of operability
  Determine whether the disease is central and resectable.
- Obtain specimen of pelvic fluid or pelvic washings for cytologic examination.
- Incise the lateral margins of the infundibulopelvic ligaments, and clamp and divide the ovarian vessels.
- Separate the loose areolar tissue between the uterosacral ligaments and the lateral aspect of the levator muscles and the pelvic floor to develop the pararectal space.
- Follow the course of the internal iliac artery and the obliterated hypogastric vessel on each side.
- Develop the paravesical space just lateral to the internal iliac artery. This space is bounded anteriorly by the anterior leaf of the broad ligament, medially by the lateral aspect of the bladder, laterally by the pelvic sidewall and obturator muscle, and inferiorly by the levator ani muscles.
- Perform pelvic and paraaortic lymphadenectomy. (Pelvic lymphatics follow the course of the pelvic vessels; see Chapter 22.)
- Paraaortic lymphatics are located on the inferior vena cava on the right side and lateral to the aorta on the left side; remove this lymphatic tissue carefully to avoid injury to the vena cava, aorta, ureters, or inferior mesenteric artery.
2. Pelvic tumor resection
- Divide the infundibulopelvic ligaments; this step may be performed earlier to facilitate nodal dissection.
- Divide and ligate the anterior division of the internal iliac artery.

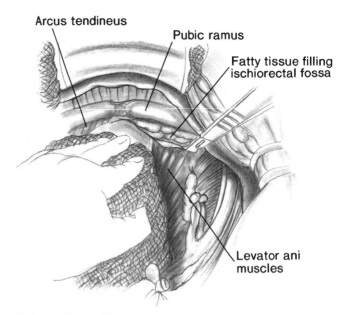

Arcus tendineus

Pubic ramus

Fatty tissue filling ischiorectal fossa

Levator ani muscles

FIG. 2. After dividing and ligating the visceral branches of the internal iliac vessels on each side, the bladder, parametrium, and pararectal regions are entirely mobilized except for their attachment to the pelvic floor. At this point, the anterior and lateral attachments of the levator muscles to the pubic rami and the obturator internis fascia are divided by sharp dissection. The underlying fatty tissue within the ischiorectal fossa is exposed.

- Divide and suture-ligate the cardinal web near the pelvic sidewall (Fig. 1).

Note: Be careful not to clamp tissue too close to the pelvic wall and thus not be able to ligate and secure the vascular bundle.

- Mobilize the bladder from the back of the symphysis, and divide the ureters. Divide the ureters outside of the irradiated field if possible.
- Mobilize the rectum by developing the retrorectal space (presacral).
- Mobilize paravaginal tissues. Resect the levator muscle if necessary to obtain tumor clearance (Fig. 2).
- Perineal phase may be necessary to remove the entire vagina, urethra, or vulva.
3. Pelvic reconstruction
- Reconstruct the pelvic floor, and reestablish the continuity of the colon if possible with hand-sewn or EEA anastomosis (Fig. 3).
- Develop an omental pedicle to cover the pelvic floor (Fig. 4). Anterior abdominal wall peritoneum or polyglactin 910 absorbable mesh can be used if the omentum is sparse (Fig. 5)
- Consider gracilis myocutaneous grafts, a modified McIndoe operation, groin fascial flaps, or sigmoid colon neovaginal reconstruction (see Chapter 11).
- Place a pelvic suction drain along the sacrum, with it exiting near the buttock or through the anterior abdominal wall.

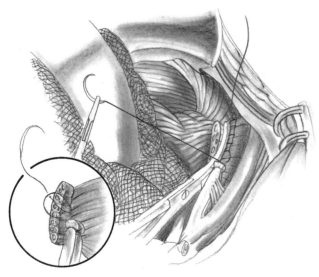

FIG. 1. Hemostasis is safely obtained by undersewing the clamp with heavy suture material (no. 1 polyglycolic acid suture). The undersewing prevents retraction of vessels between roots of the sacral plexus and can be carried back as a running locked stitch if additional hemostasis is necessary.

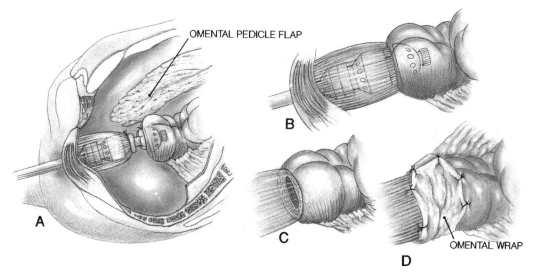

FIG. 3. A: The EEA anastomosis stapler is inserted through the anus, and the distal and proximal ends are positioned for circular stapling. **B:** The stapler is activated, and the colon anastomosed to the rectum deep in the pelvis. **C:** The EEA stapler is withdrawn. Lembert sutures may be placed to relieve tension on the staple line. **D:** Omentum may be used to cover part or all of the anastomosis.

- Close the perineal defect as appropriate (can be closed almost completely if there are no plans for neovagina).
- Perform urinary diversion by using an ileal, sigmoid, or transverse colon conduit (Fig. 6).
- Develop a colostomy if sigmoidorectostomy is not possible.

- Irrigate the abdomen and pelvis thoroughly.
- Close the abdominal wall with synthetic absorbable sutures.
4. Urinary diversion
  - Consider an ileal conduit for anterior exenteration, sigmoid conduit for total exenteration, or transverse

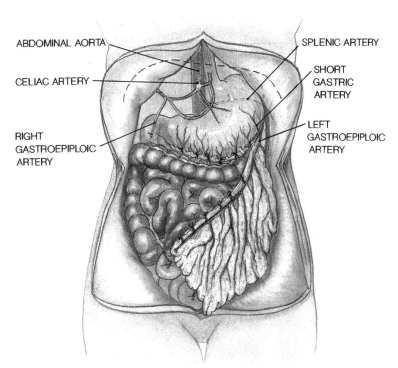

FIG. 4. Omentum is removed from the transverse colon and greater curvature of the stomach, maintaining the left gastroepiploic blood supply. Mobilized omentum can be placed in the pelvis to cover the denuded pelvic floor.

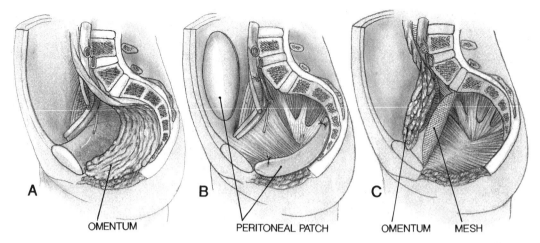

FIG. 5. Omentum (**A**), peritoneum (**B**), or a combination of absorbable mesh and omentum (**C**) is used to cover the pelvic floor.

colon conduit if sigmoid or distal ileum is heavily irradiated.

- Use either two-layered hand-sewn or stapled closure of the proximal end of the conduit to establish bowel continuity.
- Use absorbable sutures to anastomose full-thickness layers of the ureter and bowel, preferably sewn over ureteral stents (see Chapter 21).
- Suture the proximal end of the conduit to the left psoas muscle or the pelvic peritoneum to avoid anterior displacement of the conduit and potential ureteral kinking.

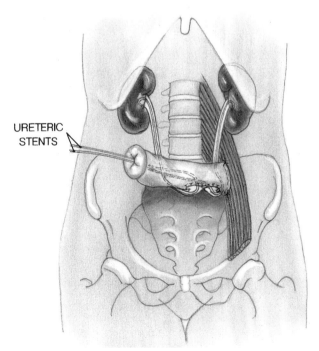

FIG. 6. Single J-stents are placed in each renal unit to protect the ureterointestinal anastomosis until edema resolves.

G. Sexual Rehabilitation
1. Gracilis myocutaneous neovaginal reconstruction
2. Labiofascial neovaginal reconstruction
3. Sigmoid colon neovaginal reconstruction
4. Immediate or delayed modified McIndoe neovaginal reconstruction (see Chapter 11)

H. Specific Postoperative Management
1. Maintenance of fluid and electrolyte balance
2. Invasive hemodynamic monitoring
3. Arterial blood gas sampling
4. Parenteral nutrition

I. Specific Postoperative Complications
1. Urinary conduit leak: detected by decreased urine output and leakage of urine from drains or through perineum; demonstrated on contrast study (excretory urogram, loopogram)

Note: If drainage is established, observe for spontaneous closure; otherwise, attempt passage of an anterograde ureteral stent through percutaneous nephrostomy and, if unsuccessful, reoperate.

2. Intestinal anastomotic leak: detected by ileus, sepsis, or perineal or cutaneous fistula

Note: When the patient's condition is stable, reoperation is the most appropriate management.

3. Sepsis: associated with anastomotic or conduit leak, pneumonia, atelectasis, pyelonephritis, wound infection, etc. Treat with appropriate antibiotics after cultures, drainage, etc.
4. Stomal necrosis: related to impairment of blood supply to stoma, due to either surgical procedure or previous irradiation. Observe if only superficial slough; however, if greater than superficial, conduit revision is indicated.
5. Neovaginal necrosis: related to poor blood supply or to previous irradiation. If only superficial, skin grafting

may be necessary; if more extensive, revision may be required.

Reading List

Pratt JH. The colon in vaginal reconstructions. *Proc Staff Meet Mayo Clin* 1961;36:34–40.

Jensen PA, Symmonds RE. The rectosigmoid urinary reservoir with anterior pelvic exenterations, an evaluation. *Obstet Gynecol* 1965;26:786–791.

Symmonds RE. Use of the colon for urinary diversion. *Clin Obstet Gynecol* 1967;10:217–226.

Symmonds RE, Pratt JH, Welch JS. Exenterative operations: experience with 118 patients. *Am J Obstet Gynecol* 1968;101:66–77.

Pratt JH. Use of the colon in gynecologic surgery. In: Sturgis SH, Taymor ML, eds. *Progress in gynecology,* vol 5. New York: Grune & Stratton, 1970:435–446.

Symmonds RE, Gibbs CP. Urinary diversion by way of sigmoid conduit. *Surg Gynecol Obstet* 1970;131:687–693.

Symmonds RE, Jones IV. Sigmoid conduit urinary diversion after exenteration. *Prog Gynecol* 1975;6:729–737.

Symmonds RE, Pratt JH, Webb MJ. Exenterative operations: experience with 198 patients. *Am J Obstet Gynecol* 1975;121:907–918.

Webb MJ, Symmonds RE. Management of the pelvic floor after pelvic exenteration. *Obstet Gynecol* 1977;50:166–171.

Symmonds RE, Webb MJ. Pelvic exenteration. In: Coppleson M, ed. *Gynecologic oncology: fundamental principles and clinical practice,* vol 2. Edinburgh: Churchill Livingstone, 1981:896–922.

Stanhope CR, Symmonds RE. Palliative exenteration—what, when, and why? *Am J Obstet Gynecol* 1985;152:12–16.

Stanhope CR, Symmonds RE, Lee RA, et al. Urinary diversion with use of ileal and sigmoid conduits. *Am J Obstet Gynecol* 1986;155:288–292.

Stanhope CR, Webb MJ, Podratz KC. Pelvic exenteration for recurrent cervical cancer. *Clin Obstet Gynecol* 1990;33:897–909.

CHAPTER 18

Radiation Injury to the Intestinal Tract

Maurice J. Webb, M.D.

I. Introduction

A. Radiation Damage

1. Radiation can produce
   - Partial or complete intestinal obstruction
   - Pseudo-obstruction
   - Intestinal necrosis and perforation
   - Intestinal fistulas
   - Ulceration and hemorrhage

   Note: Radiation fistulas rarely heal spontaneously and usually require operation.

2. For gynecologic malignancies in which pelvic irradiation is frequently administered, rectal complications (such as proctitis, ulceration, hemorrhage, stricture, and fistulas) are more common than small intestinal injuries.
3. Approximately 2% of patients who receive pelvic irradiation require operation for complications.
4. Injury can develop many years after irradiation.
5. Injury is dose related.

B. Factors Predisposing to Radiation Injury

1. Pelvic inflammatory disease with adhesions
2. Postoperative adhesions
3. Diabetes mellitus
4. Concomitant or previous chemotherapy
5. Radiation sensitizers

II. Surgical Treatment

A. Indications

1. Intestinal fistula: enterovaginal, enterocutaneous, or enterovesical

2. Intestinal obstruction: adhesions, stricture, or pseudo-obstruction (motility disorder), or recurrent malignancy
3. Intestinal hemorrhage, e.g., proctitis

B. Preoperative Investigations

1. Radiographic studies with contrast agents to define the site of the problem
2. Computed tomography to exclude recurrent tumor
3. Proctoscopy, sigmoidoscopy, or colonoscopy as indicated
4. Cystoscopy if indicated
5. Sinogram of fistula tract if present
6. Complete blood count
7. Serum chemistry
8. Chest radiography
9. Electrocardiography
10. Biopsy of fistula, stricture, etc., to exclude malignancy

C. Preoperative Preparation

1. Total parenteral nutrition, preoperatively and postoperatively
2. Bowel preparation: polyethylene glycol electrolyte solution (GoLYTELY), enemas, antibiotics, etc., depending on the diagnosis and whether obstruction is present
3. Prophylactic treatment with parenteral antibiotics

D. Surgical Techniques

1. Radiation proctitis with hemorrhage
   If conservative measures, e.g., steroid enemas, are not successful, then bypass the affected area with colostomy.
2. Rectosigmoid stricture
   - Surgical options are
     — Bypass the stricture with colostomy.
     — Resect the strictured segment and anastomose the free ends of the intestine.

Maurice J. Webb: Chairman, Division of Gynecologic Surgery, and Consultant, Department of Surgery, Mayo Clinic and Mayo Foundation; Professor of Obstetrics and Gynecology, Mayo Medical School Rochester, Minnesota.

- If resection is chosen
  — An adequate well-vascularized anorectal stump must be available for resection.
  — A temporary defunctioning colostomy is advisable to protect the anastomosis.
  — Use an omental pedicle graft to wrap around the intestinal anastomosis.
3. Recto/sigmoidovaginal fistula
  - Surgical options are
    — Vaginal approach
    — Abdominal approach
    — Combined approach
  - Vaginal approach
    — The vaginal approach is reserved for small fistulas in the lower half of the vagina.
    — A bulbocavernosus flap or gracilis flap may be used to bring in well-vascularized tissue.
    — A temporary defunctioning colostomy is advisable.
  - Abdominal approach
    — This approach is always used for fistulas high in the vagina and for complex problems.
    — It may involve resection and reanastomosis.
    — An alternative is the Bricker technique of transecting the sigmoid colon, folding over the top end, and suturing the lumen to the fistula defect. The sigmoid is reimplanted into this loop.
    — Use omental pedicle grafts or gracilis flaps to provide a well-vascularized protective layer between the bowel and the vagina.
    — Drain the site of anastomosis through an abdominal wall suction drain.
    — A defunctioning colostomy is advisable.
  - Combined approach
    A combined abdominal and vaginal approach is often necessary in complex situations.
4. Colovesical fistula
  - It may be a complicated situation combined with colovaginal fistula.
  - Resect and reanastomose the involved segment of the colon.
  - Close the defect in the wall of the bladder.
  - Place an omental pedicle graft between the bladder and the intestinal anastomosis.
  - Perform a defunctioning colostomy.
  - Drain the site of anastomosis with a suction drain through the abdominal wall.
5. Small-bowel obstruction
  - Obstruction may be caused by adhesions or recurrent malignancy.
  - Pseudo-obstruction is caused by dense fibrinous material on the serosa of the small bowel, and a significant motility disorder is produced without actual obstruction.
  - Surgical options are
    — Lysis of adhesions
    — Excision of rigid fibrinous intestinal serosal coating in pseudo-obstruction

    — Bypass
    — Resection
  - Lysis of adhesions
    — Carefully divide all the adhesions.
    — This approach should be contemplated only when a small segment of intestine is involved.
    — Repair all serosal defects, because fistula formation occurs easily in irradiated bowel.
    — It may be better to resect a densely matted segment, because lysis of the adhesions invariably produces multiple enterotomies with subsequent fistula formation.
    — Resection of segments of intestine is often necessary after attempted adhesiolysis because of intestinal trauma.
  - Excision of postradiation fibrinous serosal coating
    — Carefully peel the white fibrinous layer off the serosal surface of the small bowel.
    — This allows the narrowed, rigid small bowel to spring open and to regain motility.
    — In practice, this usually is performed in combination with lysis of the adhesions and, occasionally, resection.
    — This technique is most important in cases in which large segments of the small intestine are involved and resection would produce short-bowel syndrome.
  - Intestinal bypass
    — Advantages
      · Avoids tedious dissection
      · Shortens operating time
      · Avoids damage to adherent organs, e.g., the urinary tract
      · Avoids contamination of the peritoneal cavity
    — Disadvantages
      · Blind loop syndrome may develop in unresected loops.
      · Perforation may already be present or may develop later in the unresected segment, causing abscess formation.
    — Ileotransverse colostomy side-to-side is the most common bypass procedure. Ileoascending colostomy is also common (Fig. 1).
    — Technique
      · Bring a loop of ileum showing little radiation change just above the obstructed segment up to the transverse colon.
      · Make a 0.5-cm incision in the antimesenteric border of the ileum and in the tenia of the transverse colon.
      · Insert and fire a GIA stapler to create the anastomosis.
      · Close the small incision by suturing or using a TA 55 stapler.
      · Reinforce the anastomosis at the angles with interrupted 3-0 silk sutures.
      · A hand-sewn anastomosis can also be constructed.

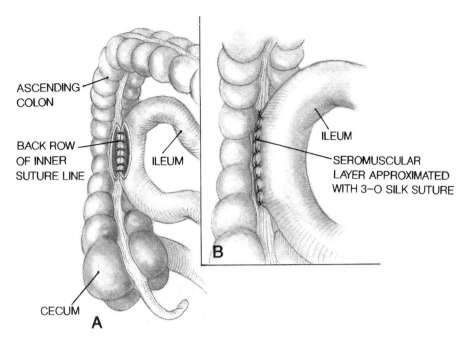

FIG. 1. A and **B:** Side-to-side ileoascending colostomy as bypass of small-bowel obstruction. (Redrawn from Lee RA. *Atlas of gynecologic surgery.* Philadelphia: WB Saunders, 1992:335, with permission.)

· As a general rule, small bowel should not be reanastomosed to small bowel, especially because the terminal ileum has usually been irradiated.

· An end-to-side enterocolic anastomosis can also be used.

· Bypass can also be accomplished by transecting the ileum above and the colon below the obstruction and directly anastomosing the ileum to the colon and completely isolating the obstructed segment by means of a mucus fistula.

• Intestinal resection

— It must be performed if perforation, fistula, necrosis, or abscess is present.

— In the absence of these complications, carefully judge whether to resect or to bypass.

— When deciding whether to proceed with resection or bypass, all the following are taken into consideration: the extent and location of the lesion, the viability of the bowel, the condition of the patient, and the surgeon's experience.

— During resection, care must be taken not to jeopardize the irradiated bladder, ureters, or rectum.

— Resection and bypass produce approximately the same incidence of anastomotic dehiscence.

— Whether undergoing resection or bypass at the initial operation, approximately the same number of patients require reoperation for subsequent fibrosis, obstruction, devascularization, and fistula formation.

— With resection, small bowel enteroenterostomy should be avoided.

— Use frozen sections of the proximal end of the small bowel to confirm that radiation change is absent and that resection has been adequate.

— The usual site of radiation-induced obstruction or fistula is the terminal ileum.

— Resection of this area should include resection of the cecum and the ascending colon.

— Then, end-to-end anastomosis between the ileum and transverse colon can be accomplished.

6. Small-bowel fistula and perforation

• Resection using the previously mentioned principles is preferred.

• Bypass with total isolation of the fistula may be an alternative if the patient is unable to withstand the more complete operation.

• In debilitated patients, especially in the presence of recurrent malignancy, a simple ileostomy above the site of the obstruction/fistula provides significant symptomatic palliation.

E. Specific Postoperative Management

1. Nothing by mouth until patient passes flatus.
2. Nasogastric suction until there are signs of return of intestinal function (jejunostomy may be used).
3. Prophylactic treatment with antibiotics perioperatively
4. Suction drainage of left colonic or rectal anastomosis until bowel function returns
5. Administration of total parenteral nutrition

F. Specific Postoperative Complications

1. Ileus: common with irradiated intestine
2. Anastomotic leak: requires reoperation because it is unlikely to heal with conservative management

3. Obstruction: may require reoperation if conservative management fails
4. Intraabdominal abscess: caused by anastomotic leak or intestinal necrosis. If it is caused by anastomotic leak and there is no fistula, the abscess may be drained percutaneously under ultrasonographic guidance.
5. Short-bowel syndrome: caused by resection or bypass of an excessively long segment of intestine
6. Chronic diarrhea: caused by resection/bypass of the terminal ileum and the ileocecal valve

Reading List

Schier J, Symmonds RE, Dahlin DC. Clinicopathologic aspects of actinic enteritis. *Surg Gynecol Obstet* 1964;119:1019–1025.

Shamblin JR, Symmonds RE, Sauer WG, et al. Bowel obstruction after pelvic and abdominal radiation therapy: factitial enteritis or recurrent malignancy? *Ann Surg* 1964;160:81–89.

Wijchulis AR, Pratt JH. Sigmoidovaginal fistulas: a study of 37 cases. *Arch Surg* 1966;92:520–524.

Russell JC, Welch JP. Operative management of radiation injuries of the intestinal tract. *Am J Surg* 1979;137:433–441.

Schmitt EH III, Symmonds RE. Surgical treatment of radiation induced injuries of the intestine. *Surg Gynecol Obstet* 1981;153:896–900.

Webb MJ, Weaver EW. Intestinal surgery in gynaecological oncology. *Aust NZ J Obstet Gynaecol* 1987;27:299–303.

Podratz KC, Symmonds RE, Hagen JC. Intestinal resection and ostomy care. *In:* Gusberg SB, Shingleton HM, Deppe G, eds. *Female genital cancer.* New York: Churchill Livingstone, 1988:589–619.

Garton GR, Gunderson LL, Webb MJ, et al. Intraoperative radiation therapy in gynecologic cancer: an update of the Mayo Clinic experience. *In:* Schildberg FW, Willich N, Kramling HJ, eds. *Intraoperative radiation therapy.* Essen, Germany: Verlag Die Blane Eule, 1993:407–410.

CHAPTER 19

Urinary Incontinence

Raymond A. Lee, M.D.

I. Anterior Colporrhaphy

A. Introduction
1. Anterior colporrhaphy is usually performed in the presence of a significant cystourethrocele with associated stress incontinence.
2. Normally, it is part of a vaginal hysterectomy and repair operation.
3. It is not usually performed without a simultaneous vaginal hysterectomy if the uterus is present.

B. Indication
Stress urinary incontinence

C. Preoperative Investigations
It is important to exclude urinary infection, bladder disorders, and fistulas before undertaking surgical treatment.
1. Detailed history and rectovaginal pelvic and abdominal examination to decide appropriate operative technique
2. Urinalysis and Gram stain with culture if indicated
3. Cystoscopy if indicated
4. Urodynamic studies if indicated
5. Voiding videocystography if indicated

D. Preoperative Preparation
1. Treat urinary infection if present.
2. Instruct patient to lose weight if obese.
3. Instruct patient to stop smoking; treat chronic respiratory disorders.
4. Give instruction about the proposed type of catheter drainage (e.g., urethral, suprapubic, self-catheterization).
5. Prophylactic treatment with antibiotics
6. Povidone-iodine vulval and vaginal preparation

Raymond A. Lee: Consultant, Departments of Obstetrics and Gynecology and Surgery, Mayo Clinic and Mayo Foundation; Professor of Obstetrics and Gynecology, Mayo Medical School, Rochester, Minnesota.

E. Surgical Technique
1. Lithotomy position
2. General or regional anesthesia
3. Bimanual rectovaginal examination to assess pelvis and mobility of pelvic structures
4. Vaginal hysterectomy (if uterus is present) or correction of any relaxation of vaginal vault in absence of uterus (enterocele) before beginning anterior Kelly-Kennedy repair
5. Place a Kocher clamp at each corner of the vaginal vault and a third clamp on the anterior vaginal wall just inferior to the urethral meatus.
6. The assistants provide traction by placing tension on the anterior vaginal wall in a triangular fashion.
7. In the midline, separate the vaginal wall carefully from the underlying pubocervical fascia covering the bladder and urethra by using Metzenbaum scissors.
8. Place the tips of the scissors immediately adjacent to the undersurface of the anterior vaginal wall, and direct the points of the scissors away from the bladder.
9. This dissection is best accomplished by spreading the tips of the scissors to aid in separating the vaginal mucosa from the pubocervical fascia.
10. As each segment (2 to 3 cm) is freed, incise the vaginal wall in the midline.
11. Dissection of the incision is continued all the way to the Kocher clamp fixed just below the external urethral meatus.
12. Place two Allis clamps on each side of the cut edge of the vaginal wall.
13. As the assistant applies spreading traction on the Allis clamps on the anterior vaginal wall, the surgeon, with toothed forceps in the left hand, applies countertraction on the bladder.
14. With Metzenbaum scissors, sharply dissect the bladder with its pubocervical fascia from the vaginal mucosa.
15. Continue the dissection laterally and superiorly adjacent to the left descending pubic ramus.

16. The anterior vaginal wall is more intimately attached to the endopelvic fascia at the level of the bladder neck and urethra.
17. Adequate mobilization is important to ensure the freedom to perform plication of the pubocervical fascia underlying the bladder neck and urethra and to provide the proper angular relationships between the urethra and base of the bladder, thus allowing urinary control.
18. A similar dissection is repeated on the right side: the surgeon holds the Allis clamps in the left hand and places the fingers on the outside of the vaginal wall.
19. The assistant applies traction on the bladder with long Russian forceps to facilitate sharp, accurate, and wide dissection.
20. After the bladder neck and urethra have been fully mobilized laterally to the pubic ramus, place the imbricating sutures.
21. Use interrupted 2-0 monofilament synthetic absorbable suture in the initial layer.
22. Place the first suture parallel and adjacent to the external urethral meatus on each side, sufficiently cephalad to incorporate the inferior aspects of the base of the posterior pubourethral ligament.
23. Place each suture so that each succeeding suture is slightly more lateral than the previously placed suture.
24. Excellent support is thereby obtained beneath the urethra, the bladder neck, and the base of the bladder.
25. Additional sutures of delayed absorbable suture may be placed in the area of the proximal urethra and bladder neck to plicate further the supporting tissues in the area most critical for urinary control.
26. Remove the Allis forceps from the edges of the vaginal wall.
27. Carefully resect redundant vaginal wall with scissors, ensuring that the resultant suture line will be in the midline and free of tension.
28. Approximate the vaginal edges with 2–0 interrupted synthetic absorbable sutures.
29. Each suture of the vaginal wall may be approximated to a small portion of the underlying pubocervical fascia to avoid dead space.
30. Inspect the suture line carefully to ensure that complete hemostasis has been obtained.
31. Place a small vaginal pack in the vagina.
32. Place a no. 16 Foley catheter in the urethra (another option is to place a suprapubic catheter before the procedure).

F. Postoperative Management

The suprapubic catheter is clamped or the urethral catheter is removed on the third morning postoperatively, and residual urine volumes are measured.

G. Specific Intraoperative Complications
1. Cystotomy
   • Mobilize the tissues adequately.
   • Close in layers with extramucosal synthetic absorbable sutures.
2. Laceration of the urethra
   • It occurs with misdirection of the dissection separating the vaginal wall from the urethra.
   • Adequate mobilization is required.
   • The urethra is closed with fine interrupted synthetic absorbable sutures.
3. Transection of unrecognized urethral diverticulum
   • Excise the rest of the diverticulum.
   • Close the defect with 3-0 synthetic absorbable sutures.

H. Specific Postoperative Complications
1. Various degrees of urinary retention are managed by suprapubic catheter or intermittent self-catheterization.
2. Bladder infection
   • Urine culture
   • Appropriate antibiotic management after catheter removal
3. Urethrovaginal fistula
   • Catheter drainage and cystoscopic examination
   • Perform immediate repair if appropriate.
   • Delayed repair of 8 to 12 weeks is preferred.
4. Vesicovaginal fistula
   • If the fistula is recognized promptly, immediate repair may be attempted if tissues are healthy.
   • Continuous bladder drainage with catheter and a delay of 8 to 12 weeks before undertaking repair are preferred.

II. Marshall-Marchetti-Krantz Operation

A. Introduction

This may be the primary operation in the absence of uterovaginal prolapse or in which significant pulmonary disease or lifestyle make a retropubic approach preferable to obtain long-term benefit.

B. Indication

Stress incontinence

C. Preoperative Investigations

Same as for anterior colporrhaphy or paravaginal defect repair

D. Preoperative Preparation

1. Same as for anterior colporrhaphy
2. The patient is supine with a Foley urethral catheter in place, legs slightly apart, and the vagina and inner thighs prepared and draped to allow insertion of the surgeon's fingers into the vagina intraoperatively.

E. Surgical Technique

1. Make a small midline or transverse incision to enter the space of Retzius.
2. Use curved forceps to carefully and bluntly mobilize the loose areolar tissue on either side of the midline vein.
3. Identify, elevate, clamp, cut, and tie the midline vein.
4. After the loose areolar tissue has been removed, the underlying fascia and the right and left pubourethral ligaments (thick, white condensation of the fascia) can be easily identified.
5. Elevate the dome of the bladder with Russian forceps, and make a 3-cm incision in the midline 2 to 3 cm superior to the bladder neck.
6. The cystotomy allows direct inspection and palpation of the bladder neck and proximal urethra.
7. A curved forceps can be used to define the open bladder neck, which may be patulous about a 20-F urethral catheter previously placed in the urethra.
8. Insert the left hand into the vagina, with the index and middle fingers on either side of the Foley catheter (Fig. 1).
9. This maneuver assists in defining the lateral borders of the urethra.
10. On the patient's right side, identify the posterior pubourethral ligament.
11. Insert the first suture through the posterior pubourethral ligament approximately 2 to 3 mm lateral

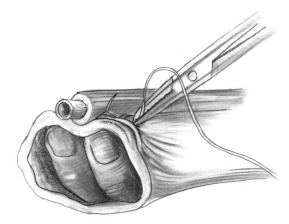

FIG. 2. Insertion of the paraurethral sutures in the Marshall-Marchetti-Krantz operation.

to the urethra with a O Ethibond suture on a Mayo 6 needle (Fig. 2).

12. With the left hand, elevate the anterior vaginal wall toward the symphysis to determine where the suture should be placed so that when it is tied, the vaginal wall will be fixed to the back of the symphysis pubis free of tension.
13. Place the suture securely and deeply in the fibrocartilage of the pubic symphysis, *not* in the periosteum (Fig. 3).
14. Place the companion suture just lateral to the urethra on the opposite side through the posterior or pubourethral ligament.

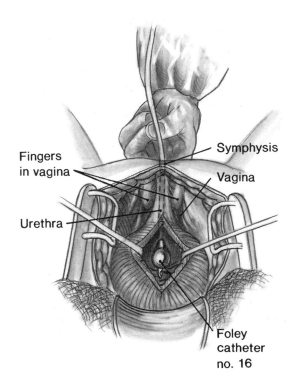

FIG. 1. Insert two fingers of the left hand into the vagina to elevate the paraurethral tissue before inserting the sutures.

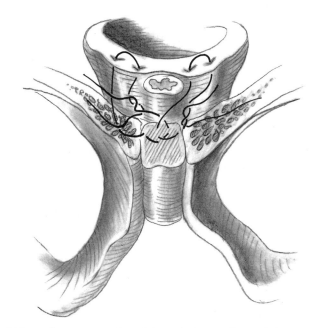

FIG. 3. Sutures are placed through the cartilage of the symphysis pubis and almost full thickness through the vaginal wall in the Marshall-Marchetti-Krantz operation.

15. With the bladder open, evaluate the location of the next set of sutures.
16. Place the first suture of the second set approximately 0.5 cm distal to the bladder neck on the right side of the urethra.
17. Place a second companion suture at the same level, with the needle placed 2 to 3 mm lateral to the urethra, incorporating essentially the full thickness of the anterior vaginal wall.
18. Elevate the anterior vaginal wall, and insert the suture into the cartilage of the symphysis pubis.
19. Tie each suture in the order in which it was placed.
20. Thus the paraurethral tissues are pulled snugly about the urethra.
21. Remove the Foley catheter.
22. Inspect and palpate the doughnut-like ring of paraurethral supporting tissues about the bladder neck.
23. Inspect and palpate the snugly closed bladder neck.
24. The bladder neck should be circular and not slit-like, which suggests that the sutures are too tight.
25. Insert a no. 16 Foley catheter with a 5-mL balloon through the cystotomy, which is closed in two layers with 3–0 running synthetic absorbable suture.
26. Bring the catheter out through a stab wound lateral to the midline incision, and close the incision in the customary fashion.

F. Postoperative Management

The suprapubic catheter is clamped on the sixth morning postoperatively, and the residual urine volumes are measured.

G. Specific Intraoperative Complications

1. Retropubic bleeding is controlled with interrupted sutures and is usually self-controlled after the paraurethral sutures have been tied.
2. Inappropriate placement of sutures causes ligation of the intramural portion of the ureter. With cystotomy, one can identify the bladder neck, determine the proper placement of paraurethral sutures, and evaluate urine flow from the ureteral orifices.
3. Sutures may be mistakenly placed in the bladder or urethral lumen. This is avoided by palpating the urethra and its catheter with the left hand in the vagina and by inspecting the interior of the bladder through the cystotomy.

H. Specific Postoperative Complications

1. Inability to void
   • This is managed with a suprapubic catheter clamping routine and passage of time. Return of function may take many weeks in some patients.
   • Interference with takedown of the suspension, urethral dilation, and so forth should be avoided.
2. Osteitis pubis
   • This occurs in approximately 3% of cases.

• It is managed with physical therapy and antiinflammatory agents.
• Radiographic changes that confirm the diagnosis may be a delayed finding.

III. Paravaginal Defect Repair

A. Indication
1. Urinary stress incontinence
2. Minor degree of anterior vaginal wall relaxation

B. Preoperative Investigations
Same as for anterior colporrhaphy

C. Preoperative Preparation
Same as for Marshall-Marchetti-Krantz operation

D. Surgical Technique
1. Make a midline lower abdominal incision.
2. Perform a dissection to develop the retropubic space.
3. Remove fat from the lateral aspect of the anterior vaginal wall; the area superior to the urethra may be left undisturbed.
4. With two fingers of the left hand in the vagina, elevate the lateral vaginal fornix on each side.
5. The paravaginal defect is the sulcus between the lateral aspect of the vagina and the arcus tendineus ("white line") at the junction of the levator and obturator muscles on the pelvic sidewall.
6. Palpate the urethrovesical junction by feeling for the balloon of the urethral catheter.
7. Place the first (key) stitch of 0 Ethibond lateral and slightly distal to the urethrovesical junction almost full thickness through the anterior vaginal wall, with fingers in the vagina to elevate the vaginal wall.
8. Bring this suture through the arcus tendineus of the lateral pelvic wall approximately 1 to 1.5 cm cephalad to its placement in the vaginal wall.
9. Insert one or two additional sutures above this first suture, fixing the lateral aspect of the vagina to the arcus tendineus and avoiding the obturator nerve, which lies anterior to the area of fixation.
10. Place another one or two sutures caudad and below the "key" stitch, placing the most distal one through the pubourethral ligament and, again, anchoring it to the arcus tendineus laterally.
11. Place a similar set of sutures on the contralateral side.
12. As the ureter comes cephalad and laterally from the bladder, it usually can be palpated between the vaginal finger and an abdominal finger.
13. Tie the sutures in order on each side, reattaching the vaginal fascia to its pelvic wall attachments.
14. This creates a platform effect, supporting the urethra and bladder neck.
15. Check for hemostasis, and close the incision in the routine fashion.

E. Specific Postoperative Management

1. The urethral catheter is removed in 24 to 48 hours.
2. The residual urine volume is measured if the patient has any difficulties with voiding.
3. Straining, lifting, and coitus are avoided for 6 weeks.

F. Specific Postoperative Complications

1. Placement of suture in the lumen of the urethra or bladder
2. Bleeding from paravaginal veins
3. Incorporation of the obturator nerve in the most cephalad suture

IV. Special Problems of Patients with Recurrent Incontinence

1. These patients should always have a complete workup, including urodynamic studies and cystoscopy.
2. They often have a mixed incontinence picture, with stress and urge incontinence.
3. The retropubic approach is always preferred to the vaginal approach.
4. If retropubic suspension has been performed previously, the bladder is often densely adherent to the back of the symphysis and has to be sharply dissected away from it.
5. Early cystotomy helps identify the anatomical layers in multioperated patients and aids retropubic dissection.
6. Occasionally, it may be necessary to release anterior vaginal scarring through a vaginal approach first to mobilize the urethra and bladder neck.
7. Often, after failed previous retropubic suspension, the surgeon finds that dissection and suturing has not been at or below the bladder neck but merely through the anterior bladder wall. Again, cystotomy enables the surgeon to place sutures at the appropriate location lateral to the urethra.

Reading List

Counseller VS, Symmonds RE. Vesicourethral suspension for urinary stress incontinence: a study of the results obtained in 82 patients. *Am J Obstet Gynecol* 1958;75:525–532.

Symmonds RE, Jordon LT. Stress incontinence of urine. *Am J Obstet Gynecol* 1961;82:1231–1237.

Williams TJ, TeLinde RW. The sling operation for urinary incontinence using mersilene ribbon. *Obstet Gynecol* 1962;19:241–245.

Lee RA. The vaginal approach to anterior vaginal relaxation. *Clin Obstet Gynecol* 1972;15:1098–1106.

Symmonds RE. The suprapubic approach to anterior vaginal relaxation and urinary stress incontinence. *Clin Obstet Gynecol* 1972;15:1107–1121.

Lee RA, Symmonds RE. Repeat Marshall-Marchetti-Krantz procedure for recurrent stress urinary incontinence. *Am J Obstet Gynecol* 1975;122:219–225.

Lee RA. Recurrent stress incontinence of urine: preoperative assessment and surgical management. *Clin Obstet Gynecol* 1976;19:661–671.

Lee RA. Abdominal operations for urinary incontinence. *In:* Sciarra JJ, McElin TW, eds. *Gynecology and obstetrics.* Hagerstown, MD: Harper & Row, 1977:1–13.

Lee RA. The modified Marshall-Marchetti-Krantz operation as a primary procedure in urinary stress incontinence. *In:* Buchsbaum HJ, Schmidt JD, eds. *Gynecologic and obstetric urology.* Philadelphia: WB Saunders, 1978:200–207.

Lee RA. Surgical procedures for recurrent stress incontinence. *In:* Buchsbaum HJ, Schmidt JD, eds. *Gynecologic and obstetric urology.* Philadelphia: WB Saunders, 1978:245–255.

Lee RA, Symmonds RE, Goldstein RA. Surgical complications and results of modified Marshall-Marchetti-Krantz procedure for urinary incontinence. *Obstet Gynecol* 1979;53:447–450.

Lee RA. Prognosis in the treatment of urinary incontinence. *In:* Slate WG, ed. *Disorders of the female urethra and urinary incontinence.* Baltimore: Williams & Wilkins, 1982:210–212.

Lee RA. Surgical management of stress incontinence. *Postgrad Obstet Gynecol* 1986;6:1–6.

Stanhope CR. Urinary incontinence. ACOG Tech Bull Jan 1987;100.

Lee RA, Barrett DM. Diagnostic approach and selective surgical management of female incontinence at the Mayo Clinic. *Clin Gynecol Obstet* 1989;6:65–71.

Kammerer-Doak DN, Cornella JL, Magrina JF, et al. Osteitis pubis after Marshall-Marchetti-Krantz urethropexy: a pubic osteomyelitis. *Am J Obstet Gynecol* 1998;179:586–590.

CHAPTER 20

Endometriosis

William A. Cliby, M.D. and Tiffany J. Williams, M.D.

I. Introduction

Surgical procedures for endometriosis can be divided basically into two categories.

A. Conservative Surgery

An attempt is made to eradicate the endometriosis and to preserve childbearing capability.

B. Definitive Surgery

The removal of the uterus, tubes, and ovaries to eliminate the source, the passageway, and the stimulus for the occurrence of endometriosis.

II. Conservative Surgery for Endometriosis

A. Principles

Conservative surgery for endometriosis should involve all the techniques that are inherent in microsurgery, in an attempt to remove by excision or by destruction, all the abnormal tissue involved with endometriosis. The potential for childbearing should be conserved (saving at least the uterus and one tube and ovary), and all efforts should be made to minimize subsequent adhesion and scar formation. In many instances, endoscopic surgical techniques can be used in the conservative surgical management of endometriosis, and the techniques outlined here should be applied regardless of an open or laparoscopic approach. The procedures for tubal reconstructive surgery are described in Chapter 9.

William A. Cliby: Consultant, Departments of Obstetrics and Gynecology and Surgery, Mayo Clinic and Mayo Foundation; Assistant Professor of Obstetrics and Gynecology, Mayo Medical School, Rochester, Minnesota.

Tiffany J. Williams: Emeritus Member, Departments of Obstetrics and Gynecology and Surgery, Mayo Clinic and Mayo Foundation; Emeritus Professor of Obstetrics and Gynecology, Mayo Medical School, Rochester, Minnesota.

B. Indications
1. Symptomatic endometriosis
2. Desire for future childbearing

C. Preoperative Investigations
Carefully review any previous operative and pathology notes.
1. Document disease and define to preserve the uterus and one tube and ovary satisfactory as well as to eradicate all areas of endometriosis (laparoscopy).
2. If there is a possibility of bowel involvement, colon radiography and proctoscopy are appropriate. These should be performed at the time of the menstrual period.
3. If urinary symptoms are present or if there is suggestion of ureteral involvement, intravenous pyelography should be performed. This is best done at the time of the menstrual period.
4. Determine the optimal route of surgical approach.

D. Preoperative Preparation
1. Povidone-iodine douche
2. Abdominoperineal shave
3. Enema
4. Thromboembolus-deterrent stockings
5. Prophylactic treatment with antibiotics
6. Preoperative bowel preparation in cases of severe endometriosis or suspected gastrointestinal tract involvement

E. Surgical Technique
1. Incision: choice is dictated by disease sites. A longitudinal incision allows adequate exposure of the upper abdomen when indicated.
2. Explore the abdominal contents.
3. Evaluate pelvic organs.
4. Carefully inspect and note all areas of endometriosis. The ureters must be definitely identified and protected during the operation.

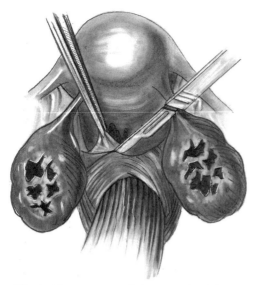

FIG. 1. Management of uterus and cul-de-sac.

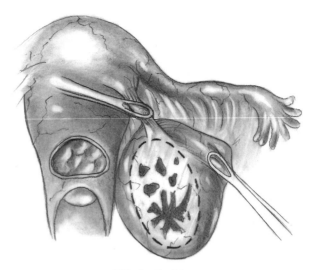

FIG. 3. Excision.

5. Completely excise or destroy endometriotic areas from the back of the uterus, broad ligaments, uterosacral ligaments, cul-de-sac, and rectosigmoid by using microcautery or laser (Fig. 1).

6. Large defects of the peritoneum may be closed with absorbable nonreactive long-acting sutures (5-0 synthetic absorbable suture).

7. After the back of the uterus, broad ligaments, cul-de-sac, uterosacral ligaments, and rectosigmoid have been cared for, pay attention to the tubes and ovaries.

8. Place packs against the cul-de-sac areas to provide hemostasis while attending to other areas.

9. Excise adhesive areas with microcautery. Electrocoagulate small areas of endometriosis or vaporize them with a laser.

10. Excise areas of endometriosis and scarring about the tubes and cornu.

11. Excise endometriomas in the ovary using microcautery, with appropriate traction and electrodissection (Figs. 2 and 3).

12. Reconstruction of the ovary is generally recommended. Use internal sutures as much as possible. These sutures may be
    - Concentric purse-string sutures
    - Subserosal sutures
    - Baseball sutures
    - Figure-of-eight sutures
    - "Snowflake" sutures (no two alike)

These are all accomplished to achieve the end result of ovarian reconstruction, to obliterate dead space, and to provide good hemostasis with the minimal amount of suture material on the peritoneal surface. Animal experiments suggest that there are fewer adhesions when the ovary is allowed to heal without external sutures. After laparoscopic excision, the ovary usually is not reconstructed.

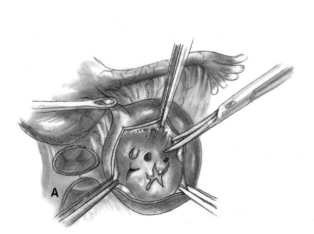

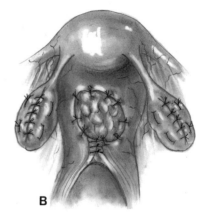

FIG. 2. A: Excision of endometrioma. **B:** Reconstructed ovaries.

13. Generally, tubal endometriosis may be excised along the area of involvement without incising the peritoneum.
14. Secure meticulous hemostasis with microcautery, laser, or bipolar cautery.
15. Similarly manage areas of endometriosis in the anterior cul-de-sac with resection and/or electrodestruction.
16. Manage peritoneal defects with approximation.
17. Tubo-ovarian suspension is recommended with cul-de-sac disease: suture the ovary to the parietal peritoneum with an absorbable suture, allowing peritonization of the cul-de-sac, thus minimizing the potential for the ovary to become adherent there.
18. Thoroughly flush the pelvis with physiologic solution and heparin, and close the incision.
19. Use an adhesion barrier if appropriate.

F. Difficulties Encountered
1. Obesity compromises exposure and delicate tissue techniques.
2. Extensive organ involvement may indicate definitive complete surgery.
3. Compromised blood supply may require oophorectomy or salpingo-oophorectomy.
4. Ovarian destruction from endometrioma may require oophorectomy.

G. Specific Postoperative Management
1. Routine postoperative care
2. Consider suppression of endometriosis medically until time of future childbearing.

III. Definitive Surgery for Endometriosis

Involves removal of the uterus, tubes, and ovaries and destruction of endometriotic tissue

A. Indications
1. Symptomatic pelvic disease
2. Dyspareunia
3. Dysmenorrhea
4. Progressive changes on examination
5. Bilateral ovarian neoplasm, persistent and enlarging
6. Completed childbearing
7. Any gastrointestinal or urinary tract involvement

B. Preoperative Investigations
1. Complete blood count
2. Serum chemistry
3. Urinalysis
4. Electrocardiography if older than 40 years
5. Chest radiography
6. Intravenous pyelography if any urologic symptoms
7. Colon radiography if gastrointestinal symptoms

C. Preoperative Preparation
1. Povidone-iodine douche
2. Abdominoperineal shave

3. Enema
4. Thromboembolus-deterrent stockings
5. Prophylactic treatment with antibiotics
6. Bowel preparation if symptoms suggest intestinal involvement or fixation of cul-de-sac

D. Surgical Technique
1. Make a low midline incision.
2. Explore abdominal contents.
3. Place patient in Trendelenburg position.
4. Pack off the intestine, and free adhesions.
5. It is strongly recommended that adhesive disease and distortion of anatomical landmarks be completely managed before initiating the hysterectomy.
6. Perform total abdominal hysterectomy and bilateral salpingo-oophorectomy as described in Chapter 7.
7. Ureteral dissection is often necessary to perform conservative or extirpative surgery safely. Meticulous sharp dissection is used to free the ureter. The uterine vessels must be dissected away from the ureter and divided (Fig. 4) to allow full mobilization.
8. Additional areas of endometriosis may be excised with the specimen.
9. Other areas of endometriosis may be electrocoagulated or excised separately if not in continuity.
10. Flush the pelvis with physiologic solution.
11. Replace the bowel, bring down the omentum, and close the incision.

E. Intraoperative Complications
1. Bleeding
   - Infundibulopelvic ligament
   - Uterine artery
   - Bladder muscularis
2. Before closure, hemostasis is ensured under direct vision by clamping and ligating.
3. Bladder or ureteral damage
4. Bowel damage

F. Specific Postoperative Management
1. Routine management
2. May elect to withhold exogenous estrogen for 6 to 9 months and treat with progesterone instead, especially if endometriosis is extensive

G. Specific Postoperative Complications
1. Ureteral damage related to difficult dissection
2. Vesicovaginal or rectovaginal fistula due to adherent organs from endometriosis
3. Ovarian remnant due to inadequate dissection and excision

IV. Ureteral Obstruction in Endometriosis

Ureteral obstruction is an uncommon complication of endometriosis; however, it may be encountered when dealing with extensive endometriosis. Definitive surgery is recom-

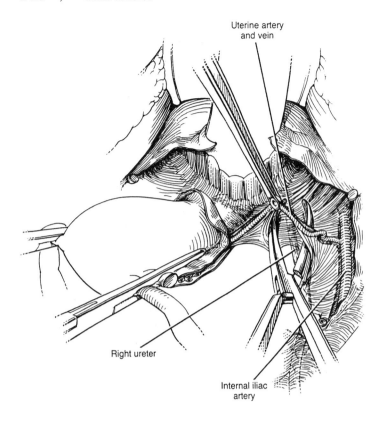

Uterine artery
and vein

Right ureter

Internal iliac
artery

FIG. 4. Lower ureteral dissection. (Redrawn from Lee RA. *Atlas of gynecologic surgery.* Philadelphia: WB Saunders, 1992:176, with permission.)

mended in addition to specific management of the endometriotic area.

A. Indications

Evidence of obstruction

B. Preoperative Investigations

1. Complete blood count
2. Serum chemistry
3. Urinalysis
4. Electrocardiography if older than 40 years
5. Chest radiography
6. Intravenous pyelography
7. Colon radiography if gastrointestinal symptoms

C. Preoperative Preparation

1. Povidone-iodine douche
2. Abdominoperineal shave
3. Enema
4. Thromboembolus-deterrent stockings
5. Prophylactic treatment with antibiotics
6. Bowel preparation if symptoms warrant

D. Surgical Technique

1. Make a low midline incision.
2. Explore abdominal contents.
3. Preoperative ureteral catheterization is not necessary, and it may increase the chance of trauma between the dissection and the catheter. It does allow identification of the ureter if cut.
4. Open the retroperitoneal space.
5. Visualize and palpate the ureter. If there is obstruction, there will be proximal dilation.
6. Continue the dissection down to the area of obstruction.
7. If the endometriosis is superficial, excise it with microcautery. If this is effective, the dilation will subside and structural resection will be avoided.
8. If there is direct luminal involvement, ureteral resection is required. In this case, open the bladder, visualize the ureteral orifice, insert a ureteral catheter, and pass it to the area of obstruction. With dissection, free the obstruction.
9. Excise the area of obstruction.
10. Perform ureteral-ureteral anastomosis with synthetic absorbable 5-0 sutures, avoiding the uroepithelium. Four or five sutures provide an appropriate anastomosis.
11. Whenever technically possible, a ureteroneocystotomy is preferable to ureteral-ureteral anastomosis. A psoas hitch is performed to relieve tension.
12. Pass a double J-ureteral-catheter through the anastomosis to serve as a stent.
13. Place a suction catheter retroperitoneally to the area of anastomosis.
14. Close the peritoneum.
15. If there is extragenital involvement, total abdominal hysterectomy and bilateral salpingo-oophorectomy are indicated.

E. Specific Postoperative Management

1. Monitor urine output.
2. A bladder catheter is left in place for 7 days to minimize suture line damage from bladder expansion with filling.
3. The ureteral stent is removed in 3 to 4 weeks via cystoscopy after normal intravenous pyelographic results.
4. If there is drainage of urine through the retroperitoneal drain, leave the catheter and stent in place for a longer time.

F. Specific Postoperative Complications

1. Ureteral fistula
2. Ureteral stenosis

V. Intestinal Obstruction in Endometriosis

A. Indications

Symptomatic intestinal symptoms:
1. Constipation
2. Diarrhea
3. Bleeding associated with the menstrual cycle
4. Symptoms of obstruction

B. Preoperative Investigations

1. Complete blood count
2. Serum chemistry
3. Urinalysis
4. Electrocardiography if older than 40 years
5. Chest radiography
6. Intravenous pyelography
7. Colon radiography at the time of the menstrual period

C. Preoperative Preparation

1. Povidone-iodine douche
2. Abdominoperineal shave
3. Enema
4. Thromboembolus-deterrent stockings
5. Prophylactic treatment with antibiotics
6. Bowel preparation

D. Surgical Technique

1. Make a low midline incision.
2. Explore abdominal contents.
3. Place patient in Trendelenburg position.
4. Locate the obstruction. Proximal dilation should be present.
5. Potential obstruction should be corrected if there appears to be significant kinking or damage from the endometriosis (i.e., more than half of the lumen is closed).
6. In many cases, the endometriosis may be excised with microcautery, allowing the bowel to open.

7. If there is significant luminal compromise by endometriosis, resection may be required.
8. Isolate the obstructed segment with noncrushing clamps.
9. Score the bowel mesentery after identifying the vascular supply.
10. Clamp, cut, and ligate the blood supply.
11. Place clamps across the obstructed segment of intestine, and incise the segment.
12. Perform anastomosis (see Chapter 24).
    - Close the back wall with interrupted inverting permanent sutures.
    - Excise the crushed areas beneath the clamps.
    - Use a continuous synthetic absorbable suture to approximate the mucosa.
    - Place inverting supporting sutures of permanent material in the anterior wall.
    - Confirm patency.
13. Approximate the mesentery.
14. Confirm the viability of the intestine and the adequacy of the anastomosis.
15. Remove the packs.
16. Perform definitive surgery (total abdominal hysterectomy and bilateral salpingo-oophorectomy).
17. Irrigate the abdomen thoroughly.
18. Drain the pelvis with suction drains if left colon or rectal resection was performed.
19. Close the incision.

E. Specific Postoperative Management

1. Nothing by mouth until flatus has been passed
2. No enemas
3. No feeding until bowel movement

F. Specific Postoperative Complication

Intestinal anastomotic leak

VI. Endometriosis of the Cul-de-sac

A. Indications

1. With extensive endometriosis, definitive surgery is recommended.

Note: Conservative management in conjunction with resection has dismal results.

2. Symptomatic intestinal symptoms
    - Constipation
    - Diarrhea
    - Bleeding associated with the menstrual period
    - Symptoms of obstruction
3. Endometriosis is often seen growing through the cul-de-sac into the vagina, in which case postcoital spotting and dyspareunia may be prominent.

B. Preoperative Investigations

1. Complete blood count
2. Serum chemistry
3. Urinalysis
4. Electrocardiography if older than 40 years
5. Chest radiography
6. Intravenous pyelography if any urinary symptoms
7. Colon radiography at the time of the menstrual period
8. Proctoscopy

C. Preoperative Preparation

1. Povidone-iodine douche
2. Abdominoperineal shave
3. Enema
4. Thromboembolus-deterrent stockings
5. Prophylactic treatment with antibiotics
6. Bowel preparation

D. Surgical Technique

1. Make a low midline incision.
2. Explore abdominal contents.
3. Place patient in Trendelenburg position.
4. Cul-de-sac involvement usually involves the rectosigmoid extensively, and resection is often required.
5. Because the involvement is anterior, a wedge resection removing only the anterior portion of the bowel and the endometriosis may work satisfactorily.
   - Accomplish the partial anastomosis by continuous mucosal closure with synthetic absorbable sutures.
   - Permanent interrupted sutures invert the muscularis and serosa.
6. The alternative: perform complete segmental resection and anastomosis of the rectosigmoid.

7. Perform a definitive operation (total abdominal hysterectomy and bilateral salpingo-oophorectomy) in the usual fashion.
8. Drain the pelvis with suction drains.

E. Specific Postoperative Management

1. Nothing by mouth until flatus has been passed.
2. Remove the pelvic suction drain after the bowels open.

Reading List

Kempers RD, Dockerty MB, Hunt AB, et al. Significant postmenopausal endometriosis. *Surg Gynecol Obstet* 1960;111:348–356.

Pratt JH. Abdominal manifestations of endometriosis. *Minn Med* 1962; 45:1103–1107.

Sheets JL, Symmonds RE, Banner EA. Conservative surgical management of endometriosis. *Obstet Gynecol* 1964;23:625–628.

Hanton EM, Malkasian GD Jr, Dockerty MB, et al. Endometriosis associated with complete or partial obstruction of menstrual egress: report of 7 cases. *Obstet Gynecol* 1966;28:626–629.

Hanton EM, Malkasian GD Jr, Dockerty MB, et al. Endometriosis in young women. *Am J Obstet Gynecol* 1967;98:116–120.

Martimbeau PW, Pratt JH, Gaffey TA. Small-bowel obstruction secondary to endometriosis. *Mayo Clin Proc* 1975;50:239–243.

Williams TJ, Pratt JH. Endometriosis in 1,000 consecutive celiotomies: incidence and management. *Am J Obstet Gynecol* 1977;129:245–250.

Pratt JH, Williams TJ. Indications for complete pelvic operations and more radical procedures in the treatment of severe or extensive endometriosis. *Clin Obstet Gynecol* 1980;23:937–950.

Williams TJ. Endometriosis. *In:* Mattingly RF, Thompson JD, eds. *Te Linde's operative gynecology,* 6th ed. Philadelphia: JB Lippincott, 1985:257–286.

Stillwell TJ, Kramer SA, Lee RA. Endometriosis of ureter. *Urology* 1986;28:81–85.

Williams TJ. Endometriosis. *Conns Curr Ther* 1987;883–886.

Lu PY, Ory SJ. Endometriosis: current management. *Mayo Clin Proc* 1995;70:453–463.

Magrina JF, Cornella JL, Nygaard IE, et al. Endometriosis involving the lower urinary tract. I. Clinical presentation. II. Results of surgical treatment. *J Pelv Surg* 1996;2:172–175;176–181.

Zanetta G, Webb MJ, Segura JW. Ureteral endometriosis diagnosed at ureteroscopy. *Obstet Gynecol* 1998;91:857–859.

CHAPTER 21

Stomas

Maurice J. Webb, M.D. and Karl C. Podratz, M.D., Ph.D.

I. Ileal Conduit

A. Indications
1. Anterior pelvic exenteration
2. To connect short transected ureter to bladder
3. Diversion of nonfunctional lower urinary tract (noncorrectable fistulas, urinary incontinence, etc.)

B. Preoperative Investigations
Depend on indication for surgery but will include
1. Intravenous pyelography
2. Serum chemistry
3. Urine culture
4. Complete blood count

C. Preoperative Preparation
1. Bowel preparation with polyethylene glycol electrolyte solution (GoLYTELY)
2. Prophylactic treatment with antibiotics
3. Patient instructed by stomal therapist
4. Marking the appropriate site of the stoma on the abdominal wall

D. Surgical Technique
1. Make a lower midline incision.
2. Proceed with pelvic exenteration (see Chapter 17).
3. Free up each transected distal ureter, leaving a flap of broad ligament peritoneum attached to the ureter.
4. With the use of transilluminated light, identify the vascular arcade of the ileocolic vessels supplying the terminal ileum.
5. Select an approximately 15- to 20-cm segment of

terminal ileum that is supplied by a major vascular bundle.
6. Divide the mesentery of the ileum perpendicular to the proximal point of the transection over a distance of about 3 to 4 cm.
7. Transect the ileum at the identified proximal end of the conduit with a GIA stapler or noncrushing bowel clamps.
8. Identify the site for distal transection of the terminal ileum, and divide the mesentery at this point over a distance of about 6 to 8 cm.
9. Greater mobility of the distal conduit is required to allow it to reach up through the abdominal wall.
10. Transect the distal margin of the conduit with the GIA stapler or with bowel clamps.
11. This isolates the ileal conduit.
12. If the proximal end has not been stapled closed, close it by oversewing in two layers with continuous 3-0 synthetic absorbable suture in the mucosal layer, supported by interrupted 3-0 silk suture in the seromuscular layer.
13. Reanastomose the terminal ileum either in an end-to-end two-layered sutured closure or as a side-to-side anastomosis using the GIA stapler (Fig. 1).
14. Perform the ileal anastomosis anterior to the conduit so the conduit can lie against the posterior abdominal wall.
15. Close (parallel rather than perpendicular to bowel) the defect in the terminal ileal mesentery, taking care not to traumatize the mesentery of the conduit.
16. Implant the ureters into the antimesenteric aspect of the ileal conduit.
17. Implant the left ureter first, because it is least accessible.
18. Grasp the antimesenteric serosa and muscularis of the conduit with fine mosquito forceps approximately 2 cm from the closed proximal end of the conduit.
19. With fine iris scissors, make a 3-mm incision into the seromuscular layer, and squeeze the conduit to make the mucosa point up into the incision.

Maurice J. Webb: Chairman, Division of Gynecologic Surgery and Consultant, Department of Surgery, Mayo Clinic and Mayo Foundation; Professor of Obstetrics and Gynecology, Mayo Medical School, Rochester, Minnesota.

Karl C. Podratz: Chairman, Department of Obstetrics and Gynecology, Consultant, Department of Surgery, Mayo Clinic and Mayo Foundation; Professor of Obstetrics and Gynecology, Mayo Medical School, Rochester, Minnesota.

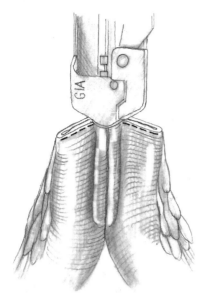

FIG. 1. Side-to-side intestinal anastomosis with the GIA stapler.

20. Next, grasp the bleb of mucosa with the mosquito forceps and incise it, opening into the intestinal conduit cavity (Fig. 2).
21. Maintain traction on the conduit mucosa with the mosquito forceps while implanting the ureter.
22. Pick up the left ureter with fine vascular forceps and trim it to the appropriate length.
23. If the lumen of the ureter is quite small, make a 2- to 4-mm incision into the cut edge of the ureter on the side opposite the attached peritoneum.
24. Next, place a 4-0 synthetic absorbable suture through the apex of this V-shaped incision, from outside to inside, full thickness through the ureter.

25. Bring the suture from inside to outside, full thickness, through the hole in the conduit in a position so that when the suture is tied, the ureter is not twisted on itself.
26. Tie this suture, thereby approximating the ureter to the conduit.
27. Place and tie two similar sutures at the top edges of the V-shaped cut in the ureter, on either side of the initial suture.
28. Insert the remaining three or four interrupted sutures in a similar fashion around the rest of the cut edge of the ureter: these sutures are held rather than tied until all sutures are in place (Fig. 3).
29. Pass a single J-ureteral-stent up the left ureter to the pelvis of the kidney, and remove the guide wire.
30. Cut the distal end of the stent to an appropriate length, and pass it into the conduit and up and out the conduit's distal end.
31. Now, tie the remaining ureteral anastomosis sutures.
32. Alternatively, use a running 5-0 delayed absorbable synthetic suture with a double-armed needle for the ureteric anastomosis.
33. Now, bring the peritoneal patch up over the anastomosis and suture it to the conduit serosa with a few interrupted 3-0 synthetic absorbable sutures (Fig. 4).
34. The peritoneal patch seals and takes tension off the anastomosis.

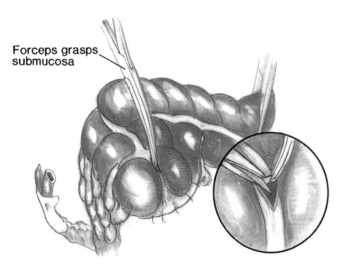

FIG. 2. Before ureteric anastomosis, a small incision is made into the seromuscular layer of the bowel wall, and the submucosa is grasped with mosquito forceps.

Forceps grasps submucosa

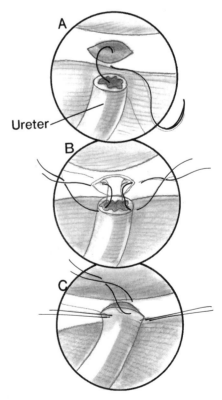

Ureter

FIG. 3. The ureter is anastomosed with multiple interrupted full-thickness sutures placed in the bowel wall.

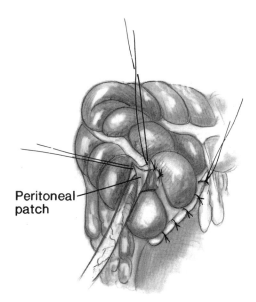

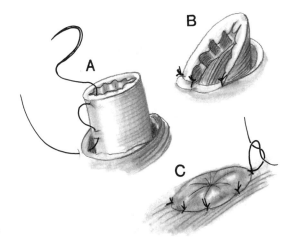

FIG. 4. A peritoneal flap (preserved on the ureter when it was divided at the level of the pelvic brim) is now attached to the bowel wall to "seal" and to relieve any "pull" on the anastomosis.

FIG. 5. In creating an ileal conduit stoma, the sutures are placed to include the subcuticular skin margins and the bowel wall 2 to 3 cm from the end (**A**) and full thickness of bowel at the end of the segment (**B**); this produces an everted "rosebud" (**C**) of bowel mucosa.

35. Implant the right ureter into the conduit in a similar fashion, approximately 2 cm distal to the left ureter.
36. Anchor the proximal end of the conduit to the mesentery of the sigmoid so that the left ureter again lies mainly on the left of the sigmoid mesentery: this prevents the ureter from kinking as it swings beneath the mesentery.
37. Excise an appropriately sized button of skin and subcutaneous fat from the abdominal wall in the previously marked right lower quadrant position.
38. Grasp the skin edge, rectus fascia, and peritoneum with straight forceps, and apply traction: this prevents subsequent shearing of the abdominal wall layers and possible obstruction of the conduit blood supply.
39. After excising the skin button, incise the rectus fascia in a cruciate fashion together with the underlying peritoneum.
40. Stretch the abdominal wall defect to at least a two-finger diameter to accommodate the conduit.
41. Draw the distal end of the conduit through the stomal site.
42. Construct the stoma as a Brooke-type nipple by folding back the distal end of the conduit on itself and then suturing it to the abdominal wall skin with multiple interrupted 3-0 synthetic absorbable sutures (Fig. 5).
43. Take care to place the sutures in the subcutaneous tissue rather than through the skin to prevent skin puckering, with subsequent leakage around the conduit appliance.
44. Suture the single J-stents to the conduit mucosa with a fine absorbable suture to prevent dislodgement.
45. Draw the cecum above and medial to the conduit, and suture it there to prevent the cecum and terminal ileum

from hanging across the mesentery of the conduit and obstructing its blood supply.

E. Specific Postoperative Management

1. A nasogastric tube may be used in the immediate postoperative period to prevent small-bowel distention.
2. Output from each ureteric stent may be measured independently and the stent irrigated if it becomes blocked.
3. The stents are removed in about 10 to 14 days in nonirradiated patients but are left for 6 weeks in irradiated patients unless the stents are expelled sooner.

F. Specific Postoperative Complications

1. Stomal necrosis
   - Viability of the conduit mucosa can be assessed by inserting a test tube into the stoma and inspecting the interior of the conduit.
   - If necrosis of the nipple only occurs, leave alone until the sloughed tissue starts to separate and then debride.
   - Subsequent stomal stenosis may occur in this situation, and surgical revision may be required later.
2. Obstruction of ureteral stent(s)
   Irrigate the stent with 5 to 10 mL of physiologic saline by using a blunt-tipped needle and syringe.
3. Conduit necrosis
   - All or part of the conduit may necrose because of interference with its blood supply.
   - This may produce a urinary perineal or other fistula.
   - Treat by reoperating and refashioning a new conduit, usually from the transverse colon.

- If there is only a small leak at the ureteral anastomosis and the stents already have been removed, it may be possible to pass an anterograde catheter through a percutaneous nephrostomy and thereby allow the leaking anastomosis to heal.
- A loopogram obtained by injecting radiopaque dye into the conduit may give more information than an excretory urogram about the integrity of the conduit.

4. Small-bowel obstruction
- Due to inadequate anastomosis or, more likely, to adhesion formation, with kinking of the intestine
- In irradiated patients, obstruction may produce intestinal fistula formation from the site of anastomosis.

5. Enteric fistula
- More common in irradiated patients
- Usually occurs at the site of anastomosis in the terminal ileum
- Often occurs because of obstruction caused by the small bowel becoming adherent in the denuded pelvis
- In irradiated patients, the fistula usually does not heal with conservative management and requires reoperation.

6. Ureteric obstruction
- Perform intravenous pyelography about 6 to 8 weeks after removal of the stents to check ureteric function.
- If it is difficult to tell whether a hydroureter is due to obstruction or is a result of poor peristalsis related to surgery, a furosemide (Lasix) "washout" radioisotope renogram or a loopogram to show free reflux up the ureters will define the situation.
- If obstruction is present, anterograde stenting may be attempted, but often reimplantation will be necessary. Ureteral balloon dilation might be attempted if stenting is unsuccessful.

7. Metabolic abnormality
Treat according to the abnormality encountered.

II. Sigmoid Conduit

A. Indication
Total pelvic exenteration

B. Preoperative Investigations and Preparation
The same as for ileal conduit

C. Surgical Technique
1. Usually a sigmoid conduit is used when a rectal resection is performed as part of a total pelvic exenteration.
2. It can be used whether bowel continuity is restored or a terminal colostomy is used.
3. A similar technique is used to construct a sigmoid neovagina, and in some instances, enough bowel is present to construct both a sigmoid neovagina and a sigmoid conduit.
4. After mobilizing the rectosigmoid and transecting it at the appropriate level in the pelvis with a TA 55 stapler, isolate a 15- to 20-cm segment by dividing the mesentery for about 3 to 4 cm at the proximal end of the proposed conduit.
5. Transect the sigmoid with the GIA stapler or with noncrushing clamps (Fig. 6).
6. The distal end of the descending colon then can be either reanastomosed to the rectal stump by using the intraluminal stapler or by a hand-sewn anastomosis or brought out as a terminal colostomy in the left lower quadrant of the abdomen.
7. Anastomose the ureters into the sigmoid conduit in a fashion similar to that described for the ileal conduit.

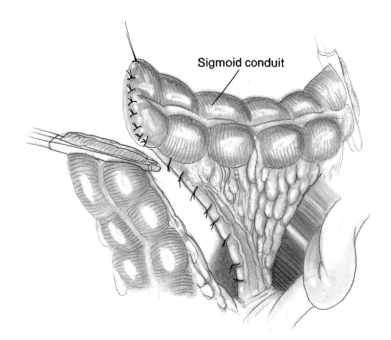

Sigmoid conduit

FIG. 6. The sigmoid conduit is isolated on its blood supply, and the proximal end is closed.

8. It is best to locate the implantation site on the antimesenteric aspect of the conduit, along one of the tenia.

9. Anchor the proximal end of the conduit to the fascia overlying the left psoas muscle to minimize tension on the ureterosigmoid anastomosis.

10. Use ureteral stents. The stomal site is in the right lower quadrant of the abdominal wall.

11. If the sigmoid is reanastomosed, it should be drained with a suction drain until bowel function returns.

D. Specific Postoperative Management and Complications

1. The same as for ileal conduit

2. Because there is no small-bowel anastomosis, obstruction and fistula formation are much less common.

III. Transverse Colon Conduit

A. Indication

Anterior or total exenteration when the terminal ileum or sigmoid colon has been heavily irradiated and does not appear suitable for conduit construction; may also be used where ureteral length is limited.

B. Preoperative Investigations and Preparation

The same as for ileal conduit

C. Surgical Technique

1. Reflect the omentum off the transverse colon, leaving the omentum still attached to the stomach.

2. Identify the middle colic artery by palpation and transillumination through the mesentery.

3. Select a 15- to 20-cm segment of transverse colon supplied by this vessel, and create a window in the mesentery adjacent to the points of transection.

4. Transect the colon proximally and distally with the GIA stapler or over bowel clamps.

5. Reanastomose the transverse colon with two layers of hand-sewn suturing or with stapling technique, keeping the conduit below the transverse colon.

6. Prepare the ureters, and implant them into the colon using the technique described above for ileal conduit.

7. This may require drawing the ureters through the defects created in the mesentery.

8. Anchor the proximal end of the conduit to the posterior abdominal wall peritoneum to prevent tension on the ureters.

9. Close the defect in the mesentery of the transverse colon.

10. Suture the stoma of the conduit as before through the right anterior abdominal wall.

D. Specific Postoperative Management and Complications

1. The same as for ileal conduit

2. Because the transverse colon usually has not been irradiated, conduit and bowel anastomosis problems are less frequent.

3. The stoma may need to be brought out at a higher and less ideal position on the abdominal wall in some patients because of the length of the transverse colon mesentery.

IV. Continent Urinary Stoma

A. Indication

Techniques are still being refined, and malfunction is more common than with free-draining conduits; therefore, patients need to be informed of choices. Also, patients need to be selected carefully for such a procedure in association with pelvic exenteration. Most techniques use the cecum and right colon, but transverse and left colon conduits have been described.

B. Preoperative Investigations and Preparation

The same as for ileal conduit

C. Surgical Technique

1. Mobilize the cecum and the terminal ileum.

2. Transect the ileum 10 to 12 cm from the ileocecal valve.

3. Transect the transverse colon at a point immediately beyond the middle colic artery.

4. Remove the appendix if present.

5. Reanastomose the distal ileum to the transverse colon.

6. Open the colon conduit longitudinally along a tenia on the antimesenteric surface using the cautery.

7. Fold the opened transverse colon down beside the cecum, and anastomose the posterior wall edges of the conduit with absorbable staples.

8. Pass a 14-F catheter along the segment of the terminal ileum and through the ileocecal valve.

9. Place a row of Allis or Babcock clamps along the antimesenteric border of the terminal ileal segment, and while applying traction on the clamps, narrow the terminal ileal lumen by stapling alongside the catheter between the catheter and the clamps with a GIA stapler.

10. This increases the pressure in the lumen of the bowel, thus assisting continence.

11. Excise the excess portion of the wall of the ileum.

12. Insert three purse-string sutures of 2-0 silk in the seromuscular layer around the ileocecal valve.

13. These purse-string sutures also aid continence.

14. Bring out the ileal stoma in the right lower quadrant of the abdomen, and suture it to the skin with multiple interrupted 3-0 synthetic absorbable sutures.

15. Anastomose the ureters into the posterior wall of the conduit in a nonrefluxing type of anastomosis (tunneled beneath the mucosal layer or lying on its surface), and suture them in place with multiple 4-0 synthetic absorbable sutures.

16. Place a few additional sutures, and peritoneal patch if present, on the exterior surface of the conduit to support the ureters further.

17. Insert a single J-ureteral-stent up each ureter, and bring them out through the anterior abdominal wall separate from the stomal site and the skin incision.
18. Close the anterior wall of the conduit with absorbable staples.

D. Specific Postoperative Management
1. Perform intravenous pyelography and radiographic contrast studies of the reservoir approximately 3 weeks postoperatively to check for leaks and ureteric obstruction.
2. If the results are satisfactory, remove the ureteric stents. The ureteric stents may be left for 6 weeks if the conduit has been heavily irradiated.
3. Teach the patient self-catheterization of the reservoir.
4. Initially, catheterize every 4 hours.
5. Repeat reservoir contrast studies and excretory urography in 6 months.

E. Specific Postoperative Complications
1. Fistula from pouch or ureteric anastomosis: treat as for urinary conduit
2. Ureteric stenosis: treat as for urinary conduit
3. Obstruction of ureteric stent: irrigate with sterile saline
4. Incontinent urinary stoma: may need surgical revision
5. Intestinal fistula from bowel anastomosis
6. Metabolic abnormalities from absorption of electrolytes from the bowel mucosa: treat according to the abnormality

V. Colostomy

May be either a permanent or a temporary defunctioning type

A. Indications
1. To protect a distal large-bowel anastomosis
2. To protect repair of a large-bowel fistula
3. For relief of colonic obstruction
4. Associated with abdominoperineal resection in pelvic exenteration
5. As a temporary Hartmann procedure with rectosigmoid resection
6. As a permanent diversion of the fecal stream in the presence of an irreparable sigmoid or rectal fistula

B. Preoperative Investigations
1. Routine laboratory tests depending on the indication
2. Colonoscopy and/or contrast studies of the colon may be indicated preoperatively to define the site and nature of the obstruction or fistula.

C. Preoperative Preparation
1. Bowel preparation (if bowel not obstructed) with polyethylene glycol electrolyte solution (GoLYTELY)
2. Prophylactic treatment with antibiotics

3. Patient instructed by a stomal therapist
4. Marking the stomal site on the abdominal wall

D. Surgical Technique
1. End colostomy
   • Grasp the skin, fascia, and peritoneal edges of the incision near the site of the stoma with straight Kocher forceps, and apply traction.
   • Grasp the skin at the site of the stoma with a straight Kocher forceps, and excise a 2-cm button of skin and underlying fat.
   • Make a cruciate incision in the rectus fascia, and open the peritoneum.
   • Enlarge the hole so it is two fingers in diameter.
   • Pass a noncrushing intestinal clamp through the hole, grasp the distal cut end of the colon, and draw it through the hole.
   • Suture the full thickness of the colonic wall to subcutaneous tissue with multiple interrupted 3-0 synthetic absorbable sutures.
   • A few extra supporting sutures may be placed internally between the bowel wall and the anterior abdominal wall peritoneum.
   • Apply a collecting device to the stoma.
2. Loop colostomy
   • Make a separate transverse or vertical incision over the site selected for the stoma.
   • Free up the loop of colon to be brought out as a loop colostomy.
   • This involves reflecting part of the omentum for a transverse colostomy or dividing the lateral paracolic peritoneum to mobilize the descending colon or sigmoid.
   • Create a small defect in the mesentery of the colon adjacent to the bowel wall, and pass a small drain through the defect.
   • Grasp the drain loop through the colostomy incision, and draw the loop of bowel through this wound.
   • Insert a rod or bridge beneath the loop of colon, and remove the drain.
   • Suture the rod or bridge to the skin.
   • Open the intestine (after the wound has been closed) by making a cruciate incision in the bowel wall with the cautery (Fig. 7).
   • Use a few interrupted 3-0 synthetic absorbable sutures to approximate the everted bowel wall to the skin edge.
3. Precolostomy
   • Precolostomy is useful when subsequent bowel obstruction is likely but has not occurred.
   • It is usually performed in cases of inoperable pelvic malignancy.
   • Bring a loop of colon out over a rod or bridge as described above.
   • Insert a few interrupted 3-0 synthetic absorbable sutures to approximate the colonic wall to the skin.

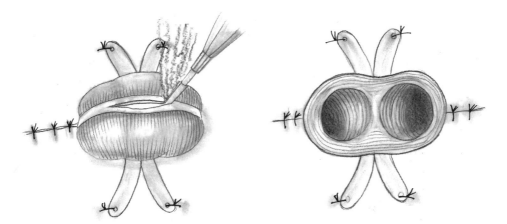

FIG. 7. The loop colostomy is opened by using the cautery.

- Do *not* open the intestinal lumen.
- After the bridge or rod is removed in 5 days, the bowel loop then retracts level with the skin and slowly epithelializes over.
- Keep a white petrolatum (Vaseline) dressing over the exposed bowel loop to protect it.
- If obstruction develops, the precolostomy can be opened under local anesthesia.

E. Specific Postoperative Management
1. Remove the rod or bridge on the fifth postoperative day, and fit a regular appliance.
2. Instruct the patient in how to apply and to remove the appliance.

F. Specific Postoperative Complications
1. Stomal necrosis: debride the necrotic tissue; revision may be required later.
2. Retraction of the stoma: due to poor adhesion of the bowel to the abdominal wall, or to excessive tension on the exteriorized bowel, or to necrosis of the stoma
   - Make a circular incision around the stoma.
   - Free it from the abdominal wall.
   - Lift it up to be resutured to the skin.
3. Parastomal hernia: herniation of abdominal contents through too large a stomal defect in the abdominal wall
   - Make an incision over the hernia.
   - Dissect the sac free and excise it.
   - Dissect the rectus fascia back to the intact fascia.
   - Repair the fascial defect with delayed synthetic absorbable or nonabsorbable interrupted sutures with some overlapping of layers if possible.
4. Prolapse of the colostomy: the bowel intersuscepts on itself and protrudes through the stomal orifice.
   - Carefully mobilize the segment of protruding colon along the mucocutaneous junction.
   - Resect the prolapsed colon and mesentery.
   - Refashion the stoma with interrupted sutures.

VI. Ileostomy and Jejunostomy

A. Indications
1. Terminal end ileostomy: performed after total colonic resection
2. Loop ileostomy: usually a temporary procedure to divert the fecal stream after difficult small-bowel fistula repair; occasionally used in the presence of inoperable small-bowel obstruction with carcinomatosis as a palliative measure
3. Feeding tube jejunostomy: used for enteral feeding or for patients likely to require prolonged intestinal suction drainage, e.g., postirradiation enteritis/obstruction/fistula problems

B. Preoperative Investigations
1. Routine laboratory tests depending on the indication
2. Radiographic contrast study of the small bowel may help define the site of obstruction or fistula preoperatively.

C. Preoperative Preparation
1. Bowel preparation if not obstructed
2. Prophylactic treatment with antibiotics
3. Parenteral nutrition may be indicated depending on the diagnosis and the surgical procedure contemplated.

D. Surgical Technique
1. End ileostomy
   - The technique is similar to that of end colostomy, except for the fashioning of the stoma.
   - Construct a Brooke-type nipple by folding the small bowel back on itself and suturing it in place, as explained in the section on ileal conduit.
2. Loop ileostomy
   The technique is similar to that for loop colostomy.
3. Catheter jejunostomy
   - Select a loop of jejunum that will reach up to the left upper quadrant of the abdominal wall.

- Place a purse string of 3-0 synthetic absorbable suture on the antimesenteric border of the jejunum.
- Make a small incision in the skin, and insert the jejunostomy catheter through the abdominal wall into the peritoneal cavity.
- Make a small opening into the jejunum within the purse string, insert the catheter tube, and tie the purse string.
- Overlap the catheter with jejunum to create a short tunnel with the use of interrupted absorbable sutures.
- Approximate the jejunum to the peritoneum of the anterior abdominal wall in the region of the catheter entry, to seal the catheter entry and to prevent the catheter from pulling out of the bowel.

E. Specific Postoperative Management

1. Remove the bridge or rod of the loop ileostomy in 5 days.
2. Fit the ileostomy with an appropriate appliance, and instruct the patient in how to apply it.
3. With catheter jejunostomy, apply low intermittent suction if required or commence enteral feeding through the catheter.
4. Remove the jejunostomy catheter when bowel function returns or when enteral feeding is no longer required.

F. Specific Postoperative Complications

1. Stomal necrosis, stenosis, retraction, and herniation, as for colostomy
2. Dehydration and electrolyte disturbances from excessive intestinal output: treatment may involve use of natural vegetable fiber, cholestyramine, diphenoxylate, and atropine sulfate.

VII. Gastrostomy

A. Indications

High small-bowel or gastric outlet obstruction that cannot be relieved surgically, e.g., as in ovarian carcinomatosis.

B. Preoperative Investigations

1. Routine laboratory tests
2. Upper gastrointestinal tract radiographic studies with contrast agents to assess site of obstruction

C. Preoperative Preparation

1. Empty stomach with nasogastric tube.
2. Prophylactic treatment with antibiotics

D. Surgical Technique

1. Open
   The technique is similar to that for catheter jejunostomy except that a large tube (14 F) usually is used.
2. Subcutaneous
   - Distend the stomach with air.
   - With the patient under local anesthesia and sedated, use computed tomographic or ultrasonographic scanning (occasionally with a gastroscope in the stomach) to pass a catheter into the stomach percutaneously.
   - Inflate the balloon, pull the stomach up to the abdominal wall, and suture the catheter to the skin.

E. Specific Postoperative Management

Gastrostomy allows patients to eat and drink and then to aspirate the stomach contents rather than vomit, thus improving the quality of life for patients who cannot be treated surgically.

F. Specific Postoperative Complications

1. Leak of gastric contents causing peritonitis
2. Bleeding from stomach incision
3. Blocked tube may need irrigation

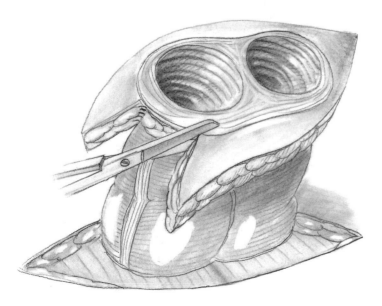

FIG. 8. The attached skin is excised before closure of the colostomy.

VIII. Closure of Colostomy or Ileostomy

A. Indication
After healing of more distal fistula or anastomosis for which the defunctioning stoma was constructed

B. Preoperative Investigation
Radiographic studies with contrast agents to confirm bowel continuity and healing at the site of the anastomosis/fistula

C. Preoperative Preparation
1. Bowel preparation with polyethylene glycol electrolyte solution (GoLYTELY)
2. Prophylactic treatment with antibiotics

D. Surgical Technique
1. After a Hartmann procedure, it is necessary to perform a laparotomy with takedown of the colostomy and reanastomosis to the closed rectal stump.
2. This is accomplished by a hand-sewn or intraluminal stapled anastomosis.
3. After a loop colostomy or ileostomy, make an elliptical incision around the stoma, and dissect the bowel free of the subcutaneous fat and abdominal wall fascia.

4. Resect the attached skin from the stoma to freshen the edges of the opened bowel (Fig. 8).
5. Next, close the defect in the bowel in two layers with a running 3-0 synthetic absorbable suture in the mucosal layer and interrupted 3-0 silk in the seromuscular layer (Fig. 9).
6. Push the closed loop of bowel back into the peritoneal cavity, and close the abdominal incision in layers over a subcutaneous drain.

E. Specific Postoperative Management
1. Nothing by mouth until flatus is passed
2. No laxatives or enemas for 6 weeks

F. Specific Postoperative Complications
1. Wound infection is not uncommon at stomal site.
2. Leaking of anastomosis

Reading List

Symmonds RE. Use of the colon for urinary diversion. *Clin Obstet Gynecol* 1967;10:217–226.

Symmonds RE, Pratt JH, Welsh JS. Exenterative operations: experience with 118 patients. *Am J Obstet Gynecol* 1968;101:66–77.

Pratt JH. Use of the colon in gynecologic surgery. *Prog Gynecol* 1970;5:435–446.

Symmonds RE, Gibbs CP. Urinary diversion by way of sigmoid conduit. *Surg Gynecol Obstet* 1970;131:687–693.

Symmonds RE, Jones IV. Sigmoid conduit urinary diversion after examination. *Prog Gynecol* 1975;6:729–737.

Symmonds RE, Pratt JH, Webb MJ. Exenterative operation: experience with 198 patients. *Am J Obstet Gynecol* 1975;121:907–918.

Raventos JM, Symmonds RE. Surgical management of acute diverticulitis in women. *Obstet Gynecol* 1981;58:557–565.

Symmonds RE, Webb MJ. Pelvic exenteration. In: Coppleson M, ed. *Gynecologic oncology: fundamental principles and clinical practice,* vol 2. Edinburgh: Churchill Livingstone, 1981:896–922.

Stanhope CR, Symmonds RE. Palliative exenteration: what, when, and why? *Am J Obstet Gynecol* 1985;152:12–16.

Stanhope CR, Symmonds RE, Lee RA, et al. Urinary diversion with use of ileal and sigmoid conduits. *Am J Obstet Gynecol* 1986;155:288–292.

Webb MJ, Weaver EW. Intestinal surgery in gynaecological oncology. *Aust NZJ Obstet Gynecol* 1987;27:299–303.

Podratz KC, Symmonds RE, Hagen JV. Intestinal resection and ostomy care. In: Gusberg SB, Shingleton HM, Deppe G, eds. *Female genital cancer.* New York: Churchill Livingstone, 1988:589–619.

Stanhope CR, Webb MJ. Pelvic exenteration. In: Donohue JH, Van Heerden J, Monson JRT, eds: *Atlas of surgical oncology.* Cambridge: Blackwell Science, 1995:310–318.

Morris M, Alvarez RD, Kinney WK, et al. Treatment of recurrent adenocarcinoma of the endometrium with pelvic exenteration. *Gynecol Oncol* 1996;60:288–291.

Magrina JF, Stanhope CR, Weaver AL. Pelvic exenterations: supralevator, infralevator, and with vulvectomy. *Gynecol Oncol* 1997;64:130–135.

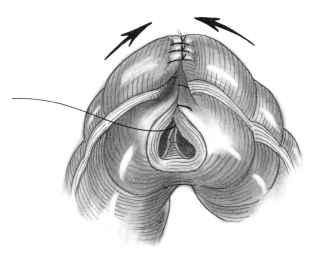

FIG. 9. The bowel is reconstituted in two layers to close the colostomy.

CHAPTER 22

Retroperitoneal Surgery

Maurice J. Webb, M.D. and Karl C. Podratz, M.D., Ph.D.

I. Introduction

Lymphadenectomy is performed as a staging procedure or as a therapeutic procedure for many gynecologic malignancies.

II. Pelvic Lymph Node Dissection

A. Indications
Pelvic lymph node dissection is performed
1. In association with radical hysterectomy in the treatment of early-stage cervical cancer
2. As a staging procedure for high-risk endometrial cancer
3. As a staging procedure for uterine sarcoma
4. As a staging, debulking, and possibly therapeutic procedure in ovarian cancer and tubal cancer
5. In association with second-look laparotomy
6. In association with pelvic exenteration for recurrent pelvic cancer

B. Preoperative Investigations
1. Routine laboratory tests depending on the diagnosis.
2. Computed tomographic scanning or magnetic resonance imaging of the abdomen and pelvis may be indicated depending on the diagnosis.
3. Cystoscopy and proctoscopy may be indicated.

C. Preoperative Preparation
1. Thromboembolus-deterrent stockings
2. Sequential calf compression devices if the patient is at high risk for deep vein thrombosis.

Maurice J. Webb: Chairman, Division of Gynecologic Surgery and Consultant, Department of Surgery, Mayo Clinic and Mayo Foundation; Professor of Obstetrics and Gynecology, Mayo Medical School, Rochester, Minnesota.

Karl C. Podratz: Chairman, Department of Obstetrics and Gynecology, Consultant, Department of Surgery, Mayo Clinic and Mayo Foundation; Professor of Obstetrics and Gynecology, Mayo Medical School Rochester, Minnesota.

3. Prophylactic treatment with antibiotics
4. Blood crossmatch depending on the operation planned

D. Surgical Technique
1. Make a midline lower abdominal incision.
2. Collect peritoneal washings for cytologic study.
3. Inspect and palpate the abdominal and pelvic contents, especially pelvic and aortic nodal areas.
4. Clamp and divide the right round ligament, and divide the peritoneum lateral to the ovarian vessels up to the pelvic brim.
5. With the index finger of each hand or with Russian forceps, dissect down into the pararectal space by retracting the medial leaf of the broad ligament peritoneum with attached ureter medially and by dissecting down the front of the sacrum medial to the internal iliac vessels.
6. Similarly dissect the paravesical space by dissecting down into the obturator fossa, retracting the obliterated hypogastric artery medially and the external iliac vessels laterally.
7. Dissect down the paravesical space until the levator muscle is exposed.
8. Insert a Deaver retractor into the paravesical space, and retract the bladder inferiorly and medially.
9. Lift up the peritoneum beneath the inguinal ligament to expose the distal end of the external iliac vessels, and insert another Deaver retractor under this peritoneal flap.
10. With long scissors and Russian forceps, divide the fatty tissue along the psoas muscle lateral to the external iliac vessels, and retract the node-bearing fatty tissue medially until the external iliac vessels are exposed.
11. Place a hemostatic clip across the lymphatic vessels where they emerge from the femoral canal, and divide the lymphatic chain flush with the femoral canal.
12. Take care to avoid the circumflex vein where it courses over the external iliac artery.

13. With a combination cutting-and-pulling technique, gradually dissect the external iliac nodes off the vessels up to the bifurcation of the common iliac artery.

14. Divide the lymphatic chain at that point, and send this group of nodes for pathologic examination marked "external iliac."

15. With the fingers of the left hand, lift up the peritoneum over the common iliac vessels, leaving the ureter attached to the peritoneum.

16. Have the assistants stand at the head end of the patient, and place two Deaver retractors beneath the upper peritoneal flap, with one retracted laterally and the other medially.

17. This exposes the common iliac vessels, lower aorta, and vena cava.

18. With scissors, separate the common iliac nodes from the lateral aspect of the common iliac vessels.

19. Separate the lymphatic tissue from the psoas muscle laterally, cauterizing or clipping the small arterial branches to the psoas muscle.

20. Lift the lymphatic chain superiorly and dissect the nodes free, placing a hemostatic clip across the perforating veins entering the vena cava and across the upper end before transecting the lymphatic tissue.

21. Retract the common and external iliac vessels medially and the psoas muscle laterally. Remove any remaining nodes deep and lateral to the common iliac vessels, and then coming inferiorly, expose the obturator nerve and lumbosacral trunk.

22. Place the retractors again inferiorly in the paravesical space and over the external iliac vessels.

23. Free the obturator nodes from the lateral pelvic wall and the obturator nerve by gentle blunt dissection with Russian forceps lateral and deep to the external iliac vessels.

24. Come medial to the external iliac vessels, place a vein retractor under these vessels, just below the bifurcation of the common iliac vessels, and retract up and laterally.

25. With scissors, free the obturator nodes from the undersurface of the external iliac vein, taking care to avoid injury to the accessory obturator vein, if present, where it enters the undersurface of the external iliac vein, traveling up from the obturator foramen through which it enters the pelvis.

26. Use a hemostatic clip to clamp the distal end of the obturator node chain, and then with two Russian forceps, lift the nodes up out of the obturator fossa and remove them.

27. Remove any remaining fatty tissue around the obturator fossa, including that over the levator muscles.

28. Dissect free the lymph-node-bearing tissue from the bifurcation of the aorta down the presacral area medial to the internal iliac vessels, taking care not to traumatize the presacral veins.

29. Repeat the same dissection on the contralateral side.

30. Drains are not usually utilized.

31. The pelvic peritoneum is left open.

E. Specific Postoperative Management

If suction drains are used, remove them when the output through individual drains is <50 mL/24 h on 2 consecutive days.

F. Specific Postoperative Complications

1. Lymphocysts
   - Most disappear with time, maybe over a period of several months.
   - Most are asymptomatic.
   - Indications for treatment include pain and pressure, ureteric obstruction, infection, or lower extremity edema.
   - Treatment can be by insertion of a suction catheter by ultrasonographic guidance, sometimes with the addition of sclerosing agents, or by laparotomy or laparoscopy, with marsupialization of the lymphocyst into the peritoneal cavity.
2. Venous thrombosis
   Caused by trauma to the pelvic sidewall venous system
3. Obturator nerve palsy produced by trauma to or transection of the nerve
   - If the nerve was not transected, there is recovery of function with time.
   - If the nerve was transected, the patient compensates by using other thigh muscles for adduction, with little residual disability.

III. Aortic Lymph Node Dissection

A. Indications

1. Involvement of common iliac nodes with malignancy during surgery for cervical carcinoma
2. In association with pelvic lymphadenectomy in cases of uterine, ovarian, or tubal cancer

B. Preoperative Investigations and Preparation

The same as for pelvic lymph node dissection

C. Surgical Technique

1. Make a midline incision from the symphysis pubis to the xiphoid process, thus opening the abdomen.
2. On the right side, a peritoneal incision extends down the right paracolic gutter peritoneum, around the cecum, up along the right common iliac vessels, and up the aorta to the root of the mesentery of the small bowel.
3. Lift the right colon, cecum, and small bowel out of the abdomen, place them in an intestinal bag or wrap them in damp sponges, and leave them on the chest.

4. Identify the right ureter and right ovarian vein, and free them from the posterior aspect of the right colon.

5. The ovarian vein may be transected and ligated or clipped where it enters the inferior vena cava.

6. With two large Deaver retractors, expose the front of the inferior vena cava and aorta by retracting the third part of the duodenum cephalad.

7. Next, dissect free the lateral and anterior caval nodes, starting at the bifurcation of the aorta and proceeding cephalad.

8. On reaching the level of the renal vessels, clip and divide the lymph node chain.

9. Likewise, remove the aortocaval nodes between the vena cava and aorta.

10. Lift the vena cava anteriorly, and remove the retrocaval nodes.

11. Occasionally, it may be necessary to clip and divide some of the lumbar veins to gain exposure.

12. Keep the right ureter in sight at all times during the dissection.

13. In a similar fashion, the nodes anterior to the aorta are removed.

14. The inferior mesenteric artery is preserved, although it normally can be sacrificed in nonirradiated patients without subsequent bowel ischemia.

15. Make an incision in the left paracolic gutter peritoneum lateral to the descending colon, and retract the left colon medially to expose the aorta.

16. Separate the left ureter and left ovarian vessels from the posterior aspect of the descending colon, and retract them laterally.

17. Remove the left lateral aortic nodes along with the retroaortic nodes up to the level of the left renal vein.

18. Secure hemostasis, and replace the bowel in the peritoneal cavity.

19. Do not close the peritoneal defects; suction drainage is not necessary.

D. Specific Postoperative Management

Because ileus is frequent after aortic node dissection, a nasogastric tube may be inserted under anesthesia and kept on suction until intestinal activity returns.

E. Specific Postoperative Complications

1. Injury to the ureter: the ureter, usually the left, may be traumatized or ligated inadvertently where it runs quite close to the aorta.

2. Lymphocyst: usually disappears with time

3. Minor trauma to the vena cava or aorta during dissection should be oversewn with 5–0 monofilament (Prolene) sutures.

IV. Paraaortic Lymph Node Sampling

A. Indications

A full dissection provides a more accurate assessment of nodal status than node sampling does, but sampling may be indicated

1. If the suspected node is palpable

2. Before extensive pelvic surgery, e.g., exenteration

3. As a staging procedure before definitive therapy, e.g., stage III cervical cancer

B. Surgical Technique

1. Introduction

   May be performed transperitoneally or extraperitoneally

   • The transperitoneal approach is used when the peritoneal cavity is opened to proceed with definitive surgery.

   • The extraperitoneal approach is used for cases in which other means of therapy (e.g., irradiation) are planned.

   • Intestinal complications are less common if the extraperitoneal instead of the transperitoneal approach is used before irradiation.

2. Transperitoneal approach

   • Make a midline incision extending well above the umbilicus.

   • Lift the small intestine out of the abdominal cavity, and expose the aortic area and the root of the mesentery.

   • Incise the peritoneum, extending from the right common iliac artery cephalad over the aorta to the third portion of the duodenum.

   • Insert fingers under the duodenum, and lift it away from the aorta and vena cava to expose the renal vessels.

   • Insert two Deaver retractors beneath the peritoneum, one on each side of the midline, and retract cephalad.

   • Excise any preaortic and precaval fat pad or any suspicious nodes up to the renal vessels.

   • Use hemostatic clips and cautery to obtain hemostasis.

   • The preaortic peritoneum does not need to be closed, and the retroperitoneal space does not need to be drained.

3. Extraperitoneal approach

   • Make a curved "hockey stick" type of incision that extends vertically down the left or right lateral aspect of the anterior abdominal wall and that curves medially 3 to 4 cm above the inguinal ligament.

   • Continue the dissection down to the peritoneum.

   • Dissect the retroperitoneal space posteriorly and medially, and retract the peritoneum medially with Deaver retractors to expose the front of the aorta and vena cava.

   • Identify and preserve the ureter and ovarian vessels.

   • Proceed with node sampling as described above.

   • Bilateral incisions are necessary to perform a full paraaortic node dissection.

   • Laparoscopic techniques are being investigated.

C. Specific Postoperative Management

Normally, retroperitoneal drainage is not necessary.

D. Specific Postoperative Complications
1. Injury to ureter or ovarian vessels
2. Hematoma or lymphocyst formation

V. Ovarian Remnant Syndrome

A. Definition
1. Occurs in patients who have had bilateral salpingo-oophorectomy
2. Causes pelvic pain and dyspareunia
3. Is usually associated with a palpable or visible mass on scanning
4. Usually occurs in patients who have had multiple pelvic operations or who have extensive pelvic adhesions from pelvic disease such as endometriosis
5. Should not be confused with "residual ovary syndrome" in which an ovary or part thereof has not been removed previously and becomes symptomatic

B. Preoperative Investigations
1. Computed tomographic or ultrasonographic scanning of the pelvis
2. Intravenous pyelography or computed tomography to rule out ureteric obstruction
3. Serum levels of follicle-stimulating and luteinizing hormone if the patient is not receiving exogenous estrogen therapy
4. Rule out other causes of pelvic pain.
5. Laparoscopy is not helpful in making the diagnosis because of the extensive pelvic adhesions and because most remnants are located retroperitoneally.

C. Preoperative Preparation
1. Bowel preparation with polyethylene glycol electrolyte solution (GoLYTELY)
2. Prophylactic treatment with antibiotics
3. Crossmatch 2 U blood.
4. Insertion of a vaginal pack preoperatively may aid dissection, because most remnants lie adjacent to the vaginal vault.

D. Surgical Technique
1. Make a large midline lower abdominal incision.
2. Carefully dissect the pelvic adhesions, returning the pelvic anatomy to its normal state.
3. Identify the remnant, which usually lies adjacent to the right or left angle of the vaginal vault.
4. Open the broad ligament peritoneum lateral to the ovarian vessels along the psoas muscle.
5. Develop the pararectal and paravesical spaces.
6. Identify the ureter attached to the broad ligament peritoneum.

7. Divide and ligate the ovarian vessels. These vessels may be intact right down to the remnant, which suggests that previous clamping at oophorectomy was too close to the ovary so that an ovarian remnant attached to the vessels was retained.
8. Divide and ligate the anterior division of the internal iliac artery.
9. Unroof the ureter, and free it from the broad ligament peritoneum.
10. Grasp the vaginal vault with a tenaculum, and carefully dissect the bladder off the anterior aspect of the vagina.
11. If the bladder, ureter, or sigmoid colon is adherent to the ovarian remnant, a segment may have to be excised to obtain adequate clearance.
12. The objective of the operation is to excise widely, all the tissue around the remnant so there will be no recurrence.
13. Dissect the rectosigmoid off the posterior vaginal wall.
14. Widely resect the remnant en bloc, with a segment of the vaginal vault, bladder, bowel, or ureter if necessary.
15. Resection of a segment of the bladder and/or ureter is accomplished best by performing a vertical cystotomy in the bladder to visualize the adherent bladder internally and externally and the relationship of the remnant to the ureter.
16. A ureteric stent may be placed intraoperatively to aid in the dissection of the ureter and may be left in place if an extensive ureteric dissection has produced significant trauma to the ureter.
17. Repair any vaginal, bladder, bowel, or ureteric defects in the usual fashion.
18. Carefully inspect the contralateral pelvic sidewall peritoneum, and resect any bilateral remnants.
19. Bring down an omental pedicle to cover the denuded pelvic floor and to protect the dissected ureter.
20. Place a suction drain in the pelvis.
21. Close the incision in the usual fashion.

E. Specific Postoperative Management
1. Leave the urethral catheter in place for 7 days if cystotomy is performed.
2. Remove the ureteric stent in 7 days or delay for 6 weeks if ureteric anastomosis is performed.
3. Remove the suction drain in 48 hours if drainage is minimal; leave for 7 days if ureteric anastomosis is performed or until bowel function returns if bowel resection is performed.

F. Specific Postoperative Complications
1. Ureteric or bladder fistula
2. Intestinal fistula

3. Recurrence of ovarian remnant (rare but may require reoperation)

VI. Presacral Neurectomy

A. Indications

1. In association with conservative surgical treatment for endometriosis in which dysmenorrhea is a significant symptom
2. Rarely performed as an isolated procedure for the treatment of dysmenorrhea

B. Preoperative Investigations and Preparation

Depends on the diagnosis

C. Surgical Technique

1. It is usually performed via laparotomy but can be accomplished laparoscopically.
2. Make a vertical incision in the peritoneum of the presacral area, extending from the sacral promontory to vertebra S3.
3. Retract the peritoneum laterally to expose the hypogastric nerve plexus and middle sacral vessels that course down over the anterior aspect of the sacrum.
4. Identify both ureters.
5. Starting as far laterally at the sacral promontory as possible and just medial to the common iliac vessels, lift up the nerve plexus with Russian forceps. Gently tunnel beneath the plexus with right-angled forceps, taking care to avoid the presacral veins but isolating all the nerve fibers.
6. Clamp, divide, and resect a 2-cm length of nerve plexus below the sacral promontory.
7. Check for adequate hemostasis, close the presacral peritoneum, and close the abdominal incision.

D. Specific Postoperative Management

Depends on the accompanying surgical procedure.

E. Specific Postoperative Complications

1. The failure rate to relieve dysmenorrhea is significant.
2. After neurectomy, some patients experience a significant increase in the amount of menstrual blood flow.
3. Injury to the presacral veins may cause significant hemorrhage intraoperatively that is difficult to control.
4. Injury to the ureters can occur unless they are specifically identified and avoided intraoperatively.

VII. Presacral Tumors

A. Introduction

1. Presacral tumors are relatively rare tumors of various types that arise in the presacral region.
2. They may be asymptomatic or may produce urinary or intestinal symptoms or pain.

B. Classification

1. Congenital
   - Benign
     — Teratoma
     — Epidermoid cyst
     — Meningocele
   - Malignant
     Teratoma
2. Neural
   - Benign
     — Neurofibroma
     — Periganglioneuroma
   - Malignant
     — Neuroblastoma
     — Ganglioneuroblastoma
     — Ependymoma
     — Neurofibrosarcoma
3. Osseous
   - Benign
     — Giant cell tumor
     — Osteoblastoma
     — Aneurysmal bone cyst
   - Malignant
     — Ewing sarcoma
     — Myeloma
4. Soft tissue
   - Benign
     — Leiomyoma
     — Lipoma
     — Fibroma
   - Malignant
     — Hemangiopericytoma
     — Fibrosarcoma

C. Indications

1. Because of the difficulty in making a definitive diagnosis, surgical removal is usually advised.
2. It is important to exclude an anterior sacral meningocele or meningomyelocele, in which surgery may not be performed unless the size or symptoms warrant intervention.

D. Preoperative Investigations

1. Complete blood count
2. Serum chemistry
3. Chest radiography
4. Radiographic examination of the sacrum with anteroposterior and lateral views to look for calcific deposits, lytic destruction of the sacrum, or congenital sacral defects, e.g., spina bifida
5. Sigmoidoscopy
6. Intravenous pyelography
7. Barium enema
8. Computed tomography or magnetic resonance imaging
9. Myelography if necessary to diagnose meningocele

E. Preoperative Preparation

1. Povidone-iodine douche
2. Bowel preparation with polyethylene glycol electrolyte solution (GoLYTELY)
3. Crossmatch 4 U of blood.
4. Insert a urethral catheter.
5. Consult with an orthopedic surgeon and neurosurgeon if indicated.

F. Surgical Technique

1. Introduction
   - A team approach involving orthopedic and neurosurgeons may be necessary.
   - The approach may be
     — Abdominal
     — Transsacral
     — Transperineal
     — Abdominoperineal
   - The choice of approach is dictated by the size and site of the tumor.
2. Abdominal approach
   - This is the most common technique, because most tumors are located above the midsacrum.
   - Careful dissection and visualization of the intestinal and urinary tracts are possible with the abdominal approach.
   - Develop the pararectal and paravesical spaces.
   - Ligate the anterior division of the internal iliac artery bilaterally.
   - Remove the tumor en bloc if there is a possibility of malignancy.
   - Aspiration of a cystic lesion or debulking of the center of a tumor allows better visualization and dissection of the tumor away from the pelvic vessels and nerves.

3. Transsacral approach
   - This is used with tumors ≤8 cm located over the distal 10 cm of the sacrum and coccyx.
   - Place patient in the Kratske position: prone with the buttocks elevated (Fig. 1).
   - Make a midline incision over the sacrum down to the anal ring.
   - Excise the coccyx.
   - Free the rectum from the front of the sacrum.
   - Sharply dissect the tumor from the front of the sacrum, preserving the sacral and pudendal nerves.
   - Dissect the tumor off the posterior aspect of the rectum.
4. Transperineal approach
   - Place patient in the lithotomy position.
   - The incision extends from the vagina down around one side of the anus and rectum.
   - Enter the presacral space; elevate and displace the rectum and vagina to the opposite side to gain access to the tumor.
   - Dissect the tumor free of the lower sacrum and rectum.
5. Abdominoperineal approach
   - Occasionally, a combined approach may be necessary to excise a large tumor completely.
   - When a combined approach is planned, accomplish the abdominal procedure first, and free up the tumor as much as possible by this approach.
   - Turn the patient, and use a transperineal or transsacral approach to remove the tumor.
   - Occasionally, after attempting a transperineal or transsacral approach, an abdominal incision may also be necessary to complete the resection.

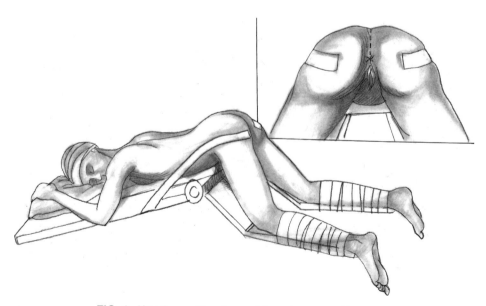

FIG. 1. Kratske position for excision of presacral tumors.

G. Specific Postoperative Management

1. Suction drainage of the presacral space
2. Urinary catheter placement, with residual check after removal, because of the possibility of urinary retention due to nerve damage

H. Specific Postoperative Complications

1. Neurogenic bladder
2. Fecal incontinence
3. Presacral hematoma/abscess
4. Recurrence/persistence of the tumor

Reading List

MacCarty CS, Waugh JM, Mayo CW, et al. The surgical treatment of presacral tumors: a combined problem. *Proc Staff Meet Mayo Clin* 1952;27:73–84.

Pratt JH. Some surgical considerations of retroperitoneal tumors. *Am J Obstet Gynecol* 1963;87:956–962.

King BJ, Pratt JH. Device for maintaining identity of lymph nodes excised in radical pelvic and abdominal surgery. *Proc Staff Meet Mayo Clin* 1964;39:273–274.

Symmonds RE. Morbidity and complications of radical hysterectomy with pelvic lymph node dissection. *Am J Obstet Gynecol* 1966;94:663–673.

Symmonds RE, Pettit PDM. Ovarian remnant syndrome. *Obstet Gynecol* 1979;54:174–177.

Webb MJ, Symmonds RE. Wertheim hysterectomy: a reappraisal. *Obstet Gynecol* 1979;54:140–145.

Lee RA. Presacral tumors: anatomy, classification, clinical features and management. *In:* Coppleson M, ed. *Gynecologic oncology: fundamental principles & clinical practice,* vol 2. Edinburgh: Churchill Livingstone, 1981:1003–1009.

Podratz KC, Symmonds RE. Radical hysterectomy and pelvic lymphadenectomy. *In:* Sarwit EA, Alberts DS, eds. *Cervix cancer,* vol. 3. The Hague: Martinus Nijhoff, 1987:67–88.

Lee RA. Ovarian remnant syndrome. *In:* Nichols DH, ed. *Clinical problems, injuries, and complications of gynecologic surgery,* 2nd ed. Baltimore: Williams & Wilkins, 1988:16–19.

Lee RA, Symmonds RE. Presacral tumors in the female: clinical presentation, surgical management, and results. *Obstet Gynecol* 1988;71:216–221.

Webb MI. Ovarian remnant syndrome. *Aust NZ J Obstet Gynaecol* 1989;29:433–435.

Cliby WA, Clarke Pearson DL, Dodge R, et al. Acute morbidity and mortality associated with selective pelvic and para-aortic lymphadenectomy in the surgical staging of endometrial adenocarcinoma. *J Gynecol Tech* 1995;1:19–25.

Lee RA. Ovarian remnant syndrome. *In:* Nichols DH, DeLancy JOL, eds. *Clinical problems, injuries and complications of gynecologic and obstetric surgery,* 3rd ed. Baltimore: Williams & Wilkins, 1995:32–35.

Garton GR, Gunderson LL, Webb MJ, et al. Intraoperative radiation therapy in gynecologic cancer: update of the experience at a single institution. *Int J Radiat Oncol Biol Phys* 1997;37:839–843.

Podratz KC, Mariani A, Webb MJ. Staging and therapeutic value of lymphadenectomy in endometrial cancer. *Gynecol Oncol* 1998;70:163–164.

CHAPTER 23

Plastic Surgical Procedures

Maurice J. Webb, M.D.

I. Introduction

Radical gynecologic surgery procedures often require reconstructive plastic surgery techniques to rehabilitate the patient (e.g., vaginal reconstruction), to cover large defects (e.g., skin or myocutaneous flaps), or to repair fistulas or areas of radionecrosis (e.g., skin or muscle flaps).

A knowledge of reconstructive techniques allows the surgeon to be as radical as necessary in resection of the tumor, with the knowledge that techniques for repairing the resulting defect are available.

II. Skin Flaps

A. Principles
1. The main types are plain skin flaps involving skin and superficial fascia or fasciocutaneous flaps when deep fascia is included.
2. Axial flaps are designed based on a specific artery and vein.
3. Random pattern flaps rely on random local vasculature and thus are less robust and must be smaller.
4. Vascularity is better in fasciocutaneous flaps, allowing greater length.

B. Indications
1. Used mainly to cover defects after resection of vulval tumors
2. Useful for covering groin or abdominal wall defects
3. Used in repair of loss of floor of urethra
4. May be used for construction of a neovagina or management of vaginal stenosis

C. Preoperative Investigations and Preparation
Depends on primary operation

Maurice J. Webb: Chairman, Division of Gynecologic Surgery and Consultant, Department of Surgery, Mayo Clinic and Mayo Foundation; Professor of Obstetrics and Gynecology, Mayo Medical School, Rochester, Minnesota.

D. Surgical Techniques
1. Rotation flap
   - The flap is designed to rotate about a point on the edge of the defect.
   - This flap is best suited to close triangle-shaped defects; therefore, trim defects to a triangular shape.
   - Extend the base of the triangle to one side (Fig. 1).
   - Make sure the base is wide enough to support the vascularity of the flap.
   - Undermine the flap until it rotates easily without tension.
   - Suture the flap in place; no secondary defect should result.
   - A back-cut may need to be made at the end of the flap if tension is excessive (Fig. 2).

Rotation flap

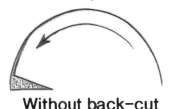

Without back-cut

FIG. 1. Rotation flap.

Rotation flap

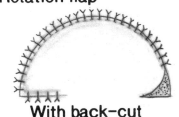

With back-cut

FIG. 2. Rotation flap with back-cut.

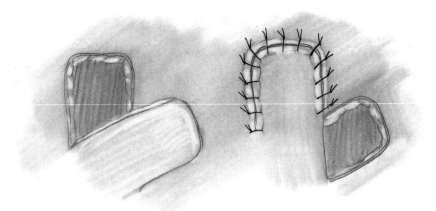

FIG. 3. Transposition flap.

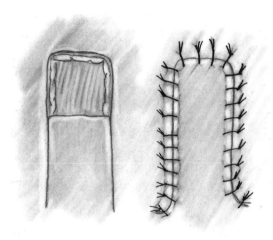

FIG. 4. Advancement flap.

2. Transposition flap
  • This flap is designed to move the skin and underlying tissue from an adjacent site to cover a defect (Fig. 3).
  • A secondary defect remains, which may be sutured or skin grafted, depending on size.
3. Advancement flap
  • This flap is used when the defect is small and the surrounding skin is mobile.

• Two parallel edges of the defect are extended, and the area between them is undermined to produce a flap.
• The flap is advanced to cover the defect and is sutured in place (Fig. 4).

E. Specific Skin Flaps
  1. Rhomboid flap
  • This flap is especially useful for closing defects in the perineum.
  • It is a type of transposition flap for covering rhomboid-shaped defects.
  • Draw a line extending out from one angle of the defect equal to the diagonal width of the defect (Fig. 5).
  • Make a back-cut parallel to one of the sides of the rhomboid defect.
  • Undermine the flap, and transpose it to fill the defect.
  • Close the secondary defect.
  • Two rhomboid flaps, one from each side, or four flaps, two from each side, can be used to cover large defects.
  • A rhomboid flap on each side of the vulva can be used to reconstruct the perineum quite adequately.
  2. Groin fasciocutaneous flap
  • Bilateral flaps based on pudendal vessels are used to form a neovagina.

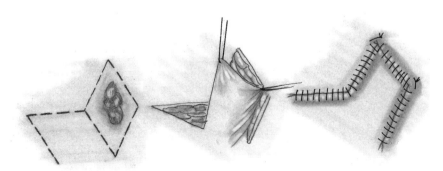

FIG. 5. Rhomboid flap.

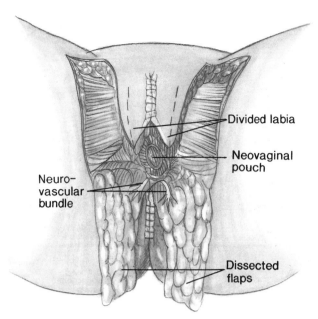

FIG. 6. Dissection of fasciocutaneous flaps from both groins to form a neovagina.

- They are long narrow flaps based posteriorly on the vulva and have good vascularity when deep fascia is left attached to the flap (Fig. 6).
- The flaps measure approximately 6 × 15 cm.
- Suture the flaps together to form a pouch.
- Rotate the pouch into the vaginal opening, and suture it to the presacral area.
- Groin wounds are closed primarily over drains.
- The advantages are good viability of flaps and that all incisions are hidden in the skin crease of the groin.

3. Z-plasty
- Z-plasty is used mainly to treat constriction rings or contracted scars.
- The aim is to gain length or diameter.
- Make three incisions in the shape of a Z, with a 60-degree angle between the incisions.
- Undermine the two flaps thus constructed.
- Transpose the flaps, and suture them in place (Fig. 7).
- Z-plasty may be used to manage vaginal or introital stenosis or strictures.

III. Myocutaneous Flaps

A. Introduction
Myocutaneous flaps have an advantage over skin flaps in that they can be larger and bulkier because of preservation of the vascular pedicle that supplies the muscle and overlying skin.

B. Indications
1. Construction of a neovagina
2. Closure of large rectovaginal or vesicovaginal fistulas
3. Covering of vulval, groin, or abdominal wall defects, whether postoperative or postradiation defects
4. Breast reconstruction

C. Preoperative Investigations and Preparation
Depend on primary operation

D. Surgical Techniques
1. Martius bulbocavernosus flap
- Its major use is to augment a vaginal mucosal defect in the repair of vesicovaginal, urethrovaginal, or rectovaginal fistula.
- Bilateral flaps may be developed from each labium major.
- The pedicle may be based anteriorly or posteriorly, depending on the site of the defect in the vagina.
- Map out on the labium major the size of the skin flap required.
- The position of the skin flap on the labium is determined by how far up the vagina it has to reach.
- Make a curved vertical incision in the labium major anterior and posterior to the skin island required.
- Undermine the vulval skin on each cut edge, and carry the dissection deeply into the fatty tissue of the labium.
- Divide the end of the pedicle, either anteriorly or posteriorly, depending on the requirements for the site to be covered.
- Tunnel beneath the labium minor and vaginal mucosa with scissors to provide a track to deliver the bulbocavernosus flap to the operative site (Fig. 8).
- Affix a suture to the distal end of the flap, and pull the flap through the tunnel.

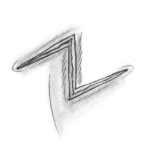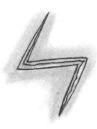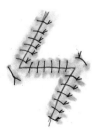

FIG. 7. Z-plasty.

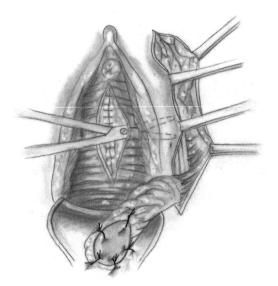

FIG. 8. Martius myocutaneous flap developed from left vulva.

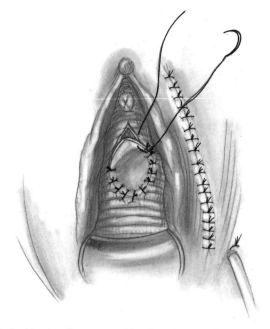

FIG. 9. Martius flap sutured in place in anterior vaginal wall.

- Suture the labial skin flap to the defect in the vaginal mucosa with multiple interrupted 2-0 synthetic absorbable sutures (Fig. 9).
- Secure meticulous hemostasis in the donor site, and close in layers over a small suction drain.
- Bilateral flaps can be used, with one turned inward to cover the bladder or rectal mucosal defect and the contralateral one turned outward to replace the vaginal mucosal defect.

2. Gracilis myocutaneous flap
   - Bilateral flaps are used to create a neovagina.
   - They are also useful for closing large vesicovaginal or rectovaginal fistulas, especially when associated with radionecrosis.

- Unilateral or bilateral flaps may be used to cover vulval, groin, or lower abdominal wall defects.
- With the patient's legs in a modified low lithotomy position, identify the surface anatomy of the gracilis muscle, extending from the adductor tubercle to the medial condyle of the tibia.
- The vascular pedicle is situated beneath the muscle, approximately 8 to 10 cm from the pubis.
- The nerve supply is from the obturator nerve.
- Map out over the line of the muscle the size of the skin flap required.
- Through an elliptical incision, carry the dissection

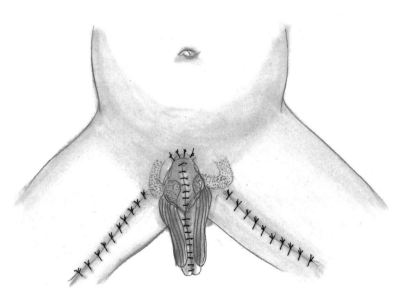

FIG. 10. Construction of neovagina using bilateral gracilis myocutaneous flaps.

down through the subcutaneous fat; identify the gracilis muscle, and detach the distal end from its tibial attachment.

- Loosely attach the skin flap to the underlying muscle with interrupted sutures to prevent separation of the skin from the muscle.
- Continue the dissection caudally until the neurovascular bundle is identified at about a quarter of the length down the gracilis muscle. (The vessels come from under the adductor longus and arise from the profunda femoris.)
- Tunnel the myocutaneous flap beneath the skin bridge adjacent to the vulva, and rotate it carefully so the vascular pedicle is not twisted.
- If a neovagina is being constructed, raise bilateral flaps, suture them together as a pouch, and then insert through the introitus and suture to the front of the sacrum (Fig. 10).
- If the flap is to cover a defect, rotate it into place and suture the skin to the edge of the defect over a suction catheter.
- Also close the leg incisions over suction catheters, and apply a compression bandage.
- Gracilis muscle alone, without overlying skin, may be used to fill large vulval, perineal, or presacral or abdominal wall defects.

3. Tensor fascia lata flap
- This is a lateral thigh flap that uses the tensor fascia lata muscle (Fig. 11).
- The flap can be up to 30 cm long; it is based on the lateral femoral circumflex artery.
- The length of the flap and its position make it particularly useful for covering groin and vulval defects.
- The anterior border of the flap runs along a vertical line just lateral to the anterior superior iliac spine.
- The vascular pedicle enters the flap at the level of the greater trochanter.
- The posterior border arises from a point about 5 cm posterior to the anterior superior iliac spine and runs inferiorly.
- The flap may extend to about 5 cm above the knee.
- Begin the dissection inferiorly; elevate the flap deep to the fascia lata and continue the dissection superiorly until the vascular hilum is identified at the level of the greater trochanter.
- The vascular pedicle extends medially, deep to the rectus femoris muscle.
- Rotate the flap to cover the groin and vulval defect, and suture it in place over a suction drain.
- The donor site is closed primarily over a suction drain.

4. Rectus abdominus flap
- This myocutaneous flap is based on the inferior or superior epigastric artery.
- The flap may be rotated upward toward the chest on the superior epigastric artery or inferiorly toward the groin and vulva on the inferior epigastric artery.

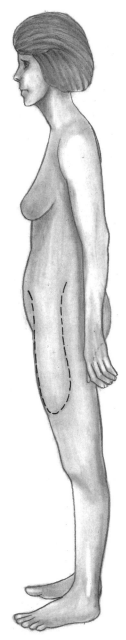

FIG. 11. Tensor fascia lata flap.

- It may be used in conjunction with a gracilis flap to cover a large vulval or perineal defect.
- The superiorly hinged flap may be used for breast reconstruction.
- The size and position of the skin flap required are mapped out over the right or left rectus abdominus muscle (Fig. 12).
- Make a vertical incision in the skin over the midline of the muscle and around the skin flap.
- Continue the incision down to expose the anterior rectus sheath.
- Incise the sheath vertically above and below the skin flap, and carefully mobilize the rectus muscle from the posterior rectus sheath, keeping the epigastric vessels with the muscle.

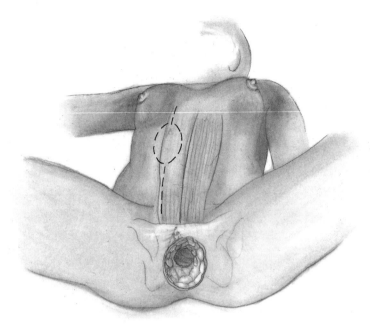

FIG. 12. Rectus abdominus flap.

- Loosely suture the skin to the underlying muscle flap.
- Divide the rectus muscle superiorly or inferiorly by using the cautery, depending on where the flap is to be positioned.
- Ligate and divide the underlying epigastric vessels at the transected end of the muscle.
- For a vulval site, bring the flap through a tunnel under the skin of the mons and suture it in place over a suction drain.
- Reapproximate the anterior rectus sheath over a suction drain, and close the skin incision.

5. Gluteus maximus flap
- It can be used to cover defects in the vulval and perineal region.
- It also can be used as a transposition flap or as a skin island flap.
- The inferior gluteal artery provides the vascular supply.
- The medial third of the gluteus maximus muscle is used together with its overlying skin.
- An island of skin may be developed over the gluteus graft, with its size designed to cover a specific defect.
- Bilateral grafts may be raised to cover a large central defect (Fig. 13).
- The advantage of using the underlying gluteus maximus muscle is that larger areas of skin may be transposed.
- Dissection may cause considerable bleeding because this is a very vascular area.

IV. Omental Grafts

A. Principles
1. The omentum is highly vascularized and may be developed into a pedicled graft and used in distant locations.

2. Because of its blood supply, the omentum is well suited for skin grafting.

B. Indications
1. To protect intestinal anastomoses
2. To protect ureteric and bladder anastomoses
3. To cover a dissected pelvic floor after radical resection, e.g., exenteration
4. To aid in the reconstruction/repair of urinary and intestinal fistulas

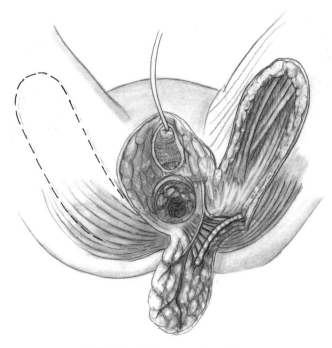

FIG. 13. Gluteus maximus flap.

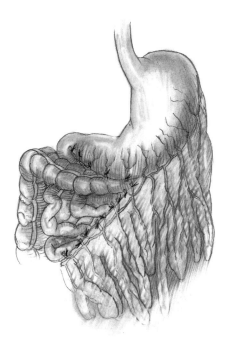

FIG. 14. Omental pedicle.

5. To aid in closure of abdominal wall defects
6. To accept a skin graft (McIndoe) for vaginal reconstruction after pelvic exenteration

C. Preoperative Investigations and Preparation

Requires laparotomy; thus routine preoperative investigations needed as dictated by the indication and other procedures to be performed.

D. Surgical Technique

1. Make a midline abdominal incision.
2. Inspect and assess the omentum regarding its adequacy for the purpose required.
3. Free the omentum from its loose attachment to the front of the transverse colon.
4. Next, free the omentum from the greater curvature of the stomach, usually basing the vascular pedicle on the right gastroepiploic vessels.
5. The pedicle can also be based on the left gastroepiploic vessels if appropriate (Fig. 14).
6. Preserve the gastroepiploic arcade of vessels close to the stomach in the omental pedicle.
7. Extra length may be gained by making an L- or J-shaped incision in the mobilized pedicle, taking care to preserve vascular continuity.

V. Skin Flaps, Myocutaneous Flaps, and Omental Grafts: Postoperative Management and Complications

A. Specific Postoperative Management of Flaps/Grafts

1. Depending on the size of the flap, immobilize the patient for a few days until the flap adheres.

2. Remove the suction drains when drainage is <20 mL/24 h.

B. Specific Postoperative Complications of Flaps/Grafts

1. Necrosis of the flap, either partial or complete, may be caused by too large a flap or interference with the vascular pedicle.
2. Hematoma under the flap is prevented by suction drainage and good hemostasis.
3. Occasionally in myocutaneous flaps, the skin will be lost but not the muscle; a split-skin graft can be applied later.

VI. Skin Grafts

A. Principles

1. A full-thickness skin graft includes the whole thickness of the dermis and epidermis.
2. A split-skin graft includes the epidermis and a portion of the thickness of the dermis.

B. Indications

1. McIndoe type of vaginal reconstruction
2. To cover an abdominal wall, vulval, or perineal defect, usually in association with a muscle or omental flap

C. Surgical Technique

1. Use either a blade or a dermatome, but an electric dermatome is preferred.
2. Lightly greased donor skin, usually over the buttock or thigh, is stretched and stabilized by use of two skin-graft boards.
3. A split-skin graft of medium thickness is about 0.3 to 0.35 mm thick.
4. Harvested skin is left to soak in isotonic saline until used.
5. The graft may be expanded by meshing so that it will cover larger areas. (Avoid this with neovaginal construction.)

D. Postoperative Management of Skin Graft

1. The grafted area is immobilized until it takes, approximately 5 to 7 days.
2. The donor-site dressings are left in place until they dry and fall off.

E. Specific Postoperative Complications of Skin Grafts

1. Failure of the graft to take: area may be prepared again and regrafted
2. Hypertrophic scar at donor site
3. Infected donor or recipient site
4. Fluid collection under graft: must be drained to allow adherence of graft

VII. Abdominoplasty

A. Principle

Abdominoplasty must never be regarded as a minor procedure, because significant morbidity can occur.

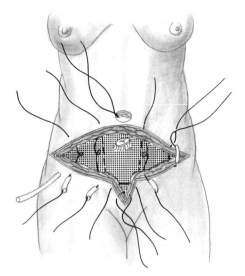

FIG. 15. Transverse elliptical incision for abdominoplasty.

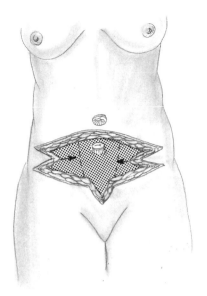

FIG. 16. W-shaped lateral ends of incision help to prevent "dog ears."

B. Indications
1. It is usually requested by patients for cosmetic reasons.
2. Occasionally, removal of a large abdominal apron allows easier access to the peritoneal cavity for abdominal surgical procedures.
3. It helps in the healing of chronically excoriated and inflamed skin beneath the abdominal fatty apron.

C. Preoperative Investigations
1. Routine laboratory tests depending on intraabdominal procedure
2. Otherwise, complete blood count and serum chemistry

D. Preoperative Preparation
Prophylactic treatment with antibiotics

E. Surgical Technique
1. Make a transverse elliptical incision designed so its size is adequate for removing the panniculus.
2. A V-shaped wedge may be excised from the lower flap to shorten the incision (Fig. 15).
3. Widely expose the rectus fascia.
4. Transplant the umbilicus cephalad through the upper skin flap.
5. A W-shaped lateral end of the incision helps prevent "dog ears" (Fig. 16).
6. Imbricate any diastasis recti.
7. Use sutures to obliterate dead space under the flaps.
8. Leave large suction drains under the flaps.
9. An alternative W-shaped incision, with undermining of the upper flap almost to the costal margins, may give a more acceptable scar (Fig. 17).

F. Specific Postoperative Management
1. Suction drainage until output is <20 mL/24 h/catheter
2. Prophylactic treatment with antibiotics
3. A jackknife position in bed for 48 hours assists adherence of the flaps to the underlying fascia.

G. Specific Postoperative Complications
1. Seroma or hematoma beneath the flaps
2. May become infected, producing an abscess beneath flaps
3. "Dog ears" at the ends of the incision

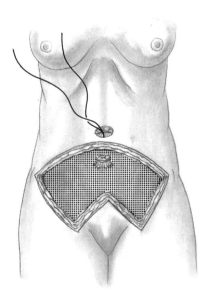

FIG. 17. W-shaped abdominoplasty incision.

Reading List

Cali RW, Pratt JH. Congenital absence of the vagina: long-term results of vaginal reconstruction in 175 cases. *Am J Obstet Gynecol* 1968;100:752–763.

Pratt JH, Irons GB. Panniculectomy and abdominoplasty. *Am J Obstet Gynecol* 1978;132:165–168.

Heath PM, Woods JE, Podratz KC, et al. Gracilis myocutaneous vaginal reconstruction. *Mayo Clin Proc* 1984;59:21–24.

Pratt JH. Panniculectomy as incidental procedure. *In:* Nichols DH, Anderson GW, eds. *Clinical problems, injuries, and complications of gynecologic surgery,* 2nd ed. Baltimore: Williams & Wilkins, 1988: 28–30.

Buss JG, Lee RA. McIndoe procedure for vaginal agenesis: results and complications. *Mayo Clin Proc* 1989;64:758–761.

Zanetta G, Welter VE, Lee RA. An unusual complication after a McIndoe procedure for vaginal agenesis. *J Pelv Surg* 1997;3:221–223.

CHAPTER 24

Miscellaneous Procedures

Maurice J. Webb, M.D.

I. Introduction

Occasionally, gynecologic patients require other general surgical procedures, either in association with or because of gynecologic surgery. Although some of these procedures may be beyond the training of a generalist gynecologic surgeon, the techniques, indications, and complications should be familiar to all pelvic surgeons.

II. Appendectomy

A. Indications
1. Acute appendicitis
2. Incidental procedure at laparotomy for another indication
3. Appendiceal abnormality discovered at laparotomy
4. Chronic pelvic pain

B. Preoperative Investigations
Depend on the indication for surgery

C. Preoperative Preparation
1. Bowel preparation is not necessary.
2. Routine preparation depending on the indications

D. Surgical Technique
1. Make a McBurney incision if the patient has appendicitis.
2. Or, make a midline lower abdominal incision if the diagnosis is in doubt.
3. Diagnostic laparoscopy or ultrasonography performed preoperatively may assist in making the diagnosis of acute appendicitis; laparoscopic removal is becoming more common.

Maurice J. Webb: Chairman, Division of Gynecologic Surgery and Consultant, Department of Surgery, Mayo Clinic and Mayo Foundation; Professor of Obstetrics and Gynecology, Mayo Medical School, Rochester, Minnesota.

4. Grasp the mesentery near the tip of the appendix with straight forceps.
5. Mobilize the appendix by dividing the lateral peritoneum if the appendix is retrocecal or otherwise adherent.
6. Perforate the mesentery with small curved forceps close to the base of the appendix.
7. Clamp, divide, and ligate the mesentery.
8. Crush the base of the appendix with straight forceps.
9. Apply straight forceps across the appendix distal to the crushed area.
10. Ligate the base with no. 1 synthetic absorbable suture flush with the cecum.
11. Transect the appendix flush with the clamp.
12. Swab the stump with povidone-iodine.
13. Leave the stump alone or bury it with a purse-string suture of 3-0 synthetic absorbable suture.

E. Specific Postoperative Management
1. Large-volume enemas are avoided for about 2 weeks, but disposable enemas and laxatives can be used.
2. Drain the appendix site if a large abscess cavity is present.

F. Specific Postoperative Complications
1. Postoperative bleeding from vascular pedicle: requires reoperation
2. Perforation of appendiceal stump; requires reoperation.
3. Abscess development without perforation: scan-guided percutaneous drainage with administration of antibiotics.

III. Right Hemicolectomy

A. Indications
1. Metastatic gynecologic cancer, usually ovarian cancer.
2. Primary carcinoma of the cecum, right colon, or appendix.
3. Obstruction from radiation or malignancy involving the terminal ileum.

4. The cecum and right colon can also be used for vaginal reconstruction and as a continent urinary reservoir.

B. Preoperative Investigations
1. Complete blood count
2. Serum chemistry
3. Colon radiography
4. Colonoscopy

C. Preoperative Preparation
1. Polyethylene glycol electrolyte solution (GoLYTELY) bowel preparation with antibiotics (see Chapter 1)
2. Intravenous fluids or parenteral nutrition as indicated

D. Surgical Technique
1. Extend a midline lower abdominal incision above the umbilicus.
2. Reflect the right colon medially by dividing the paracolic gutter peritoneum lateral to the colon.
3. Divide the hepatocolic and gastrocolic ligaments to mobilize the hepatic flexure.
4. Identify and preserve the duodenum, right kidney, right ureter, and right ovarian vessels beneath the reflected colon.
5. Clamp, divide, and ligate the ileocolic and right colic vessels in the mesentery; preserve the middle colic vessels.
6. Transect the transverse colon over clamps on the right side at a point appropriate to the vascular supply.
7. Divide the terminal ileum over the clamps approximately 20 cm from the ileocecal valve, and remove the colon (Fig. 1).
8. Next, anastomose the free ends of the ileum and transverse colon with an inner layer of continuous 3–0 synthetic absorbable suture supported by interrupted seromuscular sutures of 3-0 silk.
9. Alternatively, anastomose the ileum to the side of the transverse colon using an intraluminal stapler, and then use a TA 55 stapler to close the open end of the transverse colon.
10. Close the mesenteric defect with running 3-0 synthetic absorbable suture.

IV. Transverse Colectomy

A. Indications
1. Extensive metastatic cancer, usually ovarian, involving the omentum and adherent to the transverse colon
2. Primary carcinoma of midtransverse colon
3. If the primary lesion is in the hepatic flexure, perform a right hemicolectomy plus a transverse colectomy.
4. If the primary lesion is in the splenic flexure, perform a left hemicolectomy plus a transverse colectomy.

B. Preoperative Investigations and Preparation
The same as for right hemicolectomy

C. Surgical Technique
1. Make a midline incision above and below the umbilicus.
2. Transect the omentum at its attachment to the greater curvature of the stomach.
3. Mobilize the hepatic and splenic flexures of the colon.
4. Clamp, divide, and ligate the middle colic vessels.
5. Divide the right or left colic vessels, depending on the resection required.
6. Perform end-to-end or end-to-side colonic anastomosis as described above.
7. Repair the defect in the mesentery.

V. Left Hemicolectomy

A. Indication
Malignancy involving the proximal sigmoid colon and descending colon

B. Preoperative Investigations and Preparation
The same as for right colon resection

C. Surgical Technique
1. Divide the peritoneum lateral to the left colon in the left paracolic gutter.
2. Mobilize the splenic flexure by dividing the peritoneal reflection.
3. Clamp and divide the gastrocolic portion of the omentum on the left side.
4. Divide the greater omentum down from the point of transection of the transverse colon.
5. Reflect the left colon medially, identifying and

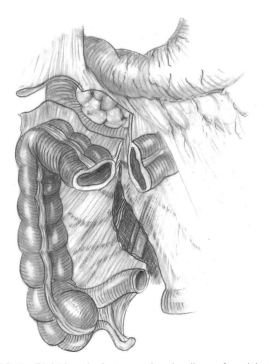

FIG. 1. Right hemicolectomy showing lines of excision.

preserving the left kidney and ureter, tail of the pancreas, and root of the mesentery.

6. Divide and ligate the inferior mesenteric vessels and the left colic vessels, and preserve the middle colic vessels.
7. Divide the transverse colon over clamps at the chosen point of resection.
8. Transect the sigmoid colon over clamps, and remove the specimen.
9. Perform end-to-end anastomosis between the cut ends of the colon, mobilizing the hepatic flexure if necessary to gain length.
10. The mesenteric defect is usually too large to close.

VI. Anterior Resection of Sigmoid / Rectosigmoid

A. Indications
1. Low sigmoid malignancy, either primary or secondary
2. Diverticular disease of the sigmoid
3. Rectosigmoid resection is common with ovarian cancer debulking surgery and exenteration.

B. Preoperative Investigations and Preparation
The same as for right colon resection

C. Surgical Technique
1. Make a lower midline incision
2. Lift the sigmoid out of the pelvis, and vertically divide the peritoneum on both sides down to the cul-de-sac.
3. Identify both ureters, and keep them under direct vision.
4. Divide and ligate the inferior mesenteric artery, preserving the left colic vessels.
5. Lift the sigmoid out of the presacral space by blunt dissection, mobilizing the sigmoid and upper rectum.
6. Make a curved incision around the front of the rectosigmoid in the cul-de-sac peritoneum, and mobilize the upper rectum from the posterior aspect of the upper vagina.
7. Transect the sigmoid over clamps above the pelvic brim.
8. Transect the lower sigmoid-upper rectum over clamps just below the peritoneal reflection, and remove the sigmoid.
9. Perform end-to-end anastomosis, mobilizing the splenic flexure to gain length if necessary (Fig. 2).
10. An alternative technique is stapled anastomosis using the intraluminal stapler (Fig. 3).

D. Specific Postoperative Management of Colonic Resections
1. Patient takes nothing by mouth until flatus is passed.
2. Parenteral nutrition if the patient is debilitated by obstruction, fistula, or malignancy.
3. Nasogastric tube suction if any abdominal distention develops.

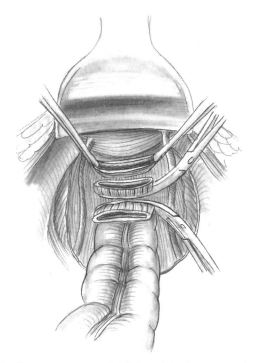

FIG. 2. Suture anastomosis of sigmoid colon to rectal stump.

4. Prophylactic nasogastric suction if extensive dissection, adhesions, multiple resections, or postradiotherapy. After flatus has been passed, the nasogastric tube is usually clamped, clear fluids are allowed, and the tube is removed if no nausea or vomiting occurs.
5. All left colon, sigmoid, or rectal resections with anastomosis should be drained with suction drains through the anterior abdominal wall.
6. Drains are removed after bowels have functioned and if there is no leakage of intestinal contents.
7. Rectal suppositories are allowed but not enemas, or laxatives in patients with intestinal anastomoses.

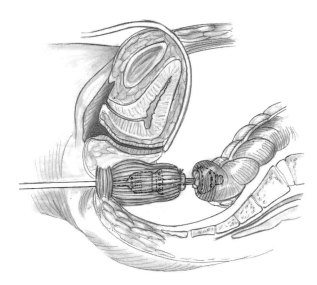

FIG. 3. Intraluminal stapled anastomosis of sigmoid colon to rectal stump.

E. Specific Postoperative Complications of Colonic Resections

1. Paralytic ileus
2. Intestinal obstruction (adhesive or at site of anastomosis)
3. Anastomotic leak causing abscess or peritonitis
4. Anastomotic leak causing intestinal-vaginal fistula
5. Sepsis without anastomotic leak
6. Diarrhea from colonic resection, loss of ileocecal valve, or resection of terminal ileum
7. Chronic diarrhea: usually managed with diphenoxylate (Lomotil), natural vegetable laxative, or cholestyramine. It usually settles within a few months.

VII. Splenectomy

A. Indications

1. Metastatic ovarian cancer
2. Trauma intraoperatively

B. Preoperative Investigations

No specific investigations

C. Preoperative Preparation

Crossmatch 3 U of blood.

D. Surgical Technique

1. Make the abdominal incision indicated for the primary operation.
2. Divide the gastrocolic omentum, and enter the lesser sac.
3. Retract the stomach cephalad and the transverse colon caudad, exposing the splenic vessels.
4. Open the peritoneum over the splenic artery, and ligate the splenic artery with silk suture.
5. Clamp, divide, and ligate the gastrosplenic ligament.
6. Next, clamp, divide, and ligate the splenocolic ligament between the spleen and the splenic flexure of the colon.
7. Roll the spleen medially, divide the splenorenal ligament, and ligate any vessels.
8. Sever any attachment of the spleen to the diaphragm.
9. Now the spleen is attached only by its vascular pedicle.
10. Lift the spleen up, identify and avoid the tail of the pancreas, ligate and divide the hilar vessels, and remove the spleen (Fig. 4).
11. Inspect the splenic bed for hemostasis.

E. Specific Postoperative Management

1. Perform platelet counts frequently; if thrombocytosis >1,000,000/mm^3 occurs, anticoagulation is indicated.
2. Patients should be treated prophylactically with antibiotics for this and future operations.
3. Pneumococcal vaccination is indicated.
4. Drainage of the splenic bed is usually unnecessary.

F. Specific Postoperative Complications

1. Hemorrhage
2. Abscess formation from collection in splenic bed

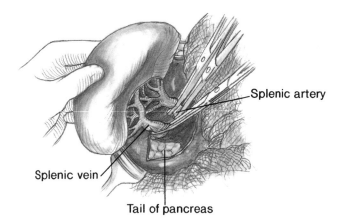

FIG. 4. Splenectomy with clamping of splenic vasculature.

3. Thrombocytosis with resulting thrombosis
4. Pulmonary atelectasis in the left lung because of poor diaphragmatic movement
5. Pancreatic fistula because of damage to the tail of the pancreas
6. Splenosis in the peritoneal cavity if the spleen ruptured
7. Arteriovenous fistula if artery and vein are ligated together

VIII. Nephrectomy

A. Indications

1. Secondary involvement with malignancy
2. Nonfunctioning kidney due to chronic ureteric obstruction caused by malignancy
3. Recurrent ureterovaginal fistula

B. Preoperative Investigations

1. Complete blood count
2. Serum chemistry
3. Urine culture
4. Intravenous pyelography and/or renography to assess function of the contralateral kidney

C. Preoperative Preparation

Crossmatch 2 U of blood.

D. Surgical Technique

1. In gynecologic surgery, most nephrectomies are performed in debulking operations for malignancy or for ureter chronically obstructed from cancer, and even then, they are rarely performed.
2. Elective nephrectomy is uncommon.
3. In view of the indications listed above, the anterior transperitoneal route is usually used.
4. Variations in the renal vasculature are very common.
5. On the *right side,* mobilize the hepatic flexure of the colon by dividing the peritoneum above and lateral to the colon.
6. Expose the right kidney by retracting the transverse

colon inferiorly and the stomach and duodenum medially.

7. Divide the posterior peritoneum over the vena cava and aorta, and expose the renal artery and vein.
8. Clamp, divide, and ligate the artery (or arteries) and vein.
9. Divide the ureter; mobilize the kidney posteriorly, superiorly, and laterally, and remove it.
10. Secure hemostasis in the renal bed, and leave a suction drain in place.
11. On the *left side,* mobilize the splenic flexure and paracolic peritoneum, and retract the left colon medially to expose the kidney.
12. Proceed with the left nephrectomy as on the right side.

E. Specific Postoperative Management

1. Monitor urine output and serum level of creatinine.
2. A transient increase in the creatinine level occurs in 24 to 48 hours.

F. Specific Postoperative Complications

1. Hemorrhage
2. Collection in renal bed

IX. Cystectomy

A. Indications

1. Segmental resection (partial cystectomy) or total cystectomy is usually performed in gynecologic surgical practice during resection of pelvic malignancy.
2. Partial cystectomy with intestinal augmentation is occasionally performed for the management of intractable urinary urgency with incontinence.

B. Preoperative Investigations

1. Routine laboratory tests depending on the primary diagnosis
2. Cystoscopy: to define the extent of bladder involvement and the proximity to the ureteric orifices
3. Intravenous pyelography: to assess ureteric patency

C. Preoperative Preparation

1. Bowel preparation is necessary if total cystectomy is likely because of the need for an intestinal conduit.
2. Prophylactic treatment with antibiotics

D. Surgical Technique

1. Partial cystectomy
   - Open the retropubic space, and free the bladder from its loose attachments to the back of the symphysis pubis.
   - Open the bladder at its dome but well away from any infiltrating tumor.
   - Visualize the ureteric orifices, and pass ureteric catheters if the ureters are close to the line of resection.
   - Excise the segment of the bladder wall, and close the defect in two layers with continuous 3–0 synthetic absorbable suture, the first layer being submucosal (Fig. 5).
   - If the tumor involves the ureter, it will be necessary to excise a segment of ureter and to perform ureteroneocystostomy (see Chapter 4).
2. Total cystectomy
   - It is usually performed as part of anterior or total pelvic exenteration.
   - Free up the bladder from its retropubic attachments to the pubis.
   - Develop the paravesical spaces bilaterally.
   - Divide the obliterated hypogastric artery near the anterior abdominal wall.
   - Divide the anterior division of the internal iliac artery at its origin.
   - Transect the urethra beneath the symphysis pubis.
   - For the remainder of the exenterative procedure and urinary tract reconstruction, see Chapters 17 and 21.

E. Specific Postoperative Management

1. Urinary catheter drainage for 7 days after partial cystectomy
2. Drainage for 6 weeks in cases of previously irradiated bladder

F. Specific Postoperative Complications

1. Vesicovaginal fistula from partial cystectomy (more common if postirradiation)
2. Ureteric obstruction due to incorporation of distal ureter in bladder closure suture

X. Liver Biopsy / Wedge Resection

A. Indications

1. Incidental discovery of liver nodule or other abnormalities at operation

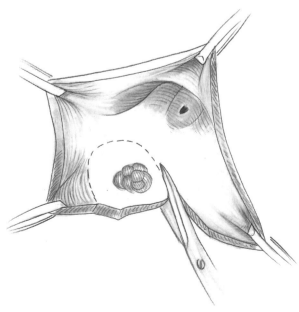

FIG. 5. Partial cystectomy for tumor invading the wall of the bladder.

2. Known liver disease (opportunity for biopsy is taken during laparotomy)
3. As part of resection of metastatic malignancy

B. Preoperative Investigations
1. Complete blood count
2. Coagulation profile

C. Preoperative Preparation
1. Correction of any coagulation defects
2. Typing and crossmatching of blood

D. Surgical Technique
1. Needle biopsy
   - Technique most commonly used for biopsy of liver parenchyma or nodule
   - Intraabdominally, steady the liver with one hand, and pass the Trucut needle through the biopsy site.
   - After withdrawing the needle, apply compression to the biopsy site with a sponge for 5 minutes to obtain hemostasis.
   - In areas of the liver that are inaccessible for intraabdominal needle biopsy, steady the liver and pass the needle through the abdominal wall directly into the liver.
2. Wedge biopsy/excision
   - Useful for biopsy of nodules along the edge of the liver or for obtaining a large piece of parenchyma for histology
   - Steady the liver, and resect a wedge with a scalpel and cautery.
   - Reapproximate the edges of the liver with interrupted no. 1 synthetic absorbable mattress sutures on a tapered needle.

XI. Fine Needle Aspiration

A. Indications
1. To confirm presence of malignant cells in a nodule
2. Nodule may be palpable or visible only on scan

B. Preoperative Preparation and Investigations
Ultrasonography or computed tomography may be needed to locate the nodule and to guide insertion of the needle.

C. Surgical Technique
1. Steady the nodule between the finger and thumb of one hand.
2. Attach a needle of appropriate length to a 20-mL syringe, and insert it into the nodule.
3. Apply suction to the syringe while making a number of passes through the nodule.
4. Release the suction *before* withdrawing the needle from tissue so that cellular material stays in the needle and is not drawn into the syringe.
5. Separate the needle and syringe. Fill the syringe with air, and reattach it to the needle.
6. Sharply depress the plunger of the syringe to expel the contents of the needle onto a cytology slide.

7. Either spray the slide with fixative or dip it into fixative and send it for processing.

D. Specific Postoperative Complications
1. Bleeding from the needle track: usually controlled by temporarily applying pressure
2. There usually are no complications when the needle is passed through the intestine to reach the biopsy site.

XII. Trucut Needle Biopsy

A. Indication
Used to obtain tissue sample rather than cytologic specimen of suspicious nodule

B. Preoperative Investigations and Preparation
1. No specific investigations required
2. Coagulation profile if suggested by medical history

C. Surgical Technique
1. The wide-bore needle contains an obturator, with a portion of the shaft hollowed out to contain the specimen.
2. The needle is particularly useful for taking biopsy samples from inaccessible areas, e.g., liver, retroperitoneal masses, and parametrium.
3. The needle may also be used transvaginally or transrectally to obtain biopsy samples from a pelvic sidewall or parametrial mass.
4. Insert the needle, with the obturator withdrawn inside the shaft, just into the mass.
5. Advance the obturator, allowing tissue to fall against the hollowed-out section.
6. Steady the obturator, and advance the needle to cover the obturator, thus cutting off a core of tissue.
7. Withdraw the needle and obturator, and send the specimen for histology.

D. Specific Postoperative Complications
1. The needle may be passed through the intestine without causing any complications.
2. A vein may be lacerated and produce hemorrhage, especially in the pelvic sidewall or paraaortic region.

XIII. Inguinal Lymph Node Biopsy

A. Indication
Enlarged inguinal lymph node to be assessed with regard to malignancy

B. Surgical Technique
1. Make an oblique incision in the line of the groin crease over the node.
2. Grasp the node with Babcock or Allis forceps, and dissect it free with cautery.
3. Secure hemostasis, and close the incision with interrupted deep sutures and subcuticular skin suture.

C. Specific Postoperative Complications

1. Hematoma: due to inadequate hemostasis
2. Lymphocyst: usually disappears
3. Infection: groin incisions frequently become infected.

XIV. Inguinofemoral Lymphadenectomy

A. Indications

1. Usually performed in association with vulval malignancy (see Chapter 12)
2. May be unilateral or bilateral, depending on the location and size of the primary lesion
3. May be performed en bloc with vulvectomy or through separate incisions

B. Preoperative Investigations

1. Complete blood count
2. Serum chemistry
3. Urine culture
4. Chest radiography
5. Computed tomography of the abdomen and pelvis

C. Preoperative Preparation

1. Prophylactic treatment with antibiotics
2. Thromboembolus-deterrent stockings and sequential calf compression device
3. Prophylactic treatment with subcutaneous injections of heparin in high-risk patients
4. Patient placed in "ski" position if vulvectomy is to be performed concurrently

D. Surgical Technique

1. Make an oblique incision about 1 cm below a line extending from the anterior superior iliac spine to the pubic tubercle.
2. Continue the incision, with cautery, down through subcutaneous fat to expose the inguinal ligament.
3. Dissect down under the lower skin flap to the level of the apex of the femoral triangle.
4. Identify the adductor longus fascia medially, and incise it to expose the muscle.
5. On the lateral aspect of the skin incision, incise the fascia over the sartorius muscle where the muscle runs from the anterior superior iliac spine down to the medial condyle of the tibia.
6. With a finger, tunnel beneath the fascia from lateral to medial until the finger appears in the incision in the fascia of the adductor muscle.
7. With cautery, divide the subcutaneous fat anterior to the fascia until the saphenous vein is identified.
8. Clamp, divide, and ligate the saphenous vein at the apex of the femoral triangle.
9. Retract the subcutaneous tissue, fascia, and superficial nodes superiorly, and open the fascia over the femoral artery by making a vertical incision over the artery.
10. Dissect the deep lymph nodes and pectineus fascia from the apex of the femoral triangle superiorly toward the inguinal ligament.
11. Dissect up along the femoral artery to the place where the superficial external pudendal artery courses medially across the femoral vein.
12. This vessel lies at the level of the saphenofemoral junction and is used to locate the origin of the saphenous vein.
13. Divide and ligate the superficial external pudendal artery. Identify the origin of the saphenous vein, and clamp, divide, and ligate it.
14. Continue to dissect superiorly to the inguinal ligament, and remove the deep and superficial lymph node tissue with the pectineus fascia.
15. If the node of Cloquet is present, remove it from the femoral canal.
16. Close the femoral canal and external inguinal ring with interrupted no. 1 synthetic absorbable sutures to prevent hernia from developing.
17. Secure hemostasis, and close the incision in layers over a suction catheter.

E. Specific Postoperative Management

1. Continue suction drainage until <50 mL of fluid is collected per 24 hours for 2 consecutive days.
2. Do not apply pressure dressings, because they can cause skin necrosis.
3. Debride the wound if skin necrosis occurs.
4. Actively mobilize the patient to prevent deep vein thrombosis.

F. Specific Postoperative Complications

1. Lymphocyst formation
   - Occurs when drains are removed prematurely and primary healing of skin incision prevents drainage
   - If small, aspirate with a syringe or leave alone.
   - If large, open the incision over the lymphocyst and insert a drain.
2. Skin necrosis
   - Groin incisions often develop skin-edge necrosis.
   - Débride and pack wound if necessary.
   - If it is a large area, it can be grafted with a split-skin graft.
3. Deep vein thrombosis
   - Caused by operation around the femoral vein and by immobility
   - Prevention involves support stockings, sequential calf compression device, prophylactic treatment with heparin, and active mobilization postoperatively.

XV. Supraclavicular Lymph Node Biopsy

A. Indications

1. Palpable node in patients with pelvic malignancy
2. To assess possible metastatic spread of malignancy before embarking on an extensive pelvic operation

B. Preoperative Investigations and Preparation

Depend on the indication

C. Surgical Technique

1. Make a transverse incision in the skin crease above the clavicle.
2. Turn the patient's head to the opposite side.
3. Continue the incision through the platysma muscle and deep cervical fascia.
4. Retract the sternomastoid muscle medially, and expose the scalene fat pad.
5. Remove the palpable node or the whole scalene fat pad.
6. Take care to avoid the internal jugular vein medially and the subclavian vessels inferiorly.
7. Approximate the deep fascia, and then close the skin with a subcuticular suture.

D. Specific Postoperative Complications

1. Damage to the phrenic nerve
2. Damage to the internal jugular vein

XVI. Paracentesis Abdominus

A. Indications

1. Malignant ascites, usually from ovarian cancer
2. Diagnostic procedure to collect fluid for cytologic examination
3. Therapeutic procedure to drain off fluid and to relieve symptoms of distention

B. Preoperative Investigations and Preparation

1. No specific preparation is necessary.
2. Occasionally, it may be difficult to differentiate ascites from other causes of abdominal distention; ultrasonography can help make the distinction.

C. Surgical Technique

1. Select the site of puncture to avoid major organs and abdominal wall vessels. Ultrasonography may be helpful.
2. Infiltrate the site with a local anesthetic agent.
3. Make a small incision in the skin.
4. Insert a trochar, and drain off the fluid.
5. The volume and rate of fluid removed do not have to be restricted with malignant ascites.

D. Specific Postoperative Management

May be performed as an outpatient procedure, with no specific requirements

E. Specific Postoperative Complications

1. Perforation of a viscus
   - Patient should be observed and treated prophylactically with antibiotics.
   - If peritonitis develops, laparotomy is required.

2. Hemorrhage
   If a major vessel is traumatized, laparotomy may be required.

XVII. Thoracentesis

A. Indications

1. To obtain pleural fluid for cytology for staging of pelvic malignancy
2. To remove fluid preoperatively that may interfere with ventilation intraoperatively
3. For symptomatic treatment

B. Preoperative Investigations

Chest radiography

C. Preoperative Preparation

Patient sits upright with trunk flexed.

D. Surgical Technique

1. The usual site of puncture is just below the tip of the scapula in the seventh intercostal space.
2. Infiltrate the area of puncture with local anesthetic through to the parietal pleura.
3. Advance a large-bore needle that is attached to a syringe and a three-way stopcock through the pleura, applying suction to the syringe until effusion is reached.
4. Aspirate the effusion, and withdraw the needle.

E. Specific Postoperative Management

Chest radiography to check for amount of residual effusion and any evidence of pneumothorax

F. Specific Postoperative Complications

1. Pneumothorax
   - Caused by the needle lacerating the lung
   - If significant, insertion of a chest tube and underwater sealed drainage are needed.
2. Hematothorax
   - Caused by the needle lacerating the lung
   - If severe, thoracotomy may be needed.

Note: Closed tube drainage of the pleural space may be the best method for draining a large effusion. It is also used for decompression of pneumothorax. The tube is placed anteriorly in the second or third intercostal space in the midclavicular line or posteriorly if fluid is present in this region.

XVIII. Insertion of Peritoneal Catheter

A. Indications

1. For administration of ^{32}P intraperitoneally
2. For administration of chemotherapy intraperitoneally

B. Preoperative Investigations and Preparation

Empty the patient's bladder.

C. Surgical Technique

1. Make a transverse upper abdominal incision over the rectus muscle.
2. Retract this muscle medially, and make a small opening into the peritoneal cavity.
3. Check that there are no adhesions locally in the peritoneal cavity.
4. Insert a catheter, and bring it out through the wound in an indirect course to prevent leakage.
5. Close the rectus fascia and the skin.
6. Instill radiopaque dye through the catheter, and check fluoroscopically that the dispersion is satisfactory.
7. A permanent catheter device may be inserted if repeated treatments are indicated. The metal device is inserted in a pocket over the lower anterior ribs, and the catheter is tunneled subcutaneously until it is inserted through the fascia into the peritoneal cavity.

D. Specific Postoperative Complications

Intestinal obstruction due to adhesions or localized irradiation from intraperitoneal ^{32}P.

XIX. Perineal Hernia

A. Introduction

1. Perineal hernia usually develops after pelvic exenteration.
2. It may also occur after total vaginectomy.
3. It usually protrudes through the perineum, between the levator muscles.
4. Occasionally, a hernia may develop laterally through the levator plate.
5. It usually contains small intestine but may also contain rectum, sigmoid, or bladder (if present).

B. Preoperative Investigations

1. Routine preoperative laboratory tests
2. Radiographic studies of the intestinal tract with contrast agent or magnetic resonance imaging may outline the contents of the hernia.

C. Preoperative Preparation

1. Prophylactic treatment with antibiotics
2. Patient placed in lithotomy position

D. Surgical Technique

1. Make a vertical incision over the skin of the hernia, extending from the symphysis pubis anteriorly to the coccyx posteriorly (or anus if present).
2. Undermine the skin and subcutaneous tissue laterally to expose the inferior pubic rami periosteum.

3. Take care not to traumatize the bowel, which is usually adherent to the hernial sac.
4. Suture synthetic nonabsorbable mesh with interrupted nonabsorbable sutures from the ischial tuberosity on one side, up the inferior aspect of the inferior pubic ramus to the symphysis pubis, and then down the other side to the opposite ischial tuberosity.
5. Anchor the mesh posteriorly to the coccyx and to the tissue between the coccyx and the ischial tuberosities.
6. Secure hemostasis, excise redundant skin, and close the incision over a small suction drain.

E. Specific Postoperative Management

1. Have the patient avoid straining, vomiting, and coughing in the immediate postoperative period.
2. Remove the suction drain when the output is <20 mL/24 h.

F. Specific Postoperative Complications

1. Enterotomy: due to adherent bowel
2. Hematoma: avoid with suction drainage and good hemostasis
3. Infected mesh: needs to be removed

XX. Ventral Hernia

A. Introduction

1. Develops after a previous abdominal incision
2. More common with midline incisions
3. Wound infection, obesity, and cachexia predispose to wound herniation.

B. Indication

All hernias should be repaired if there is a risk of incarceration of the intestine with obstruction.

C. Preoperative Investigations

Routine laboratory tests

D. Preoperative Management

1. Weight loss if patient is obese
2. Prophylactic treatment with antibiotics if mesh is to be used

E. Surgical Technique

1. Make a vertical or elliptical incision in the skin of the hernia.
2. Undermine the skin to dissect around the sac.
3. Continue the dissection above, below, and lateral to the sac until encountering the anterior rectus sheath.
4. Widely expose the anterior abdominal wall fascia around the hernia.
5. Make an incision in the hernial sac, and free any adherent intestine.

6. Excise the peritoneum of the hernial sac with any attenuated fascia back to intact abdominal wall.

7. Overlap the intact fascial edges of the defect in a "vest-over-pants" fashion, using two layers of interrupted horizontal mattress no. 0 monofilament (Prolene) sutures.

8. Insert a suction drain in the subcutaneous space, and close the skin with subcuticular 3-0 synthetic absorbable suture.

9. If the fascial edges are too far apart to be overlapped, use a synthetic nonabsorbable mesh to cover the defect.

F. Specific Postoperative Management

1. Remove the suction drain when the output is <20 mL/24 h.

2. Have the patient avoid heavy lifting and straining for 8 weeks.

G. Specific Postoperative Complications

1. Hematoma

2. Wound infection (or mesh infection)

3. Intestinal fistula because of inadvertent enterotomy or because suture was placed through the bowel.

4. Recurrent herniation

XXI. Umbilical Hernia

A. Indications

1. Routinely repaired when performing other abdominal operations

2. Elective repair when the hernia is large, symptomatic, or contains bowel

B. Preoperative Investigations

No specific tests

C. Preoperative Preparation

Weight loss if patient is obese

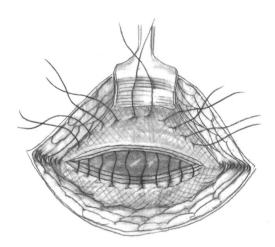

FIG. 6. Overlapping of fascial layers with repair of umbilical hernia.

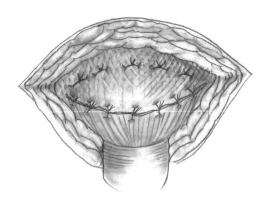

FIG. 7. Completed umbilical hernia repair.

D. Surgical Technique

1. Make a transverse incision above or below the umbilicus (occasionally, the umbilicus can be excised).

2. Dissect down to the rectus sheath all around the hernia.

3. Free the sac from the surrounding fascia.

4. Open the sac, and reduce the contents.

5. Excise any redundant peritoneum of the sac, and close the peritoneum.

6. Insert horizontal mattress sutures of synthetic nonabsorbable material (e.g., Prolene) to bring the lower fascial flap under the upper flap ("vest-over-pants") (Fig. 6).

7. Next, suture the upper flap to the lower flap with another row of nonabsorbable sutures (Fig. 7).

8. Anchor the skin of the umbilical dimple to the fascia to invert the umbilicus.

9. Close the skin incision with subcuticular 3-0 synthetic absorbable suture.

Note: If an umbilical hernia is noted at the time of laparotomy, the midline incision is extended cephalad into the defect. The sac is excised, the fascial edges trimmed, and the hernia repaired as a continuation of the routine abdominal wall closure.

E. Specific Postoperative Complications

1. Wound infection

2. Recurrences are rare.

Reading List

Pratt JH, Souders JC. A review of ventral hernia in gynecology patients. *Minn Med* 1962;45:714–717.

Raventos JM, Symmonds RE. Surgical management of acute diverticulitis in women. *Obstet Gynecol* 1981;58:557–565.

Stanhope CR. Complications of parenteral and oral alimentation, subclavian catheter insertion, thoracentesis, and paracentesis. In: Delgado G, Smith JP, eds. *Management of complications in gynecologic oncology.* New York: John Wiley & Sons, 1982:255–263.

Webb MJ, Weaver EW. Intestinal surgery in gynaecological oncology. *Aust NZJ Obstet Gynaecol* 1987;27:299–303.

Webb MJ. Proctectomy and bowel surgery in gynecologic malignancies. *Magyar Noovoork Lapja (Hungarian J Gynecol)* 1995; Suppl 2, Evfolyam Kulonsgam:1–94.

Webb MJ. Small bowel urinary diversion. *CME J Gynecol Oncol* 1996; 98:80–83.

CHAPTER 25

Hysteroscopy

Bobbie S. Gostout, M.D.

I. Diagnostic Hysteroscopy

A. General Principles

1. Hysteroscopy is a valuable tool in the evaluation of abnormal uterine bleeding. It can also be useful in the evaluation of suspected uterine anomalies and infertility.
2. Diagnostic hysteroscopy can be performed as an office procedure or in the surgical suite as an adjunct to dilation and curettage.
3. Hysteroscopy is not a reliable diagnostic tool for differentiating endometrial hyperplasia from endometrial cancer.

B. Preoperative Investigations

1. Pregnancy test, if appropriate
2. Rule out or treat genital tract infection, if appropriate

C. Preoperative Preparation

1. Povidone-iodine douche
2. Microenema to facilitate examination under anesthesia

D. Surgical Technique

1. Select an appropriate uterine distending medium: normal saline for diagnostic hysteroscopy; D$_5$W or 1.5% glycine if operative hysteroscopy is anticipated. Flush air from the tubing and hysteroscope.
2. Sound the endometrial cavity, and dilate the cervix.
3. Insert the hysteroscope with the distention media flowing. Whenever possible, the cervix should be dilated well enough so that the distending medium can flow out of the cavity around the hysteroscope.
4. If more than 1 L of distending medium is anticipated, collect the effluent to maintain an estimate of the

volume of fluid delivered into the peritoneal cavity via the fallopian tubes.
5. Limit the fluid deficit to <1 L in healthy women and about half that in older women with cardiovascular compromise, thereby decreasing the chance of volume overload.
6. Examine the endometrial cavity systematically. Sweep from one tubal ostium to the other to examine the fundus (Fig. 1). Next, withdraw the hysteroscope from the fundus to the endocervix, examining the anterior, posterior, right, and left lateral walls of the cavity sequentially (Fig. 2).
7. Perform dilation and curettage if indicated by patient symptoms or by hysteroscopic findings.
8. Reinsert the hysteroscope, and reexamine the endometrial cavity to ensure that all surfaces have been evaluated and that removal of tissue is complete.

E. Specific Postoperative Management

1. Same as for dilation and curettage

F. Specific Postoperative Complications

1. Fluid overload can result from absorption of intraperitoneal fluid. The symptoms should respond well to diuretics. Observe oxygen saturation closely, and provide supplemental oxygen as needed until fluid balance has been restored. Prevention is important.
2. Dilutional hyponatremia can result if significant transperitoneal absorption of D$_5$W or glycine occurs. Treatment with fluid restriction and diuretics usually restores the serum sodium level to a safe range. Consider hypertonic saline in addition to these measures if hyponatremia is severe.
3. Uterine perforation is not usually associated with adverse effects. The possibility of infection or bowel injury must be kept in mind and the patient counseled appropriately. In the absence of symptoms or heightened suspicion by the surgeon, the patient may be dismissed according to the usual routine.

Bobbie S. Gostout: Consultant, Departments of Obstetrics and Gynecology and Surgery, Mayo Clinic and Mayo Foundation; Assistant Professor of Obstetrics and Gynecology, Mayo Medical School, Rochester, Minnesota.

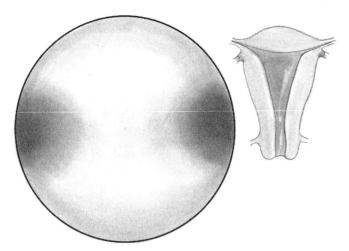

FIG. 1. Hysteroscopic view of normal endometrial space, fundal region. The orifices of the fallopian tubes can be visualized by directing the hysteroscope into each cornual recess. If curettage is not performed before hysteroscopy, the characteristics of the endometrial surface will vary with the menstrual cycle.

II. Hysteroscopic Resection of Uterine Fibroids

A. General Principles

1. Hysteroscopic resection of submucous fibroids should be considered when the fibroids might be contributing to symptoms of abnormal uterine bleeding. Hysteroscopic resection affords the potential advantages of avoiding a major surgical procedure and preserving the option of future fertility. The disadvantage of hysteroscopic resection compared with hysterectomy is that amelioration of bleeding symptoms is less certain and additional symptomatic fibroids may develop with time.

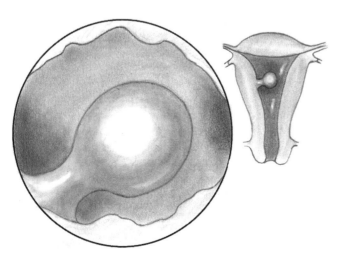

FIG. 2. An endometrial polyp appears as a fleshy intraluminal rounded or tongue-shaped projection. The point of attachment can be identified if the hysteroscope is maneuvered around all sides of the polyp.

2. Fibroids may contribute to problems with infertility, and hysteroscopic resection of asymptomatic submucous fibroids may be indicated in the presence of infertility. The overall success of myomectomy alone as a treatment for infertility is low, and the preoperative discussion should include the limitations of this surgical procedure as a treatment for infertility.

3. Planning the procedure so that it is performed immediately after the menstrual period will minimize artifact due to the endometrial lining.

4. Resection of the fibroids may require more than one hysteroscopic procedure. Prevention of intravascular volume overload may require limiting what can be accomplished in a single operative procedure.

B. Preoperative Investigations

1. The same as for diagnostic hysteroscopy

2. Diagnostic hysteroscopy, ultrasonography, or hysterosalpingography to demonstrate submucous fibroids

C. Preoperative Preparation

1. The same as for diagnostic hysteroscopy

2. Preoperative preparation using a gonadotropin-releasing hormone agonist for 2 to 3 months may enhance visibility of submucous fibroids by inducing an atrophic endometrium. The obvious disadvantage is that it may also shrink some submucous fibroids so they are no longer easily identified.

D. Surgical Technique

1. Perform preliminary dilation and curettage.

2. Begin as for diagnostic hysteroscopy, inserting a two-channel operating hysteroscope. Use a nonionic distention medium. Use a draping system that allows the efflux of fluid around the cervix to be measured. An assistant is assigned the task of continuously monitoring inflow and output of distending fluid.

3. Identify the location and apparent size of the fibroids (Fig. 3). Consider laparoscopic guidance of the resection if large fibroids are to be resected or if fibroids are near the tubal ostia, where the uterine wall is thin. (If laparoscopic guidance is to be used, see Chapter 26.)

4. Use a cautery loop that allows the wire to be well applied to the exposed surface of the fibroid, usually an angled loop for the sidewalls and a straight loop for the fundal region. Begin with cautery set at blended cut and coagulation currents at 40 W.

5. Systematically resect and cauterize strips of the exposed surface of the fibroid until the surface is level with the surrounding myometrium. Each pass should begin at the most cephalad point of the myoma; the resecting instrument is drawn toward the cervical end. If laparoscopic guidance is used, an assistant watches the serosal surface overlying the site of resection.

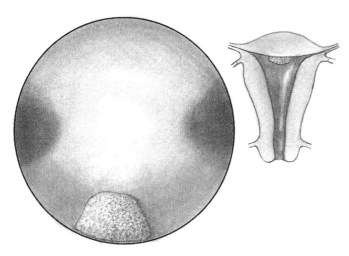

FIG. 3. Submucous uterine fibroids appear as irregular intra-luminal projections. The surface often appears ragged or rough after curettage removes overlying endometrium.

Adjacent structures such as fallopian tubes or bowel loops should be moved as far from the resection site as possible.

6. Continue to resect additional fibroids until all surfaces are reduced to normal or until the retained distending fluid reaches the maximal safe volume.

7. Secure hemostasis at resection sites using additional cautery without additional resection.

E. Specific Postoperative Management

The same as for diagnostic hysteroscopy

F. Specific Postoperative Complications

1. The same as for diagnostic hysteroscopy; the risk for fluid overload is greater than with diagnostic hysteroscopy alone.

2. As with other forms of myomectomy, attempt to esti-mate the risk of uterine rupture if the patient becomes pregnant. The operative note should include a statement recommending a trial of labor or cesarean section, based on the observations made at the time of resection.

3. Bleeding from the site of resection is usually minimal. If significant postoperative bleeding occurs, examine the patient for cervical lacerations before assuming an intrauterine source. Bleeding from the endometrial surfaces can be controlled with a Foley catheter balloon for tamponade. Use a large Foley catheter with a 30-mL balloon. Pass the catheter through the cervical os. Distend the balloon until moderate resistance is encountered. Leave the catheter and balloon in place for 24 hours.

III. Hysteroscopic Resection of Uterine Septa

A. General Principle

Resection of a uterine septum may be indicated in the treatment of infertility.

B. Preoperative Investigations

1. The same as for diagnostic hysteroscopy

2. A uterine septum must be distinguished from a bicornuate uterus. Laparoscopic visualization of the serosal surface of the uterus will clarify the diagnosis.

C. Preoperative Preparation

The same as for diagnostic laparoscopy

D. Surgical Technique

1. Begin with a two-channel operating hysteroscope. Laparoscopic guidance should be considered. Laparoscopic evaluation is necessary if a bicornuate uterus has not been ruled out as the cause for the intrauterine abnormality.

2. Sharply incise the presenting edge of the septum in the midline (Fig. 4). The two edges may retract toward the anterior and posterior uterine walls.

3. Excise the remnants of the septum using scissors if bleeding is minimal or a cautery resecting loop if necessary to control bleeding. Reduce the tissue to the level of the surrounding myometrium.

4. Repeat steps 2 and 3 until the septum has been completely excised.

5. Use cautery to establish hemostasis as needed.

E. Postoperative Management

The same as for hysteroscopic resection of fibroids

F. Specific Postoperative Complications

The same as for hysteroscopic resection of fibroids

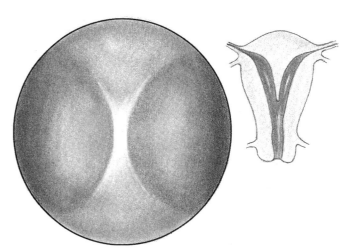

FIG. 4. Hysteroscopic view of an incomplete uterine septum. With the scope positioned low in the endometrial cavity, the septum appears as a band or ridge between the two tubal os-tia. If the scope is positioned above the septum, the cavity may appear normal except that only one tubal ostium can be identified. Gradual withdrawal of the scope will allow the lim-its of the septum to be defined and the opposite half of the en-dometrial cavity to be examined.

IV. Endometrial Ablation

A. General Principle

The techniques used are designed to destroy the endometrium down to the basal layer so that regeneration does not occur.

B. Preoperative Investigations

1. The same as for diagnostic hysteroscopy
2. Evaluate the patient for intrinsic blood clotting abnormalities if the history indicates. Isolated menometrorrhagia does not suggest an intrinsic defect.

C. Preoperative Preparation

The same as for diagnostic hysteroscopy

D. Surgical Technique

1. Cautery and resectoscope
   - Begin with dilation and curettage to ensure that no underlying malignancy is the cause of menorrhagia.
   - Insert the operating hysteroscope that has been flushed with nonconducting distention medium. Use a ball-tipped cautery, a resecting cautery loop, or a combination of the two to destroy the entire surface of the endometrium sequentially to a myometrial depth of approximately 2 to 4 mm. The cautery is set at 40 to 80 W. The cornual and fundal regions can be difficult to treat and require careful attention to ensure that treatment is complete. The ball-tipped cautery is preferred for treatment in the cornual regions.
   - Avoid treating the endocervical region to prevent problems with cervical stenosis.
2. Thermal ablation
   - Begin with dilation and curettage to ensure that no underlying malignancy is the cause of menorrhagia. Determine the approximate size of the uterine cavity. Consider alternative treatment if the uterine depth sounds to >10 cm or <6 cm.
   - Insert the balloon catheter. Verify connections to the controller unit and syringe.
   - Fill the balloon to achieve a pressure of 160 to 180 mm Hg (unless recommended otherwise by the manufacturer of the balloon device).
   - Activate the heat cycle.
   - After the heating cycle has been completed, aspirate the balloon fluid and withdraw the balloon.

E. Specific Postoperative Management

Nonsteroidal antiinflammatory agents to manage cramping

F. Specific Postoperative Complications

1. The same as for hysteroscopic resection of uterine fibroids
2. Uterine synechia may develop and result in hematometra if destruction of the endometrial tissue was erratic.
3. Persistent abnormal bleeding results in the need for additional treatment in approximately 25% of women after a single hysteroscopic endometrial ablation treatment. Recurrent bleeding may be less frequent after balloon thermal ablation of the endometrium.

Reading List

Corfman RS. Indications for hysteroscopy. *Obstet Gynecol Clin North Am* 1988;15:41–49.

Good AE. Diagnostic options for assessment of postmenopausal bleeding. *Mayo Clin Proc* 1997;72:345–349.

CHAPTER 26

Laparoscopy

Bobbie S. Gostout, M.D.

I. Diagnostic Laparoscopy

A. Indications
1. Indeterminate pelvic mass
2. Pelvic pain
3. Congenital anomalies
4. Unexplained infertility

B. Principles
1. The patient must always be prepared for the possibility that the laparoscopic procedure may diagnose or result in conditions that will require immediate laparotomy.
2. Laparoscopy may clarify diagnoses in many clinical settings, but especially in the case of chronic pelvic pain, the patient must be prepared for the possibility that all the pelvic organs will look entirely normal.

C. Preoperative Investigations
1. Physical examination to exclude conditions that warrant proceeding directly to laparotomy
2. CA-125 if procedure is performed for suspicious pelvic mass
3. Review history of abdominal or pelvic operations to evaluate risk of adhesions.
4. Review menstrual history if a tubal dye study is planned so that the procedure may be performed in the follicular phase of the menstrual cycle.

D. Preoperative Preparation
1. Povidone-iodine douche
2. Microenema
3. Limited shave at site of suprapubic trocar

Bobbie S. Gostout: Consultant, Departments of Obstetrics and Gynecology and Surgery, Mayo Clinic and Mayo Foundation; Assistant Professor of Obstetrics and Gynecology, Mayo Medical School, Rochester, Minnesota.

E. Surgical Technique
1. Place patient in modified lithotomy position, and allow enough flexion at the hips and abduction of the thighs to permit access to the vagina, without compromising movement of instruments.
2. Place a tenaculum on the anterior cervix, and secure a uterine manipulator in the cervical canal. Empty the bladder with a catheter.
3. Make a 10-mm transverse or longitudinal incision in the subumbilical region, including skin and subcutaneous tissue. Grasp the abdominal wall on each side of the umbilicus to stabilize. Insert the Veress needle as near the umbilical cleft as possible, and advance the needle at a 45-degree angle as soon as the tip is felt to pop through the fascia. The fascia and peritoneum should be well attached if the needle was positioned near the umbilicus, and one or two "pops" may be felt as the needle enters the peritoneal cavity. Verify alarm settings on the insufflation device.
4. Verify the position of the Veress needle by at least one of the following methods:
   - Instill 2 to 5 mL of sterile water or saline. Attempt to withdraw. If the needle is in the peritoneal cavity, you should not be able to withdraw the fluid. Next, place a drop of water at the hub of the needle. Grasp and elevate the abdominal wall; the drop should flow freely through the needle.
   - Connect the Veress needle to the gas insufflator to evaluate the pressure at the needle tip. When the abdominal wall is grasped and elevated, the pressure transducer should indicate negative pressure.
   - Begin insufflation if at least one of the above tests appears to confirm an intraperitoneal position of the needle. After 0.5 L of gas has been instilled, percussion over the liver should produce tympany.
5. Insufflate with CO_2 until the abdominal wall is full to palpation or until the intraabdominal pressure reaches a maximum of 18 mm Hg.
6. Withdraw the Veress needle, and insert a 10-mm trocar

at a 45-degree angle, with the tip pointed toward the pelvis.

7. Reconnect the insufflation device. Insert the laparoscope. Inspect the upper abdomen.

8. Place the patient in the Trendelenburg position. Briefly inspect the pelvis. Establish a second port site in the suprapubic region or lateral abdominal wall, depending on anticipated needs (Figs. 1 and 2). Create a 5- to 10-mm skin incision two fingerbreadths above the symphysis pubis. Use the laparoscope to verify that the site is above the bladder reflection. Insert the trocar under direct visualization with the laparoscope. Aim the tip toward the pelvis after the peritoneal cavity has been entered.

9. If laparoscopy is being performed for a pelvic mass, use a hollow probe or suction/irrigation device to collect a sample of fluid or wash for cytologic examination.

10. Use a blunt probe to sweep bowel loops over the sacral promontory.

11. Inspect the pelvic organs, including the uterus, fallopian tubes, and ovaries (Fig. 3). Use the blunt probe to evaluate mobility of the ovaries and to elevate the ovary for inspection of the inferior surface as well as the peritoneum of the ovarian fossa.

12. Sequentially examine all anterior and posterior peritoneal surfaces, including the round and uterosacral ligaments. Aspirate all fluid from the cul-de-sac to evaluate the most dependent peritoneal surfaces.

13. Visualize the appendix if possible.

14. Withdraw the lower trocar under direct visualization. Inspect the trocar site for hemostasis. If a fascial suture is indicated, place that suture with the laparoscope still in place. In thin patients, this stitch may be placed using a curved needle; however, for a thicker abdominal wall, several specialized needles are available to assist with accurate placement of fascial sutures.

15. Withdraw the laparoscope. Allow the pneumoperitoneum to escape from the trocar. A blunt probe through the trocar may slip bowel loops away, allowing more complete evacuation of the CO_2. Remove the trocar.

16. Place a single suture to close the subumbilical fascial defect.

17. Use subcuticular sutures to close the skin incisions.

F. Special Considerations

The initial incision may be made in the midclavicular line of the left subcostal region if midline scarring is likely. After the umbilical region has been visualized and freed, a port and the laparoscope can be placed in the usual site. If the decision is made to proceed to laparotomy, the trocars may be left in place to maintain the pneumoperitoneum until the laparotomy incision is made. If laparotomy is likely, plan the laparoscopic incisions so they might be incorporated into the laparotomy incision whenever possible.

G. Specific Postoperative Management

1. Patient may resume full activity as soon as symptoms allow; it is usually about 2 weeks before vigorous activity can be resumed without discomfort.

2. Pain between the scapulae and shoulder tips is frequent, because of irritation of the diaphragm from retained CO_2. The discomfort usually is relieved if the patient lies down.

H. Specific Postoperative Complications

1. Trocar site hematoma: primarily a problem at lateral trocar sites where the epigastric vessels may have been traumatized. These hematomas respond poorly to attempts to control with pressure dressings. Consider extending the skin incision to identify the bleeding vessel. Ligate the vessel on the superior and inferior margins of the incision. Use of special suture applicators through the trocar site may be advantageous if the hematoma is recognized intraoperatively.

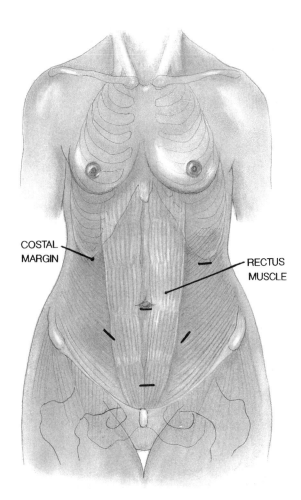

COSTAL MARGIN

RECTUS MUSCLE

FIG. 1. Usual sites for laparoscopic trocar placement and their anatomical relationships with the anterior abdominal wall.

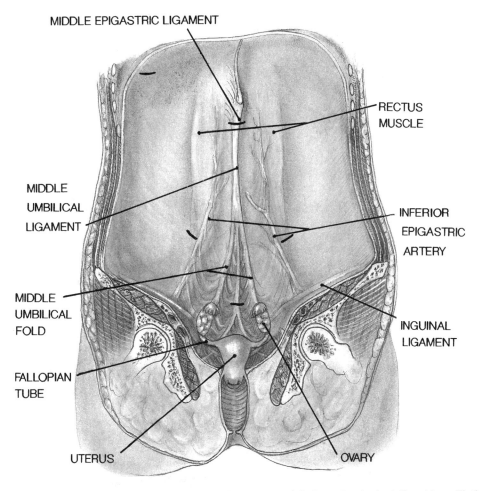

MIDDLE EPIGASTRIC LIGAMENT

RECTUS MUSCLE

MIDDLE UMBILICAL LIGAMENT

INFERIOR EPIGASTRIC ARTERY

MIDDLE UMBILICAL FOLD

FALLOPIAN TUBE

INGUINAL LIGAMENT

UTERUS

OVARY

FIG. 2. The same laparoscopic trocar sites as in Figure 1, and their anatomical relationships with the inner surface of the anterior abdominal wall.

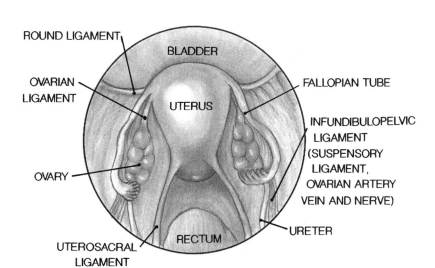

ROUND LIGAMENT

BLADDER

OVARIAN LIGAMENT

UTERUS

FALLOPIAN TUBE

OVARY

INFUNDIBULOPELVIC LIGAMENT (SUSPENSORY LIGAMENT, OVARIAN ARTERY VEIN AND NERVE)

UTEROSACRAL LIGAMENT

RECTUM

URETER

FIG. 3. Laparoscopic view of pelvic structures. With anterior traction on the uterus, the most common sites involved with endometriosis can be examined. The ovaries must be individually elevated to verify mobility and to examine the peritoneal surface of the ovarian fossa. The cul-de-sac can be seen by retracting the rectum cephalad.

2. Trocar site hernias are managed in the same way as any abdominal wall hernia. Prompt surgical repair is usually indicated because the hernia opening is small and poses a risk for strangulation of the contents.

3. Unrecognized bowel injury: be alert for this complication if patient does not appear to be doing well 24 hours after laparoscopy.

4. Carbon dioxide embolism is a rare but potentially fatal complication of laparoscopy. Management includes positioning the patient head down on her left side to attempt to trap the gas in the right side of the heart. Aspiration of the gas may be attempted through a central catheter or needle inserted through the chest wall. Respiratory support is provided as needed. If available, a hyperbaric chamber may facilitate recovery.

II. Laparoscopic Tubal Ligation

A. Indications
1. Patient desires permanent contraception.
2. Medical conditions associated with need for permanent contraception

B. Preoperative Preparation
1. Counseling about contraceptive alternatives
2. Review of recent menstrual history and contraceptive practices

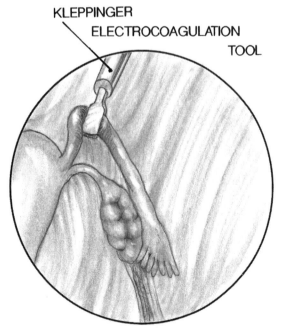

KLEPPINGER
ELECTROCOAGULATION
TOOL

FIG. 4. The fallopian tube is grasped and cauterized using a bipolar electrocoagulation tool. Beginning 2 cm from the uterine cornua and extending distally, a 2-cm section of the isthmus is cauterized.

C. Preoperative Investigations
1. Pregnancy test if indicated
2. Pelvic examination and Pap smear

D. Surgical Technique
1. Follow general instructions for diagnostic laparoscopy; use a single 5-mm suprapubic port for instruments.
2. With electrocautery forceps, grasp the isthmic portion of the fallopian tube at least 2 cm from the uterine cornua (Fig. 4).
3. Elevate the tube away from the ovary, pelvic vessels, and any bowel loops that remain in the region.
4. Activate bipolar cautery, applying 30- to 35-W current until the thermal tissue reaction has been completed.
5. Again, grasp the tube distal to the first cautery site and continue to treat until 2 cm of tube has been treated. Include the mesosalpinx immediately adjacent to the tube.
6. Use laparoscopic scissors to transect the tube in the center of the cauterized area. Verify that the cauterized ends of the tube fall freely away from each other after the cut has been carried completely through the tube and into the adjacent mesosalpinx.
7. Repeat on the contralateral side.
8. Check hemostasis, and remove trocars, as for diagnostic laparoscopy.

E. Specific Postoperative Management
The same as for diagnostic laparoscopy

F. Specific Postoperative Complications
The same as for diagnostic laparoscopy

III. Laparoscopic Ovarian Cystectomy

A. Indications
1. Persistent adnexal cyst with very low suspicion for malignancy
2. Benign-appearing cyst incidentally identified during diagnostic laparoscopy

B. Principle
Laparoscopic cystectomy is associated with a high risk of cyst rupture. The cyst must appear benign by all measures, and the patient and surgeon must accept the risk of rupture of a malignant cyst.

C. Preoperative Investigations
1. Ultrasonography to evaluate the cyst for benign or malignant characteristics
2. Preoperative blood sample for CA-125

D. Preoperative Preparation
The same as for diagnostic laparoscopy

E. Surgical Technique

1. Follow general instructions for diagnostic laparoscopy; use two lateral ports or one suprapubic port and one port contralateral to the cyst.
2. Collect peritoneal washings for cytologic study.
3. Use spinal needle and syringe or suction irrigation device to aspirate cyst contents if rupture appears likely and cyst appears to be benign.
4. Use needlepoint cautery and/or laparoscopic scissors to excise the cyst wall from the ovary. Peel any remaining fragments of the cyst wall from the ovary using a grasping instrument.
5. Establish hemostasis, using cautery sparingly
6. If fertility is a concern, apply an adhesion barrier to the treated surface of the ovary.
7. Withdraw trocars, as described for diagnostic laparoscopy.

F. Specific Postoperative Management

1. Consider oral contraceptives to suppress further cyst formation, if indicated.
2. Consider further medical therapy for endometriosis, if indicated.

G. Specific Postoperative Complications

A patient with a hemorrhagic corpus luteum may have pain for several months after resolution or removal of the cyst. Reassurance and suppression of ovulation are the best treatments.

IV. Laparoscopic Oophorectomy

A. Indications

1. Ovarian neoplasm requiring removal for pathologic evaluation: the neoplasm must be cystic, so that aspiration of cyst fluid will result in a small mass that can be removed through laparoscopic ports, or a small solid neoplasm.
2. Hereditary ovarian cancer syndromes

B. Principle

The principle of minimizing risk of injury by identifying adjacent organs is followed for laparoscopic surgery in the same manner as for laparotomy. In the case of oophorectomy, this means that the ureter is identified before the infundibulopelvic ligament is transected.

C. Preoperative Investigation

1. The same as for diagnostic laparoscopy
2. Blood sample for preoperative CA-125

D. Preoperative Preparation

The same as for diagnostic laparoscopy

E. Surgical Technique

1. Follow general instructions for diagnostic laparoscopy; use two lateral ports and/or one suprapubic port and one port contralateral to the cyst.
2. Collect peritoneal washings for cytologic study.
3. Grasp the round ligament at the uterine cornua. Retract toward the midline to put traction on the anterior leaf of the broad ligament.
4. Use endoscopic scissors with cautery as needed, and open the anterior peritoneum of the broad ligament to create a 5- to 6-cm opening lateral to the adnexa.
5. To allow selective incision of a single layer of peritoneum, use the lower blade of the scissors to elevate the anterior peritoneum.
6. Retract the infundibulopelvic ligament toward the midline, and use a blunt probe to open the broad ligament and identify the ureter (Fig. 5).
7. Use endoscopic scissors to create an opening in the posterior leaf of the broad ligament well above the level of the ureter.
8. Transect the infundibulopelvic ligament with an endoscopic stapling device, tripolar cautery, or argon beam coagulator (Fig. 6).
9. Incise the remaining posterior peritoneal attachments to the level of the uterine cornua.
10. Transect the fallopian tube and utero-ovarian ligaments with an endoscopic stapling device, cautery, or argon beam coagulator (Fig. 7).
11. Place the specimen in the cul-de-sac, and repeat the procedure on the other side if indicated.
12. Small atrophic ovaries may be withdrawn directly through 10-mm trocars. Larger specimens are placed in an endoscopic pouch and withdrawn through 10-mm incisions after the trocar has been withdrawn. If both ovaries are removed, withdraw the smaller one first.

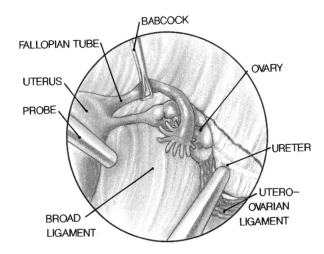

FIG. 5. With the anterior leaf of the broad ligament opened, the infundibulopelvic ligament can be retracted medially. The ureter can be visualized attached to the medial leaf of the broad ligament.

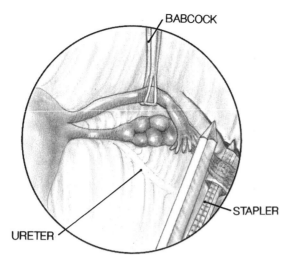

FIG. 6. With endoscopic scissors, a defect is created in the posterior broad ligament above the level of the ureter. The infundibulopelvic ligament is then transected in a hemostatic fashion (in this figure, through the use of an endoscopic stapling device).

13. The cyst may be aspirated to decrease specimen size. Bring the endoscopic pouch through a 10-mm incision as far as possible, so that the ovary is pulled up snug against the abdominal wall and the pneumoperitoneum is maintained. Open the bag, and aspirate the cyst using a spinal needle and syringe or suction irrigation device. Use continuous laparoscopic guidance to ensure that the intraabdominal portion of the bag is not punctured. Finally, if the incision must be enlarged to remove the ovary, complete all remaining surgery (securing hemostasis, washing blood from cul-de-sac, closure of the contralateral incision) before enlarging the incision, because it will be difficult to maintain a

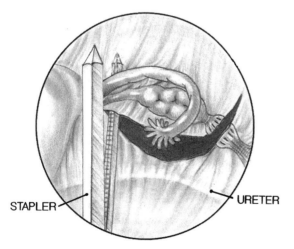

FIG. 7. The utero-ovarian ligament and proximal tube are transected, freeing the tube and ovary for extraction.

pneumoperitoneum after the incision has been enlarged.

14. Proceed with closure as described for diagnostic laparoscopy.

F. Specific Postoperative Management
Initiate hormone replacement therapy if indicated.

G. Specific Postoperative Complications
1. The same as for diagnostic laparoscopy
2. Ureteric injury

V. Laparoscopic Treatment of Endometriosis

A. Indications
1. Endometriosis with associated infertility or pain
2. Incidentally encountered endometriosis at time of diagnostic laparoscopy

B. Principles
1. Laparoscopic treatment is appropriate for mild-to-moderate endometriosis.
2. Laparoscopic surgery for severe endometriosis is a lengthy procedure associated with risk of recurrent disease that requires additional surgery. Therefore, for patients with severe endometriosis, laparotomy is preferred for conservative management. If future fertility is not desired, consideration should be given to hysterectomy with bilateral salpingo-oophorectomy.

C. Preoperative Investigation
The same as for diagnostic laparoscopy

D. Preoperative Preparation
1. The same as for diagnostic laparoscopy
2. If pelvic examination, symptoms, or previous procedures suggest severe endometriosis, consider preoperative bowel preparation with polyethylene glycol electrolyte solution (GoLYTELY).
3. Careful attention to intraoperative positioning is essential, because operating time may be long, with the attendant risk of nerve compression injuries.

E. Surgical Technique
1. Follow the general instructions for diagnostic laparoscopy.
2. Additional techniques will depend on the location and severity of the endometriosis.
3. Lyse adhesions with laparoscopic scissors. Strive for accurate identification of surgical planes to minimize the need for cautery. Free all adhesions until the pelvic organs are well visualized to allow accurate assessment of the feasibility of laparoscopic surgery.
4. Obtain biopsy specimens from several endometriotic sites to verify the diagnosis. Use a toothed grasping

instrument to pick up the peritoneum in the region of an endometriotic implant. Elevate the tissue gently to verify that only a thin layer of tissue is in the jaws of the instrument. Next, with a quick lift and twist motion, excise the tissue. Ovarian cyst walls may be similarly sampled.

5. Ovarian cysts (endometriomas) may be removed as described for laparoscopic ovarian cystectomy. Complete removal or destruction of the cyst wall is necessary. If portions of the wall remain, the area should be treated with cautery or laser for ablation.

6. Inspect the peritoneum to identify the course of the iliac vessels and the ureter. Unless the patient is obese or the peritoneum is scarred, peristalsis of the ureter can usually be visualized through the peritoneum. In the region of the posterior leaf of the broad ligament, endometriotic implants often overlie the uterosacral ligaments, which is a safe region for treating with cautery.

7. Smaller powder burn, white, or red implants can be treated easily and inexpensively with needlepoint cautery unless they overlay a ureter or vessel. Begin with the cautery set at half the power output used for cautery at open laparotomy. Increase as needed. If the tissue sticks to the cautery instrument, the cautery probably is set too high.

8. Saline may be injected under the peritoneum to elevate the peritoneum away from the ureter before lasering or cauterizing endometriotic deposits in the region.

9. The undersurface of the ovary and the ovarian fossa are frequent sites of endometriosis. Be sure to elevate the ovary to inspect the undersurfaces.

10. Irrigate the treated surfaces, and inspect for hemostasis.

11. Consider application of an adhesion barrier over raw surfaces on the ovary and peritoneal surfaces in the region of the tubal fimbria.

12. Withdraw trocars as for diagnostic laparoscopy.

F. Specific Postoperative Management
Consider medical treatment aimed at suppressing further growth of endometriosis.

G. Specific Postoperative Complications
1. With the use of monopolar cautery, the possibility of occult thermal injury must be considered if the patient's postoperative course is other than normal. A flat and upright abdominal radiograph will show free air under the diaphragm if bowel perforation has occurred. Thermal injury may result in disruption of the bowel wall more than a week after laparoscopy.

2. Patients with symptomatic endometriosis frequently have had several surgical procedures, and they may have extensive adhesions, resulting in postoperative bowel obstruction.

VI. Laparoscopic Reversal of Torsion

A. Indications
Laparoscopically confirmed ovarian torsion with viable-appearing ovarian parenchyma.

B. Preoperative Investigations
1. The same as for diagnostic laparoscopy, with the addition of tests noted below
2. Ultrasonography with Doppler flow can sometimes suggest the diagnosis preoperatively, but it is not a reliable indicator of torsion.
3. Because the preoperative differential diagnosis usually includes pelvic inflammatory disease, cervical cultures and a white blood cell count are indicated.

C. Preoperative Preparation
The same as for diagnostic laparoscopy

D. Surgical Technique
1. Follow the general instructions for diagnostic laparoscopy.
2. Evaluate the ovary for viability. A dusky or pale ovary is likely to respond well to reversal of the torsion. A deep blue- or purple-colored ovary may still have a good outcome if the torsion is reversed, as long as the tissue remains firm. A black ovary, or one with a soft consistency, should be treated with oophorectomy.
3. Gently elevate and flip the ovary until the utero-ovarian ligament assumes a normal configuration. This may require one, two, or more 180-degree flips.
4. Evaluate the ovary for the presence of a cyst or neoplasm. If a physiologic cyst may have caused the ovarian enlargement that led to torsion, then observation or drainage alone is warranted. If the cyst or neoplasm is complex, cystectomy or oophorectomy is indicated.
5. Consider tacking one or both ovaries to the pelvic sidewall to prevent future torsion. This can be accomplished with a stitch from the upper pole of the ovary to the peritoneum of the broad ligament. Care must be taken to avoid extensive manipulation of the fallopian tube in the process of placing a stitch, lest the tubal adhesions created obviate the theoretic advantage of preventing future torsion.

E. Specific Postoperative Management
1. Ultrasonographic surveillance to confirm resolution of ovarian cyst if indicated.
2. Consider oral contraceptive pills to decrease future risk of cysts and torsion if fertility is not desired immediately.
3. It may be difficult to evaluate residual ovarian tenderness and to differentiate the usual postoperative pain from recurrent torsion. However, in the immediate postoperative period, recurrent torsion is rare.

F. Specific Postoperative Complications

1. Previously, textbooks warned about reversal of torsion because it was believed that clots from the twisted ovarian vein might embolize. Currently, this complication is thought to occur rarely, if ever. The leg veins should still be considered the most likely source of postoperative pulmonary emboli should this complication arise.

2. Fever may indicate progressive necrosis of the ovary in spite of the surgical reversal of the torsion. Infection, sepsis, disseminated intravascular coagulation, and adult respiratory distress syndrome are all possible if a significant volume of ovarian tissue undergoes necrosis instead of healing after reversal of the torsion.

VII. Laparoscopic Evaluation and Treatment of Ectopic Pregnancy

A. Principle

Patients with a presumptive diagnosis of ectopic pregnancy who are hemodynamically stable may be considered for laparoscopic treatment.

B. Preoperative Investigations

1. Hemoglobin or hematocrit
2. Quantitative human chorionic gonadotropin (HCG) assay
3. Ultrasonography to evaluate for presence of intrauterine pregnancy: correlate ultrasonographic results with HCG level.
4. If tissue or clot is passed via vagina, request pathologic evaluation for presence of villi.

C. Preoperative Preparation

Because the surgical procedure is often semiurgent and the patient is in considerable pain, the usual preoperative douche and enema are not performed.

D. Surgical Technique

1. Begin as described for diagnostic laparoscopy.
2. Use a suction irrigation device to evacuate blood and clots from the pelvis. Retain all irrigation fluid and clots for possible pathologic evaluation.
3. Identify the abnormal section of the fallopian tube. If the enlargement or bleeding area appears to be on an ovary, remember that an ovarian ectopic pregnancy is much rarer than a hemorrhagic corpus luteum. Consider reevaluating the possibility of an intrauterine pregnancy.
4. If the pregnancy has ruptured the tube, tease the remaining products of conception from the rupture site.
5. If a bulge in the tube demonstrates the probable site of the ectopic pregnancy, create a longitudinal incision along the proximal half of the bulge with needlepoint cautery (Fig. 8).

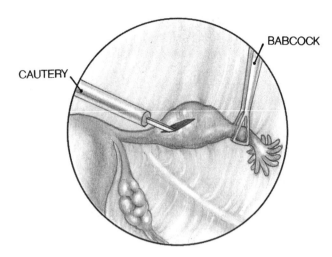

FIG. 8. Laparoscopic salpingostomy for ectopic pregnancy. The incision is made in the proximal one-half of the tubal deformity that marks the site of the ectopic pregnancy. Careful application of noncrushing instruments stabilizes the tube.

6. Tease the clot and products of conception from the fallopian tube. Bleeding will slow or stop when the products have been cleared from the tube.
7. Remove products of conception through a laparoscopic port. If no obvious sac or placenta is seen, carefully collect all clots and debris for pathologic evaluation.
8. Use needlepoint cautery sparingly to establish hemostasis at the salpingostomy site.
9. If bleeding persists or if tubal damage is extensive, consider salpingectomy. Elevate the tube, placing traction on the mesosalpinx. Use cautery, followed by scissors or tripolar cautery, to divide the mesosalpinx and to secure hemostasis. (This may not be needed if the ectopic pregnancy is in the distal portion of the tube.) Additional cautery and sharp dissection, a suture loop, or a stapling device can be used to transect the tube and the remaining mesosalpinx proximal to the ectopic site. Remove the fallopian tube through a laparoscopic port.
10. Complete the procedure as described for diagnostic laparoscopy.

E. Specific Postoperative Management

Follow with serial HCG levels until the value normalizes.

F. Specific Postoperative Complications

1. The risk of persistent ectopic pregnancy is greater with a laparoscopic approach than with an open approach, unless laparoscopic salpingectomy was performed. Following HCG levels until a normal value is reached allows early detection and the possibility of medical treatment of a persistent ectopic pregnancy. HCG levels may be elevated only mildly or even be normal with a persistent ectopic pregnancy.
2. The patient should be counseled both preoperatively

and postoperatively about the risk of recurrent ectopic pregnancy. For a subsequent pregnancy, early prenatal care is advised, with the goal of early detection if ectopic pregnancy recurs.

Reading List

Damario MA, Holcomb K, Bodack MP. Bilateral femoral neuropathy complicating a combined laparoscopic-vaginal procedure. *J Am Assoc Gynecol Laparosc* 1966;4:69–72.

Ory SJ. Pelvic endometriosis. *Obstet Gynecol Clin North Am* 1987; 14:999–1014.

Leach RE, Ory SJ. Modern management of ectopic pregnancy. *J Reprod Med* 1989;34:324–338.

Lu PY, Ory SJ. Endometriosis: current management. *Mayo Clin Proc* 1995;70:453–463.

Damario MA, Rock JA. Classification of endometriosis. *Semin Reprod Endocrinol* 1997;15:235–244.

Magrina JF, Cornella JL. Office management of ovarian cysts. *Mayo Clin Proc* 1997;72:653–656.

Hanson MA, Dumesic DA. Initial evaluation and treatment of infertility in a primary-care setting. *Mayo Clin Proc* 1998;73:681–685.

Subject Index

Page numbers followed by f indicate illustrations; t following a page number indicates tabular material.